Cardiothoracic Surgery Essentials

Cardiothoracic Surgery Essentials

Edited by Daniel Willson

hayle
medical

New York

Hayle Medical,
750 Third Avenue, 9th Floor,
New York, NY 10017, USA

Visit us on the World Wide Web at:
www.haylemedical.com

ISBN: 978-1-63241-553-0

Cataloging-in-Publication Data

Cardiothoracic surgery essentials / edited by Daniel Willson.
   p. cm.
Includes bibliographical references and index.
ISBN 978-1-63241-553-0
1. Heart--Surgery. 2. Chest--Surgery. I. Willson, Daniel.
RD598 .C37 2019
617.412--dc23

Table of Contents

Permissions

List of Contributors

Index

Preface

This book has been an outcome of determined endeavour from a group of educationists in the field. The primary objective was to involve a broad spectrum of professionals from diverse cultural background involved in the field for developing new researches. The book not only targets students but also scholars pursuing higher research for further enhancement of the theoretical and practical applications of the subject.

The treatment of the conditions of the heart and lungs, and the surgical treatment of the organs inside the thorax is under the scope of cardiothoracic surgery. Blalock-Taussig shunt creation, aortic coarctation repair, closure of patent ductus arteriosus, bypass surgery, etc. are procedures that fall under the domain of cardiac surgery. Modern heart surgery scales the boundaries of off-pump bypass surgery and minimally invasive surgery or robot-assisted heart surgery. An important surgical procedure involving the removal of the pleura is called pleurectomy, which is used in the treatment of mesothelioma and pneumothorax. Some thoracic surgical procedures are lung volume reduction surgery (LVRS), segmentectomy, sleeve/bronchoplastic resection, etc. This book includes some of the vital pieces of work being conducted across the world, on various aspects related to cardiothoracic surgery. It provides significant information of this discipline to help develop a good understanding of this surgical specialty and associated fields. This book aims to equip students and experts with the advanced topics and upcoming concepts in this area.

It was an honour to edit such a profound book and also a challenging task to compile and examine all the relevant data for accuracy and originality. I wish to acknowledge the efforts of the contributors for submitting such brilliant and diverse chapters in the field and for endlessly working for the completion of the book. Last, but not the least; I thank my family for being a constant source of support in all my research endeavours.

Editor

Volume of mural thrombus plays a role in the elevation of inflammatory markers after endovascular aortic repair

Jae Hang Lee[*] ⓘ, Jin-Ho Choi and Eung-Joong Kim

Abstract

Background: Although systemic inflammatory responses are common after endovascular aortic repair (EVAR), its etiology remains uncertain. It is normally well tolerated and has a benign course. This study was undertaken to investigate the possible etiology of post-EVAR inflammation by measuring volumes of chronic mural thrombus and fresh thrombus.

Methods: The subjects of this study included 34 patients who underwent EVAR from February 2012 to July 2017. Inflammatory markers in all the patients were evaluated before surgery, using the highest value among the laboratory data up to 5 days after surgery, and postoperative computed tomographic angiography (CTA) was taken for all of them before their discharging. Volumes of mural thrombus and fresh thrombus were calculated by CTA. The mean interval from surgery to immediate postoperative CTA was estimated as 6.8 ± 4.0 days.

Results: After undergoing EVAR, white blood cell (WBC) ($p < 0.01$), C-reactive protein (CRP) ($p < 0.01$) and erythrocyte sedimentation rate (ESR) ($p = 0.01$) were significantly elevated. Two groups were defined according to the post-implantation syndrome (PIS) by the criteria of systemic inflammatory response syndrome (SIRS);no significant differences were observed in any factors between the two groups. Classification of two groups by the criteria of increasing WBC and CRP revealed that inflammatory markers were significantly enhanced as the volume of mural thrombus increased ($p = 0.03$). However, no significant risk factor was found in view of aneurysmal growth after EVAR.

Conclusion: Volume of mural thrombus is an important risk factor for the elevation of inflammatory markers after EVAR.

Keywords: Aortic aneurysm, Endovascular aortic repair, Inflammation, Thrombus

Background

It is relatively common for a systemic inflammatory response to occur after endovascular aortic repair (EVAR). This phenomenon, known as post-implantation syndrome (PIS), was first described in 1999 [1]. PIS is defined when fever and leukocytosis occur in the absence of any suspected infections after undergoing EVAR; its incidence has been reported from 14 to 60% [2–4]. PIS is known to be transient, self-limiting and benign, but current the methods and needs of management are controversial.

The hypotheses of the etiologies for the development of PIS are varied, and the typical presumed causes are foreign body reaction and thrombus formation. Of these, there is a general consensus regarding the role of materials on PIS. Numerous studies showed that PIS occurred in endografts made of polyester rather than expanded polytetrafluoroethylene (ePTFE) [2, 5, 6]. Conversely, the relation with thrombus formation remains uncertain. Few study outcomes reportedly measured the volumes of mural thrombus and fresh thrombus for comparison.

This study aims to investigate the probable causative factors of PIS including thrombus volume in aneurysm, and to understand the relationship with aortic aneurismal growth after EVAR.

* Correspondence: truemed@hotmail.com
Department of thoracic and cardiovascular surgery, Dongguk University Ilsan Hospital, Goyang, Gyeonggi, South Korea

Methods

Study design and patient population

A single-center, retrospective, observational study was undertaken to review the medical records of patients. A total of 61 patients underwent aortic intervention at this hospital from February 2012 to July 2017. Of these, 34 patients were included as the study subjects, whereas exclusions comprised of thoracic endovascular aortic repair (TEVAR) (n = 24), ruptured abdominal aortic aneurysm (AAA) (n = 2), and infected AAA (n = 1).

Variables of interest

Demographics (age, gender), risk factors (hypertension, diabetes mellitus, coronary artery occlusive disease, cerebrovascular accident, chronic renal failure), preoperative medications (antiplatelet agent, statin), computed tomographic findings (maximum aneurysm diameter, volume of fresh and pre-existing mural thrombus, gas formaiton) were checked for each patient. Clinical course (mortality and morbidity, intensive care unit (ICU) and hospital stay, the occurrence of PIS) and laboratory findings (white blood cell (WBC), platelet (PLT), C-reactive protein (CRP) , and erythrocyte sedimentation rate (ESR)) were also recorded for each patients. The study patients were divided into two groups with regard to the various factors (PIS versus non-PIS, low WBC versus high WBC, low CRP versus high CRP, decreased AAA versus no change or increased AAA).

Perioperative procedure

All the patients underwent EVAR under general anesthesia. Prophylactic antibiotics (1st generation cephalosporin) were administered 30 min before incision, along with intravenous heparin (body weight (kg) × 100 unit). Surgical approach included two inguinal incisions performed without pre-closing device. After exposure of both femoral arteries, purse-string suture was performed using 5–0 Prolene, according to the Seldinger technique. Endurant (Medtronic Inc., Santa Rosa, CA, USA) endograft made of polyester was used for the stent graft. Patients were administered aspirin (100 mg) from the day after surgery. All the surgeries were performed by a single surgeon.

Blood samples and volume measurement

Inflammatory markers were evaluated in all patients before surgery, and laboratory data were used up to 5 days after the surgery with the highest value. All patients underwent postoperative computed tomographic angiography (CTA). The volume measure was calculated by assessing the area in axial view and multiplying by thickness. When the aneurysm extends to the iliac arteries, the volume of each iliac arteries were measured and added with the abdominal aortic aneurysmal sac. Mural thrombus was measured by preoperative CTA.

The volume is measured by first obtaining the volume of the entire aneurysmal sac, and then subtracting the area filing the contrast. The volume of fresh thrombus was calculated by the volume of contrast filling in preoperative CTA and subtracting the graft volume observed in the immediate postoperative CTA (Fig. 1).

Mean interval from surgery to immediate postoperative CTA was 6.8 ± 4.0 days. PIS was defined as 1) fever over 38.0 °C and 2) leukocytosis, assessed at ≥ 12,000 white blood cell (WBC). These values were obtained as per the definition of systemic inflammatory response syndrome (SIRS).

Statistical analysis

Continuous variables were expressed as mean ± standard deviation, whereas dichotomous variables were presented as counts and percentages. Comparisons of continuous variables were performed by Student t test for normally distributed variables, and Mann-Whitney U test for abnormally distributed variables. Chi-square test was used for categorical variables. All statistical analyses were performed using SPSS for Windows version 19.0 (SPSS Inc., Chicago, IL, USA), and statistical significance was considered for differences of 0.05 ($p < 0.05$).

Results

Patient characteristics and peri-operative clinical data are presented in Table 1. There were no incidences of perioperative mortality or any major complications. Type 2 and type 1 endoleaks were observed in 4 and 1 patient, respectively. No open conversion was performed, and 2 patients underwent thrombectomy and stent insertion the day after surgery due to postoperative limb occlusion. CTA was performed for all patients before discharge, at postoperative day 6.8 ± 4.0.

Postoperative elevations of inflammatory markers are presented in Table 2. There were no changes in the platelet counts; however, significant elevations of white blood cell (WBC), C-reactive protein (CRP), and erythrocyte sedimentation rate (ESR) were observed. Although they were not statistically evaluated, increasing trends were observed for WBC at postoperative 1–2 days, and for CRP at postoperative 3–4 days (Figs. 2 and 3).

Table 3 shows the comparative results of two groups based on the definition of PIS. According to this, only WBC and fever showed statistical significance, other characteristics and CT findings did not show significant difference between the two groups. In addition, no statistically significant difference was found between the two groups during the clinical course of the patients.

However, differences were statistically significant when WBC and CRP were considered as the inflammatory markers (Table 4). WBC was elevated as the patient's age increased, and volume of mural thrombus was also greater.

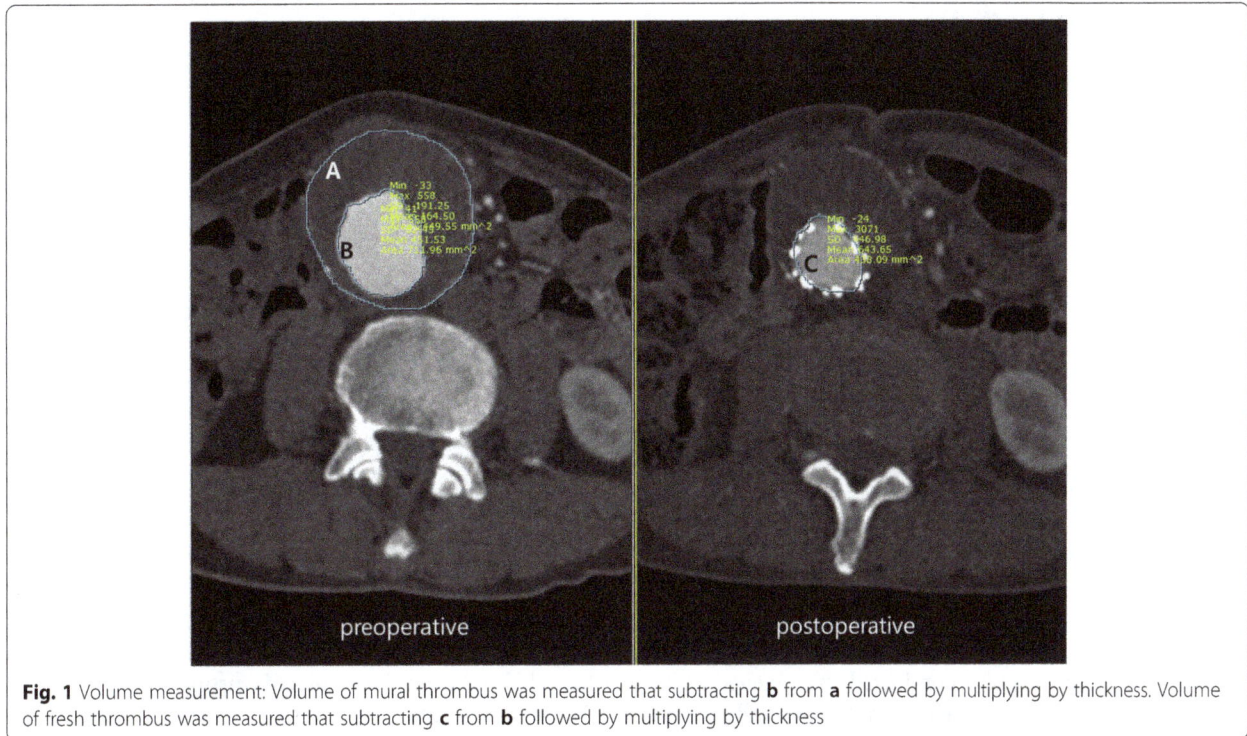

Fig. 1 Volume measurement: Volume of mural thrombus was measured that subtracting **b** from **a** followed by multiplying by thickness. Volume of fresh thrombus was measured that subtracting **c** from **b** followed by multiplying by thickness

CRP was elevated with larger volume of mural thrombus. In general, the elevated inflammatory markers did not occur in accordance to fresh thrombus, but was proportional to the volume of mural thrombus. However, these criteria did not extend the hospital and intensive care unit (ICU) stays.

Lastly, we reviewed the risk factors of aneurysmal growth and compared them with the last follow up CTA. The interval from the surgery to the last follow up CTA was 12.5 ± 13.8 months. We observed a decrease in the aneurysm size in 22 of the 34 patients, and an increase in 4 patients after the EVAR. The remaining 8 patients did not show any changes in the aneurysm size. As seen in Table 5, no correlation was found between any of the characteristics, including thrombus volume and inflammatory markers, upon reviewing the two groups of decreased aneurysm size and non-decreased aneurysm size.

Discussion

Since EVAR is a popular method for the treatment of abdominal aortic aneurysm, studies on PIS have been widely conducted. Its incidence varies due to the ambiguity of PIS definition. For example, some authors defined PIS with regards to fever and leukocytosis, while others consider fever and elevated CRP [2, 5]. In this study, PIS was defined according to the SIRS definition by considering fever and leukocytosis. However, inflammatory markers such as CRP are also considered to be strongly related to PIS. In fact,

Table 1 Baseline characteristics and peri-operative clinical data of patients

Patients' characteristics	Number of patients ($n = 34$)
Age, years	75.7 ± 8.5
Male gender, n (%)	25 (74)
HTN, n (%)	25 (74)
DM, n (%)	5 (15)
CAOD, n (%)	6 (18)
CVA, n (%)	7 (21)
CRF, n (%)	2 (6)
Antiplatelet agent, n (%)	19 (56)
Statin, n (%)	16 (47)
Diameter of AAA, mm	57.2 ± 9.4
ICU stay, hours	22.4 ± 14.2
Hospital stay, days	9.9 ± 12.6

HTN: Hypertension; DM: Diabetes mellitus; CAOD: Coronary artery occlusive disease; CVA: Cerebrovascular accident; CRF: Chronic renal failure; AAA: Abdominal aortic aneurysm; ICU: Intensive care unit

Table 2 Preoperative and postoperative laboratory data

Variable	Preoperative value	peak postoperative value	p
WBC, × 10³/μl	7.8 ± 3.1	13.7 ± 4.6	< 0.01
PLT, ×10³/μl	226.2 ± 61.8	226.9 ± 6.5	0.93
CRP, mg/dL	2.5 ± 3.1	11.6 ± 5.4	< 0.01
ESR, mm/h	34.1 ± 31.6	83.1 ± 29.9	0.01

WBC: White blood cell; PLT: Platelet; CRP: C-reactive protein; ESR: Erythrocyte sedimentation rate

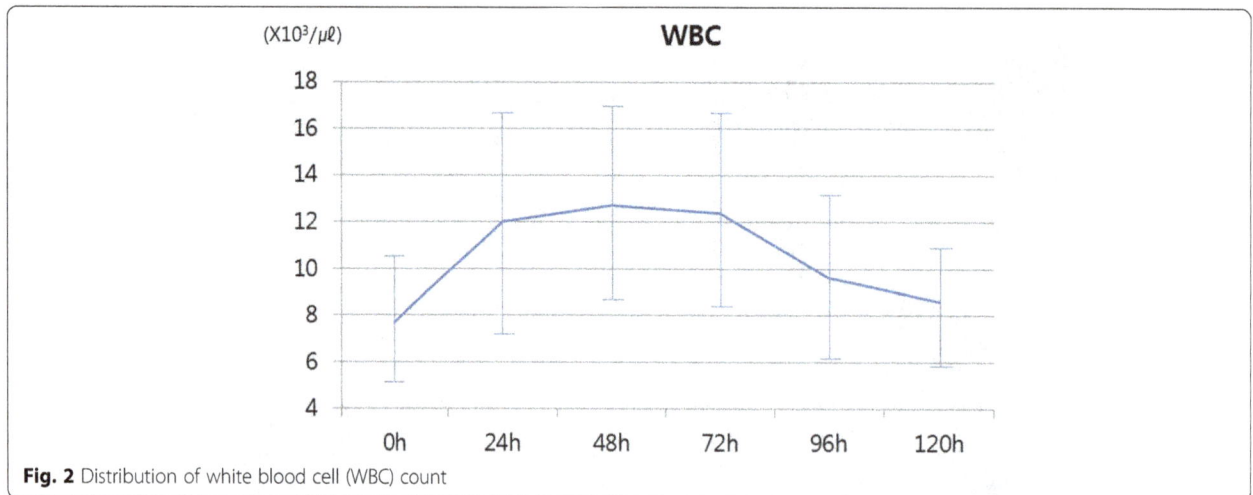

Fig. 2 Distribution of white blood cell (WBC) count

many investigators have studied not only on WBC, CRP, and PLT, but also on various types of inflammatory markers including interleukin 6 and 8 (IL-6, IL-8), tumor necrosis factor α (TNF-α), and interferon gamma (IFN-γ) [6–9]. Moreover, a study was also conducted using genetic tests such as messenger ribonucleic acid (RNA) and protein analyses [10]. The common conclusion of these studies was that EVAR causes a systemic inflammatory reaction.

The associations between PIS and patient outcomes have been well established in most studies. Although PIS causes prolonged hospitalization and difficulty in postoperative recovery, most of the cases are known to be benign and self-limiting [2, 5–7, 11, 12]. On the other hand, several reports have alerted severe complications [13–15]. The authors of these studies revealed that PIS was associated to adverse events such as pulmonary dysfunction, cardiovascular events, renal insufficiency, multisystem organ failure, etc. Especially, Arnaoutoglou et al. reported a significant number of adverse events including major cardiovascular events, renal failure, and death, being 25.

9% in the PIS group and 2.9% in the non-PIS group at 30 days after surgery [6]. However, in this study, major complications were not reported for all the patients; moreover, hospital and ICU stays were not extended, which differed from the results of existing studies.

Numerous studies have also been conducted on the etiology of PIS. Some consistency was observed in the relationship between the materials of endograft and PIS. Most of the studies reported frequent occurrences of PIS in the stent graft made of polyester than that made of ePTFE [2, 5–7]. In particular, Arnaoutoglou et al. claimed polyester endograft a 10 times higher independent predictor of PIS. Another theory on the etiology of PIS is the possibility of bacterial translocation by transient colonic ischemia [16]. This may result from occlusion or microembolism in the inferior mesenteric artery (IMA) or internal iliac artery (IIA). In addition, although it is believed that the operation time and contrast volume could possibly contribute to the etiology, the evidences are not sufficient.

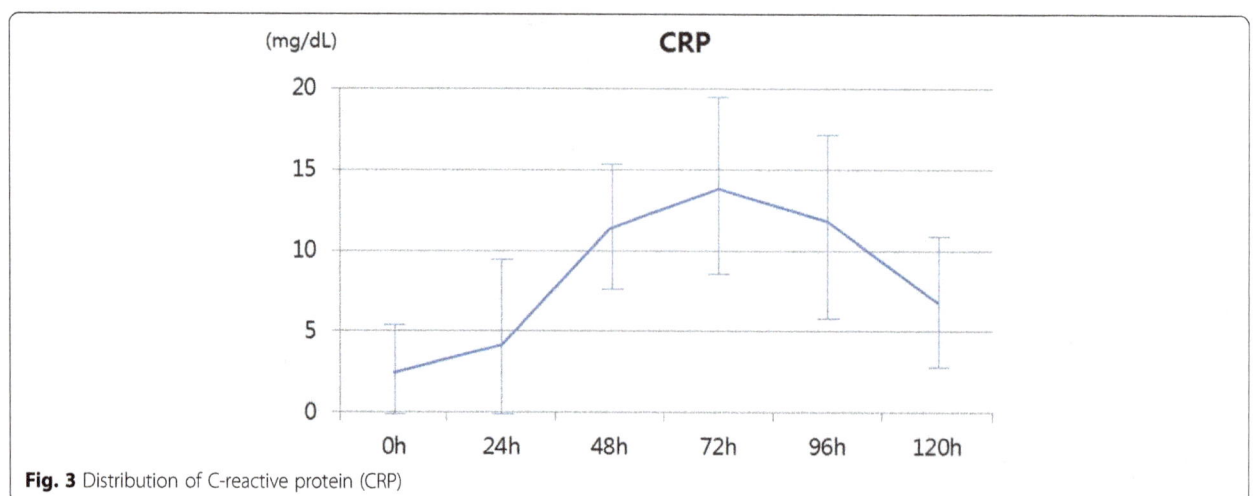

Fig. 3 Distribution of C-reactive protein (CRP)

Volume of mural thrombus plays a role in the elevation of inflammatory markers after endovascular aortic...

5

Table 3 Patient characteristics, risk factors, and clinical data according to the presence or absence of postimplantation syndrome (PIS) after endovascular aortic repair (EVAR)

	PIS, n = 8	Non-PIS, n = 26	P
Age, years	78.8 ± 8.5	74.8 ± 8.4	0.25
Male gender, n (%)	6 (75)	19 (73)	1.00
HTN, n (%)	5 (63)	20 (77)	0.65
DM, n (%)	1 (13)	4 (15)	1.00
CAOD, n (%)	1 (13)	5 (19)	1.00
CVA, n (%)	1 (13)	6 (23)	1.00
CRF, n (%)	0 (0)	2 (8)	1.00
Antiplatelet agent, n (%)	4 (50)	15 (58)	1.00
Statin, n (%)	2 (25)	14 (54)	0.23
Mural thrombus, ml	64.8 ± 50.2	81.6 ± 69.1	0.53
Fresh thrombus, ml	65.8 ± 56.5	35.7 ± 34.1	0.19
Gas formation, n (%)	5 (63)	12 (46)	0.69
Fever, n (%)	8 (100)	3 (12)	< 0.01
WBC, ×10³/μl	17.1 ± 3.6	12.7 ± 4.5	0.02
PLT, ×10³/μl	258.4 ± 64.4	217.2 ± 63.4	0.12
CRP, mg/dL	12.7 ± 3.1	10.4 ± 7.0	0.22
ESR, mm/h	84.8 ± 25.4	69.3 ± 28.8	0.29
ICU stay, hours	25.0 ± 17.1	21.6 ± 13.5	0.57
Hospital stay, days	10.8 ± 6.3	9.6 ± 14.0	0.82

PIS: Post-implantation syndrome; HTN: Hypertension; DM: Diabetes mellitus; CAOD: Coronary artery occlusive disease; CVA: Cerebrovascular accident; CRF: Chronic renal failure; WBC: White blood cell; PLT: Platelet; CRP: C-reactive protein; ESR: Erythrocyte sedimentation rate; ICU: Intensive care unit

Lastly, the shape and nature of the aortic aneurysm needs to be considered. One of the remarkable examples was mural thrombus formation in the aneurysm on which few studies have been conducted. Investigations tried to correlate PIS only with the maximal diameter of aneurysm or thickness of mural thrombus, but no correlation was observed [17, 18]. Very few studies tried to investigate the correlation with PIS by calculating the volume of thrombus. One study by Kakisis et al. was similar to our current study. Their results concluded that new-onset fresh thrombus might cause PIS rather than chronic mural thrombus [19]. This is interestingly inconsistent with our study. Kakisis et al. tried to explain PIS that fever occurred by absorbing blood as in deep vein thrombosis (DVT) or pulmonary embolism. Yet, they have the limitation not to consider the bias of materials since they enrolled the mixed cases with endografts made of ePTFE and polyester. This differed from our study, which has the advantage to eliminate the bias of graft materials by using a single product for all patients. The results of our study could be consistent with those in the previous studies. Swartbol et al. observed high amounts of IL-6 in mural thrombus in their study, demonstrating that released IL-6 upon the endovascular procedure stimulated to elevate WBC count [20], thereby concluding similar to our study that volume of mural thrombus can be a cause of PIS.

There were several limitations in this study. First, the study had a retrospective study design and second, the relatively small number of patients enrolled. Third, the inflammatory markers were not checked diversely, and hence we were unable to get the results of laboratory data

Table 4 Comparison of patient characteristics, risk factors, and clinical data based on the elevation of inflammatory markers

	Low WBC (< 12.0 × 10³/μl), n = 12	High WBC (< 12.0 × 10³/μl), n = 22	p	Low CRP (< 10.0 mg/dL), n = 17	High CRP (> 10.0 mg/dL), n = 17	p
Age, years	71.6 ± 5.9	77.9 ± 9.0	0.04	73.0 ± 6.6	78.4 ± 9.5	0.06
Male gender, n (%)	10 (83)	15 (68)	0.44	13 (76)	12 (71)	1.00
HTN, n (%)	10 (83)	15 (68)	0.44	14 (82)	11 (65)	0.44
DM, n (%)	1 (8)	4 (18)	0.64	3 (18)	2 (23)	0.44
CAOD, n (%)	1 (8)	5 (23)	0.40	4 (24)	2 (23)	0.66
CVA, n (%)	4 (33)	3 (14)	0.21	5 (29)	2 (23)	0.40
CRF, n (%)	1 (8)	1 (5)	1.00	2 (23)	0 (0)	0.49
Antiplatelet agent, n (%)	6 (50)	13 (59)	0.61	12 (71)	7 (41)	0.08
Statin, n (%)	6 (50)	10 (45)	0.80	10 (59)	6 (35)	0.17
Mural thrombus, ml	51.4 ± 3.2	92.0 ± 7.4	0.03	53.6 ± 6.5	101.7 ± 7.9	0.03
Fresh thrombus, ml	49.5 ± 4.4	39.1 ± 4.0	0.49	41.8 ± 3.9	43.8 ± 4.9	0.89
Gas formation, n (%)	6 (50)	11 (50)	1.00	7 (41)	10 (59)	0.30
ICU stay, hours	17.2 ± 9.0	25.3 ± 15.9	0.11	21.9 ± 15.8	23.0 ± 13.0	0.83
Hospital stay, days	6.7 ± 4.5	11.6 ± 15.1	0.28	11.1 ± 17.1	8.6 ± 5.3	0.58

WBC: White blood cell; CRP: C-reactive protein; HTN: Hypertension; DM: Diabetes mellitus; CAOD: Coronary artery occlusive disease; CVA: Cerebrovascular accident; CRF: Chronic renal failure; ICU: Intensive care unit

Table 5 Risk factor analysis for aneurysmal growth after endovascular aortic repair (EVAR)

	Decreased AAA, $n = 22$	No change or increased AAA, $n = 12$	p
Age, years	75.5 ± 9.2	76.1 ± 7.4	0.85
Male gender, n (%)	15 (68)	10 (83)	0.44
HTN, n (%)	15 (68)	10 (83)	0.44
DM, n (%)	5 (23)	0 (0)	0.14
CAOD, n (%)	4 (18)	2 (17)	1.00
CVA, n (%)	4 (18)	3 (25)	0.68
CRF, n (%)	1 (5)	1 (8)	1.00
Antiplatelet agent, n (%)	11 (50)	8 (67)	0.35
Statin, n (%)	9 (41)	7 (58)	0.33
Diameter of AAA, mm	56.7 ± 8.3	58.1 ± 11.5	0.70
Mural thrombus, ml	69.3 ± 42.6	93.0 ± 93.5	0.42
Fresh thrombus, ml	45.1 ± 40.3	38.4 ± 45.3	0.66
Gas formation, n (%)	10 (45)	7 (58)	0.47
Fever, n (%)	9 (41)	2 (17)	0.25
WBC, ×10³/μl	13.4 ± 4.5	14.3 ± 5.0	0.58
PLT, ×10³/μl	218.1 ± 70.0	243.1 ± 55.0	0.29
CRP, mg/dL	10.7 ± 6.0	11.5 ± 7.2	0.74
ESR, mm/h	80.0 ± 21.0	55.5 ± 37.9	0.07

AAA: Abdominal aortic aneurysm; *HTN*: Hypertension; *DM*: Diabetes mellitus; *CAOD*: Coronary artery occlusive disease; *CVA*: Cerebrovascular accident; *CRF*: Chronic renal failure; *WBC*: White blood cell; *PLT*: Platelet; *CRP*: C-reactive protein; *ESR*: Erythrocyte sedimentation rate

such as TNF-α or IL-6 and IL-8 as seen in other studies. Lastly, the duration of CTA follow up was too short to check aneurysmal growth. Thus, a large number of patients and long-term follow-up period are required for more complete results.

Conclusions

From this study, we showed that the volume of pre-existing mural thrombus is an important risk factor for the elevation of inflammatory markers after EVAR.

Abbreviations
AAA: Abdominal aortic aneurysm; CAOD: Coronary artery occlusive disease; CRF: Chronic renal failure; CRP: C-reactive protein; CTA: Computed tomographic angiography; CVA: Cerebrovascular accident; DM: Diabetes mellitus; DVT: Deep vein thrombosis; ePTFE: Expanded Polytetrafluoroethylene; ESR: Erythrocyte sedimentation rate; EVAR: Endovascular aortic repair; HTN: Hypertension; ICU: Intensive care unit; IFN: Interferon; IIA: Internal iliac artery; IL: Interleukin; IMA: Inferior mesenteric artery; PIS: Post-implantation syndrome; PLT: Platelet; RNA: Ribonucleic acid; SIRS: Systemic inflammatory response syndrome; TEVAR: Thoracic endovascular aortic repair; TNF: Tumor necrosis factor; WBC: White blood cell

Funding
The authors declare that they have no funding.

Authors' contributions
Lee JH is the lead surgeon and designed this study. Choi J-H and Kim E-J performed the literature review and participated in the manuscript writing. All authors have read and approved the final manuscript.

Competing interests
The authors declare that they have no competing interests.

References
1. Velazquez OC, Carpenter JP, Baum RA, Barker CF, Golden M, Criado F, et al. Perigraft air, fever,and leukocytosis after endovascular repair of abdominal aorticaneurysms. Am J Surg. 1999;178:185–9.
2. Voûte MT, Bastos Gonçalves FM, van de Luijtgaarden KM, Klein Nulent CG, Hoeks SE, Stolker RJ, et al. Stent graft composition plays a material role in the postimplantation syndrome. J Vasc Surg. 2012;56:1503–9.
3. Görich J, Rilinger N, Söldner J, Krämer S, Orend KH, Schütz A, et al. Endovascular repair of aortic aneurysms: treatment of complications. J Endovasc Surg. 1999;6:136–46.
4. De La Motte L, Vogt K, Panduro Jensen L, Groenvall J, Kehlet H, Veith Schroeder T, et al. Incidence of systemic inflammatory response syndrome after endovascular aortic repair. J Cardiovasc Surg. 2011;52:73–9.
5. Moulakakis KG, Alepaki M, Sfyroeras GS, Antonopoulos CN, Giannakopoulos TG, Kakisis J, et al. The impact of endograft type on inflammatory response after endovascular treatment of abdominal aortic aneurysm. J Vasc Surg. 2013;57:668–77.
6. Arnaoutoglou E, Kouvelos G, Papa N, Kallinteri A, Milionis H, Koulouras V, et al. Prospective evaluation of post-implantation inflammatory response after EVAR for AAA: influence on patients' 30 day outcome. Eur J Vasc Endovasc Surg. 2015;49:175–83.
7. Gerasimidis T, Sfyroeras G, Trellopoulos G, Skoura L, Papazoglou K, Konstantinidis K, et al. Impact of endograft material on the inflammatory response after elective endovascular abdominal aortic aneurysm repair. Angiology. 2005;56:743–53.
8. Gabriel EA, Locali RF, Romano CC, Duarte AJ, Palma JH, Buffolo E. Analysis of the inflammatory response in endovascular treatment of aortic aneurysms. Eur J Cardiothorac Surg. 2007;31:406–13.
9. Norgren L, Swartbol P. Biological responses to endovascular treatment of abdominal aortic aneurysms. J Endovasc Surg. 1997;4:169–73.
10. Abdul-Hussien H, Hanemaaijer R, Kleemann R, Verhaaren BFJ, van Bockel JH, Lindeman JHN. The pathophysiology of abdominal aortic aneurysm growth: corresponding and discordant inflammatory and proteolytic processes in abdominal aortic and popliteal artery aneurysms. J Vasc Surg. 2010;51:1479–87.
11. Arnaoutoglou E, Kouvelos G, Milionis H, Mavridis A, Kolaitis N, Papa N, et al. Post-implantation syndrome following endovascular abdominal aortic aneurysm repair: preliminary data. Interact Cardiovasc Thorac Surg. 2011;12:609–14.
12. Baek JK, Kwon H, Ko GY, Kim MJ, Han Y, Chung YS, et al. Impact of graft composition on the systemic inflammatory response after an elective repair of an abdominal aortic aneurysm. Ann Surg Treat Res. 2015;88:21–7.
13. Arnaoutoglou E, Papas N, Milionis H, Kouvelos G, Koulouras V, Matsagkas MI. Post-implantation syndrome after endovascular repair of aortic aneurysms: need for postdischarge surveillance. Interact Cardiovasc Thorac Surg. 2010;11:449–54.
14. Cross KS, Bouchier-Hayes D, Leahy AL. Consumptive coagulopathy following endovascular stent repair of abdominal aortic aneurysm. Eur J Vasc Endovasc Surg. 2000;19:94–5.
15. Chang CK, Chuter TA, Niemann CU, Shlipak MG, Cohen MJ, Reilly LM, et al. Systemic inflammation, coagulopathy, and acute renal insufficiency following endovascular thoracoabdominal aortic aneurysm repair. J Vasc Surg. 2009;49:1140–6.
16. Akin I, Nienaber CA, Kische S, Rehders TC, Ortak J, Chatterjee T, et al. Effect of antibiotic treatment in patients with postimplantation syndrome after aortic stent placement. Rev Esp Cardiol. 2009;62:1365–72.
17. Ferreira V, Machado R, Martins J, Loureiro L, Loureiro T, Borges L, et al. Post-implantation syndrome – retrospective analysis of 52 patients. Angiol Cir Vasc. 2015;11:204–8.

2

Video-assisted Thoracoscopic Surgery (VATS) with mini-thoracotomy for the management of pulmonary hydatid cysts

Nizar Abbas[1*], Sarah Zaher Addeen[2], Fatima Abbas[2], Tareq Al Saadi[2], Ibrahem Hanafi[2], Mahmoud Alkhatib[2], Tarek Turk[2] and Ahmad Al Khaddour[3]

Abstract

Background: Hydatid cyst is an endemic infectious disease. Various modalities have been provided to approach hydatosis. This article reports a 20-years-experience of a new minimally invasive technique for the management of solitary pulmonary hydatid cysts using video-assisted thoracoscopic surgery (VATS) with mini-thoracotomy.

Methods: We reviewed the medical records of patients who underwent unilateral or bilateral single pulmonary hydatid cyst excision using VATS with mini-thoracotomy. All patients were managed by the same surgeon over the period from January 1996 till January 2015.

Results: The study involved 120 patients aged between 11 and 74 years (median age = 30 years). The overall number of conducted surgeries was 130 (10 patients needed two surgeries). No deaths were reported during or after surgery. No recurrences were seen in the follow-up period that ranged between 10 and 30 months. Three patients (2.3% out of the 130 surgeries) developed post-operative complications: one patient had prolonged air leak and two patients developed empyema.

Conclusion: VATS with mini-thoracotomy is an effective and safe option for managing intact or ruptured solitary pulmonary hydatid cysts. Further studies in controlled prospective design are needed to compare this approach to other modalities of management.

Keywords: Echinococcosis, Echinococcus granulosus, Hydatid cyst, Video-assisted thoracoscopic surgery (VATS), Mini-thoracotomy

Background

Hydatid cyst is a parasitic infectious disease, which is endemic in many places around the world, such as the Mediterranean countries, Iran, India, Australia and South America. According to World Health Organization (WHO), the annual incidence of Cystic Echinococcus is up to 220 per 100,000 inhabitants in these countries [1].

The causal parasite of the disease is Echinococcus Granulosus. Humans can serve as intermediate hosts for this organism. It usually infects human organs separately or in groups, especially the liver and the lungs. The hydatid cyst grows slowly and asymptomatically in most of the cases to an extent that some cysts may exceed 20 cm in diameter. This expansive growth can seriously damage the tissue of the hosting organ, and makes spontaneous, traumatic, or intra-operative rupture of the cyst easier. The optimal treatment targets are: complete elimination of the parasite, preservation of the utmost of the healthy tissue, and prevention of recurrence by avoiding the spillage of the cystic fluid and dissemination of the cyst contents [1, 2].

Medical treatment attempts with Benzimidazoles to manage hydatid cysts are countless and persistent. Although this management spares patients the risks of surgery, its efficacy is still limited to specific cases such as hydatid cysts that are smaller than 6 cm, and in inoperable patients, and it is given after surgery to prevent recurrence and secondary echinococcosis [1, 3, 4]. Also,

* Correspondence: nr.abbas@scs-net.org
[1]Department of thoracic surgery, Al-Assad University Hospital, Damascus, Syrian Arab Republic
Full list of author information is available at the end of the article

aspiration of cystic fluid yields high risks and small benefits, and is still limited to liver cysts [3, 5].

Surgery with open thoracic surgery, sternotomy or right thoraco-abdominal approach, is the first and the best choice to manage large, multiple or complicated cysts in the lung or the liver [6–8]. Although this surgical approach allows delivering the cysts or removing them along with the damaged tissue without cystic rupture, it is a traumatic and highly invasive procedure for patients [6–8].

Surgical removal using video-assisted thoracoscopic surgery (VATS) has been used to minimize the risks of open surgery. However, it is limited to few clinical entities because of the high risk of postoperative complications such as cyst rupture, cystic fluid spillage and difficulties in controlling bronchial fistulas associated with cysts [9–16].

In this article, we report a series of cases of solitary pulmonary hydatid cyst managed with a new minimally invasive technique using video-assisted thoracoscopic surgery with mini-thoracotomy in order to prevent spillage and facilitate management of the residual cavity and control of the associated bronchial fistulas.

Methods

Study design

This is a case-series study. We reviewed the medical records of 120 patients with unilateral or bilateral single pulmonary hydatid cyst, whether it was intact, ruptured, or infected, and those who were managed with thoracoscopic surgery by the same surgeon, who applied the exact same technique for all patients, during the period from January 1996 till January 2015. All consecutive cases which met the inclusion criteria were included. We aimed to investigate operative time, duration of hospital stay, postoperative complications, morbidity, mortality, and recurrence rate.

Exclusion criteria:

1. Big hydatid cysts that are > 15 cm in diameter. Because it might need lung resection.
2. Multiple cysts in a single lung. Thoracotomy provides a better access in these cases.
3. Children under the age of 10 years, due to technical reasons related to anesthetic and thoracoscopic equipment.

Applied surgical procedure

The surgery is performed with the patient in the lateral decubitus position and under general anesthesia, with the use of double-lumen endotracheal tube in order to isolate the affected lung during surgery. A small entrance for camera is made in the seventh intercostal space at the posterior axillary line, and a small thoracic incision (mini-thoracotomy), with a length of approximately 5 cm, is made directly above the hydatid cyst (location is determined by the use of the scope and the patient's CT scan images) (Figs. 1 and 2). Then, a small thoracoscopic rib spreader is placed, and pleural adhesions, if present, are partially or completely removed. The pleural cavity is isolated with the use of packs soaked in 20% saline; the lung is pushed away, and the hydatid cyst is pushed closer to the incision area. A lung holder is applied to hold the lung in place.

In case of an intact hydatid cyst (Fig. 3), it is aspirated using a 14–16 gauge catheter, which is connected to a 3-ways catheter, which, in turn, is connected to both a syringe filled with scolicidal solution (20% saline), and to an empty bag used to collect the aspirated fluid. Consecutively, some fluid of the hydatid cyst is aspirated and the scolicidal solution is injected. A few minutes later this procedure is repeated several times. Then the fluid is completely aspired, and the catheter is withdrawn. The fibrous capsule is then opened and the germinal membrane is removed (Fig. 4). The remaining cavity is once more sterilized, and the bronchial fistulas are investigated and tightly closed using a 2/0 polyglactine 910; Vicryl. The fibrous capsule is debrided. Finally, the cavity of the hydatid cyst is tightly obliterated by suturing upward from the bottom (capitonnage).

In the event of bilateral hydatid cysts, surgery was performed first on the larger cysts. Preoperative chest radiography and CT scanning were performed on all patients. In patients presented with combined pulmonary and hepatic hydatid cysts, we proceeded with simultaneous combined resection of hydatid cysts in one stage through midsternotomy along with laparotomy or transdiaphragmatic removal of liver cysts in order to avoid three-stage operation of two thoracotomies and a laparotomy.

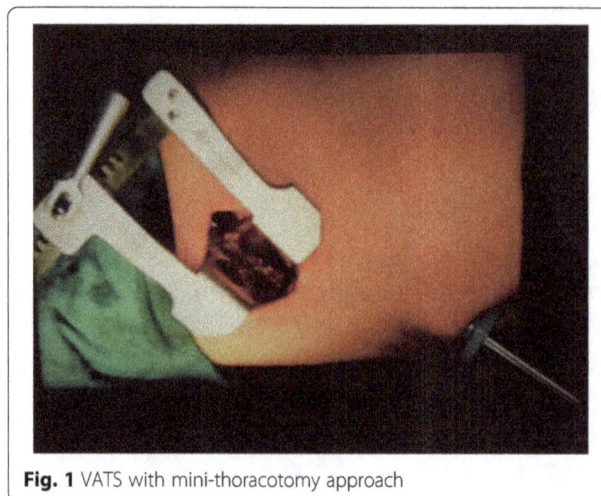

Fig. 1 VATS with mini-thoracotomy approach

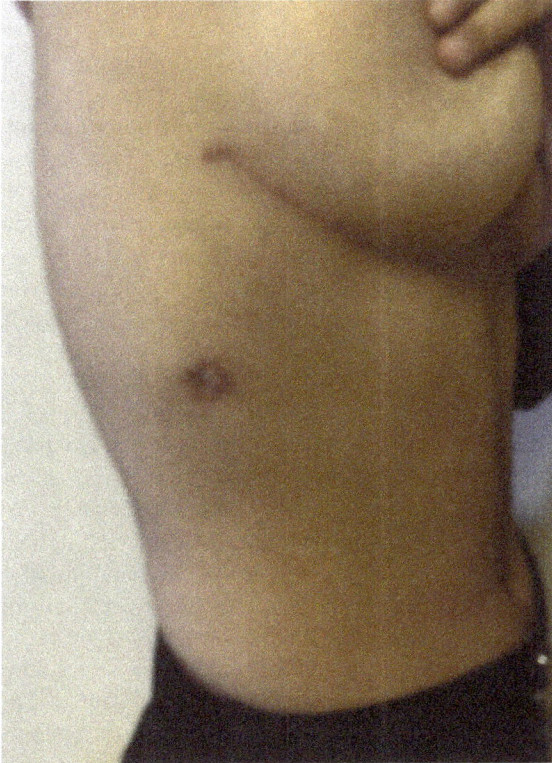

Fig. 2 Postoperative cosmetic scar

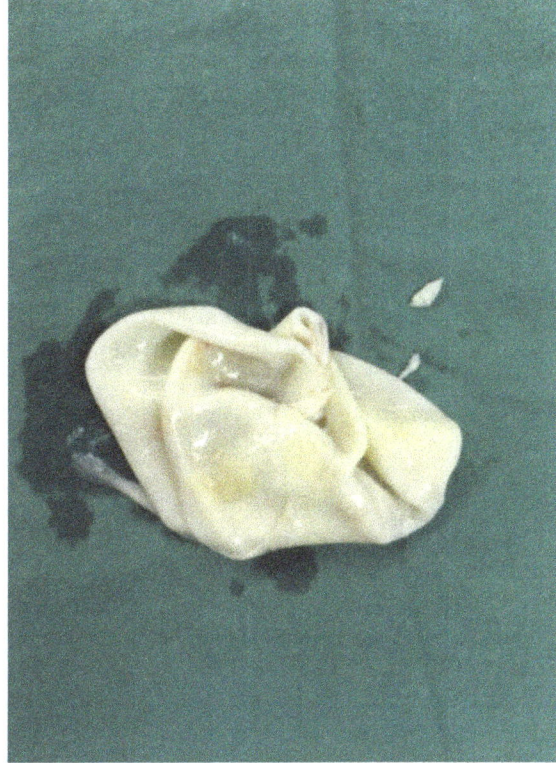

Fig. 4 Removed germinal membrane of the cyst

In cases of the ruptured hydatid cysts into the bronchi (Fig. 5) or the pleura, surgery starts by opening the fibrous capsule, followed by aspiration of the remaining fluid then removing the germinal membrane with sterilizing of the remaining cavity, followed by firm closing of the fistulas with the remaining cavity. If signs of any infection are present, the largest portion possible of the fibrous capsule is removed. Definitive diagnosis of infection was considered in the following circumstances: (i) positive culture of bacterial or fungal pathogens from drainage samples, or (ii) surgical or percutaneous drainage of purulent material from the cyst and growth of the organism in blood cultures. Probable diagnosis was defined by surgical or percutaneous drainage of purulent material and one of the following: (i) clinical data of systemic inflammatory response, or (ii) radiological settings

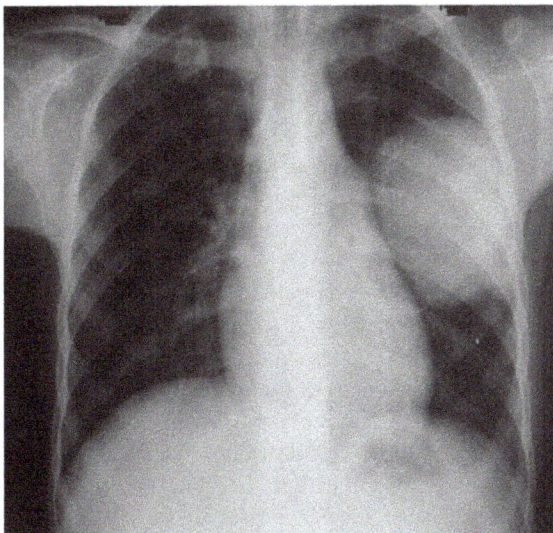

Fig. 3 Intact cyst in the left lung

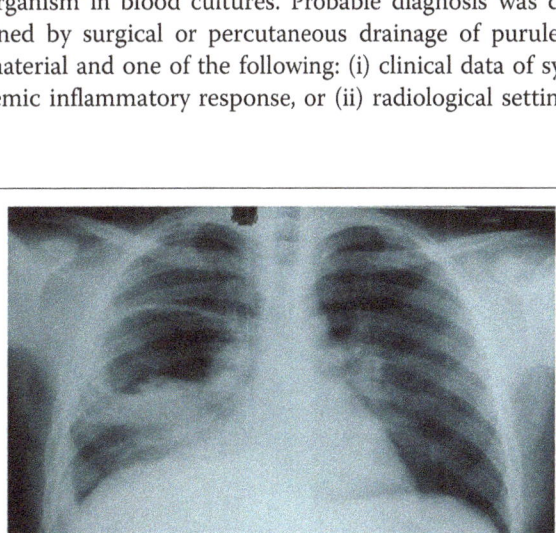

Fig. 5 Ruptured cyst

suggestive of hydatid cyst infection [17]. Continuous supportive suturing of the cyst margins is applied trying to prevent bleeding and air leak, which lasts for more than the average length of stay or 5 days according to the definition of prolonged air leak (PAL) used in the Society of Thoracic Surgeons database [18]. Cystic cavity is left opened into the pleural cavity.

In all cases, the surgery is ended by repeated washing of the pleural cavity with warm saline, and placing a chest tube for drainage through the same entrance of the camera. Albendazole is administered at a dose of 10 mg/kg continuously for three consecutive months post-surgery.

The follow up was done by chest radiography every 3 months for at least 10 months postoperatively.

Results

Clinical characteristics of study participants are summarized in Table 1. The study involved 120 patients aged between 11 and 74 years (median age was 30 years). There was no noticeable difference between the proportions of males and females, nor between patients with left- and right-sided cysts. The overall number of performed surgeries was 130; 10 patients had bilateral cysts and required a two-staged surgery for each patient (Table 1).

Mean operative time ranged from 75 to 100 min, including the time for anesthesia. Mean hospital stay was 2–3 days for all patients, except for the three patients who developed post-operative complications (2.3% out of the 130 surgeries). Prolonged air leakage (for more than 5 days) occurred in one of these three patients, and it needed an open thoracic surgery to close the bronchial

Table 1 Clinical characteristics of the patients

	Number	Percent
Gender		
Males	62	51.7%
Females	58	48.3%
Total	120	
Lung involved		
Left	58	48.3%
Right	52	43.3%
Bilateral	10	8.3%
Clinical type of cysts		
Intact	52	40%
Ruptured into the bronchi	66	50.7%
Ruptured into the pleura	8	6.1%
Infected	4	3.07%
Total	130	

fistulas. The two other patients with post-operative complications had infections: the first one had an empyema that required drainage and regular washing of the pleural cavity with antibiotic therapy according to culture and sensitivity test results, and the other one developed an abscess in the place of the removed cyst and required thoracotomy and lobectomy. The two patients who suffered from infectious postoperative complications had already had infected cysts before surgery.

No mortality was reported during or post-surgery, and no recurrences were seen during the follow-up period (10 to 36 months).

Discussion

In this case-series, we found that using video-assisted thoracoscopic surgery (VATS) with mini-thoracotomy for the management of a certain group of patients with solitary pulmonary hydatid cysts allowed for total elimination of the parasite, maximum preservation of the healthy tissue, and prevention of recurrences by avoiding the spillage of the cystic fluid.

Published studies in this field are very few and limited to a very small number of cases (Table 2). This is due to the risk of cystic rupture and the spillage of its content during operation, leading to recurrence in the future, and to the difficulty in controlling the accompanied bronchial fistulas and the residual cavity, which increases complication rates and lengthen hospital stay. Such complications may be the reason why some surgeons suggest preserving this technique for dead cysts only [19].

Our results showed that there was no cystic rupture or cystic fluid spillage during operations, which is supported by the absence of recurrences during the follow up period that lasted for up to 3 years. Moreover, the routine application of prophylactic pharmacological therapy with Albendazole after surgery had helped in preventing recurrence which reached zero in some studies [16, 20]. However, the follow up period in some of these studies was short (about 6 months) and not sufficient to detect all cases of recurrence [11, 14, 16].

The operative time in our study was shorter than that reported in some similar studies [9, 14] by virtue of the operative easiness through mini-thoracotomy. Giving the fact that those studies were limited to small cysts that are less than 7 cm in diameter, which are not usually accompanied by bronchial fistulas, while our study included large cysts that reached 15 cm in diameter.

Duration of hospital stay in our study was relatively short, due to the easiness of control over bronchial fistulas and closure of the residual cavity after cyst removal via mini-thoracotomy, and thus avoiding prolonged post-operative air leakage (a single case out of 130 operations). In some studies [2, 14, 16], where mini-thoracotomy approach was not used, prolonged post-operative air leakage

Table 2 Results of various studies of VATS for pulmonary hydatid cysts

Authors	Year and country	Patients No.	Age	Mean cyst diameter (cm)	Mean Operative time (min)	Mean Duration of hospital stay (day)	Complication %	Mean period of follow up (month)	Mortality and recurrence
Present study Abbas et al.	Syria 2016	120	Median: 30 Range: 11–74	< 15	75–100	2–3	2.3	10–36	0
Alpay et al. [9]	Turkey 2015	30	Mean: 31.7 Range: 8–85	6.5	102.6	4	13.3	21.8	0
Findikcioglu et al. [12]	Turkey 2012	12	Mean: 32.3 Range: 18–78	(2–7.5)	51.5 (30–100)	2.9 (2–6)	–	29	0
Parelkar et al. [14]	India 2009	3	≤9	< 7	150	4.5	1/3	6	–
Uchikov et al. [16]	Bulgaria 2004	11	Range: 17–55	< 6	–	5	9	6	–
Ettayebi et al. [11]	Morocco 2003	20	Children	–	60	3	–	6–36	0

was the most common complication which had led to a longer hospital stay and to an increased complications rate that reached 13.3% in Levent Alpay study [9].

The rate of infectious complications was high in our series, in which we reported two cases: empyema and abscess formation within the place of the removed cyst, in two out of four patients who already had infected cysts. This is consistent with the results of Milind study [15], and requires reconsideration of the role of thoraco-scopic surgery in such cases, and looking for a better alternative.

Conclusion

In conclusion, the case series revealed that (VATS) with mini-thoracotomy is an effective and safe option for managing intact or ruptured solitary pulmonary hydatid cysts. Further studies in controlled prospective design are needed to compare this approach to other modalities of management.

Acknowledgments
None

Funding
None

Authors' contributions
NA: developed the surgical technique, performed surgeries, and finalized the manuscript. SZ, FA, TA, IH, MA, TT: collected and analyzed the data, and participated in writing the manuscript. AA: helped NA in the surgical aspects, and participated in writing the manuscript. All authors approved the final manuscript as submitted, and agreed to be accountable for all aspects of the work.

Competing interests
The authors declare that they have no competing interests.

Author details
[1]Department of thoracic surgery, Al-Assad University Hospital, Damascus, Syrian Arab Republic. [2]Faculty of Medicine, University of Damascus, Damascus, Syrian Arab Republic. [3]Cardiothoracic surgeon, Damascus University Hospital, Damascus, Syria.

References
1. Organization WH. Guidelines for treatment of cystic and alveolar echinococcosis in humans. WHO informal working group on echinococcosis. Bull World Health Organ. 1996;74:231–42.
2. Bagheri R, Haghi S7, Amini M, Fattahi AS, Noorshafiee S. Pulmonary hydatid cyst: analysis of 1024 cases. Gen Thorac Cardiovasc Surg. 2011;59:105–9.
3. Nabarro LE, Amin Z, Chiodini PL. Current management of cystic echinococcosis: a survey of specialist practice. Clin Infect Dis. 2015;60:721–8.
4. Stojkovic M, Zwahlen M, Teggi A, Vutova K, Cretu CM, Virdone R, Nicolaidou P, Cobanoglu N, Junghanss T. Treatment response of cystic echinococcosis to benzimidazoles: a systematic review. PLoS Negl Trop Dis. 2009;3:e524.
5. Organization WH: Puncture, aspiration, injection, re-aspiration: an option for the treatment of cystic echinococcosis. 2001.
6. Biswas B, Ghosh D, Bhattacharjee R, Patra A, Basuthakur S, Basu R. One stage surgical management of hydatid cyst of lung & liver—by right thoracotomy & phrenotomy. Indian J Thorac Cardiovasc Surg. 2004;20:88–90.
7. Dezfouli AA, Arab M, Pejhan S, Kakhki AD, Shadmehr MB, Farzanegan R, Dezfouli GA. Presentation of a surgical technique and results in the treatment of lung hydatid cyst. Tanaffos. 2008;7:11–8.
8. Pejhan S, Zadeh MRL, Javaherzadeh M, Behgam M. Surgical treatment of complicated pulmonary hydatid cyst. Tanaffos. 2007;6:19–22.
9. Alpay L, Lacin T, Ocakcioglu I, Evman S, Dogruyol T, Vayvada M, Baysungur V, Yalcinkaya I. Is video-assisted thoracoscopic surgery adequate in treatment of pulmonary hydatidosis? Ann Thorac Surg. 2015;100:258–62.
10. Chowbey P, Shah S, Khullar R, Sharma A, Soni V, Baijal M, Vashistha A, Dhir A. Minimal access surgery for hydatid cyst disease: laparoscopic, thoracoscopic, and retroperitoneoscopic approach. J Laparoendosc Adv Surg Tech. 2003;13:159–65.
11. Ettayebi F, Benhannou M. Echinococcus granulosus cyst of the lung: treatment by thoracoscopy. Pediatr Endosurgery Innov Tech. 2003;7:67–70.

12. Findikcioglu A, Karadayi S, Kilic D, Hatiopoglu A. Video-assisted thoracoscopic surgery to treat hydatid disease of the thorax in adults: is it feasible? J Laparoendosc Adv Surg Tech. 2012;22:882–5.

13. Mallick MS, Al-Qahtani A, Al-Saadi MM, Al-Boukai AAA. Thoracoscopic treatment of pulmonary hydatid cyst in a child. J Pediatr Surg. 2005;40: e35-e37.

14. Parelkar SV, Gupta RK, Shah H, Sanghvi B, Gupta A, Jadhav V, Garasia M, Agrawal A. Experience with video-assisted thoracoscopic removal of pulmonary hydatid cysts in children. J Pediatr Surg. 2009;44:836–41.

15. Tullu MS, Lahiri KR, Kumar S, Oak SN. Minimal access therapy in pediatric pulmonary hydatid cysts. Pediatr Pulmonol. 2005;40:92–5.

16. Uchikov AP, Shipkov CD, Prisadov G. Treatment of lung hydatidosis by VATS: a preliminary report. Can J Surg. 2004;47:380.

17. Chen YC, Yeh TS, Tseng JH, Huang SF, Lin DY. Hepatic hydatid cysts with superinfection in a non-endemic area in Taiwan. Am J Trop Med Hyg. 2002; 67:524–7.

18. Burt BM, Shrager JB. Prevention and management of postoperative air leaks. Ann Cardiothorac Surg. 2014;3:216–8.

19. Auldist AW, Blakelock R. Pulmonary hydatid disease. In Pediatric Thoracic Surgery. London: Springer; 2009. pp. 161–167.

20. Creåu C, Codreanu R, Mastalier B, Popa L, Cordoş I, Beuran M. Albendazole associated to surgery or minimally invasive procedures for hydatid disease– how much and how long. Chirurgia (Bucur). 2012;107:15–21.

3

Should high risk patients with concomitant severe aortic stenosis and mitral valve disease undergo double valve surgery in the TAVR era?

Pey-Jen Yu[1]* (ID), Allan Mattia[1], Hugh A. Cassiere[1], Rick Esposito[1], Frank Manetta[1], Nina Kohn[2] and Alan R. Hartman[1]

Abstract

Background: Significant mitral regurgitation in patients undergoing transcatheter aortic valve replacement (TAVR) is associated with increased mortality. The aim of this study is to determine if surgical correction of both aortic and mitral valves in high risk patients with concomitant valvular disease would offer patients better outcomes than TAVR alone.

Methods: A retrospective analysis of 43 high-risk patients who underwent concomitant surgical aortic valve replacement and mitral valve surgery from 2008 to 2012 was performed. Immediate and long term survival were assessed.

Results: There were 43 high-risk patients with severe aortic stenosis undergoing concomitant surgical aortic valve replacement and mitral valve surgery. The average age was 80 ± 6 years old. Nineteen (44%) patients had prior cardiac surgery, 15 (34.9%) patients had chronic obstructive lung disease, and 39 (91%) patients were in congestive heart failure. The mean Society of Thoracic Surgeons Predicted Risk of Mortality for isolated surgical aortic valve replacement for the cohort was $10.1\% \pm 6.4\%$. Five patients (11.6%) died during the index admission and/or within thirty days of surgery. Mortality rate was 25% at six months, 35% at 1 year and 45% at 2 years. There was no correlation between individual preoperative risk factors and mortality.

Conclusions: High-risk patients with severe aortic stenosis and mitral valve disease undergoing concomitant surgical aortic valve replacement and mitral valve surgery may have similar long term survival as that described for such patients undergoing TAVR. Surgical correction of double valvular disease in this patient population may not confer mortality benefit compared to TAVR alone.

Keywords: Aortic stenosis, Aortic valve surgery, Mitral valve surgery, Transcatheter aortic valve replacement

Background

Aortic stenosis is the most prevalent valvular heart disease referred for treatment and it is frequently associated with concomitant mitral regurgitation (MR) [1]. Surgical aortic valve replacement is the standard treatment for symptomatic severe aortic stenosis, and there is general consensus that in the presence of severe MR, a double-valve operation is indicated. With the advent of the transcatheter aortic valve replacement (TAVR),

surgical aortic valve replacement has largely been replaced by TAVR for patients at high or prohibitive surgical risk. It has been estimated that the prevalence of moderate or severe MR in patients undergoing TAVR ranges from 22 to 48% [1–6]. In these patients, the concomitant significant MR is typically left untreated and is associated with increased morbidity and mortality after TAVR [3, 4, 6–9].

Given the poor outcome of TAVR patients with severe aortic stenosis and significant MR, we sought to determine the short and long term outcomes of high risk patients undergoing concomitant surgical aortic valve replacement and mitral valve surgery to determine if

* Correspondence: pyu2@northwell.edu
[1]Department of Cardiovascular and Thoracic Surgery, Hofstra Northwell School of Medicine, 300 Community Drive, 1DSU, Manhasset, NY 11030, USA
Full list of author information is available at the end of the article

open surgical approach may be preferable to TAVR only in such patients.

Methods

This study was conducted with the approval of the Hofstra Northwell Health System Institutional Review Board with specific waiver of the need for individual patient consent. A retrospective review was performed on all patients who underwent concomitant aortic valve replacement and mitral valve surgery between 2008 and 2012. Each patient's baseline surgical risk was determined using the Society of Thoracic Surgery Predicted Risk of Mortality (STS PROM) calculator. As the calculator is unable to give mortality risks for double valve surgery, the mortality risk for isolated AVR was used for each patient. Total predicted risk of mortality was calculated as the summation of the STS PROM plus any incremental risks not are not included in STS PROM [10, 11]. Patients were included in the study if their total predicted risk of mortality was greater than or equal to 8%. Patients undergoing aortic valve replacement for aortic insufficiency and/or aortic valve endocarditis were excluded. Definitions used for the preoperative risk factors and perioperative complications are standardized based on published guidelines by the New York State Department of Health for the New York State Cardiac Surgery Reporting System and the Society of Thoracic Surgeons cardiac surgery database. The following data were collected: gender, left ventricular ejection fraction, preoperative dialysis, presence of comorbidities (cerebral vascular disease, diabetes mellitus, hypertension, hyperlipidemia, congestive heart failure, chronic obstructive lung disease, peripheral vascular disease), urgency of surgery, previous myocardial infarction, preoperative arrhythmia and if this was a re-operation.

Clinical endpoint was long-term survival. Long-term survival was determined from the Social Security Death Index. All statistical analyses were performed using SAS Version 9.3 (SAS Institute Inc., Cary, NC). For categorical factors, survival from date of surgery was estimated using the Kaplan-Meier product limit method and compared using the log-rank test. For each continuous factor, Cox regression was used to determine if that factor was associated with survival. For this analysis, patients who died during surgery were counted as having survived for one day from the start of surgery. Length of stay (LOS) from day of surgery was calculated as the number of days from surgery to discharge, and patients who died during surgery were counted as having a one day LOS.

Results

A total of 43 high-risk patients underwent aortic valve replacement for aortic stenosis and mitral valve surgery between 2008 and 2012. The preoperative characteristics for the study group are listed in Table 1. The average age was 80 ± 6 years old. Nineteen (44.2%) patients had prior cardiac surgery, 15 (34.9%) patients had severe chronic obstructive lung disease, 39 (90.7%) patients had congestive heart failure and 14 (32.6%) patients had severe pulmonary hypertension with pulmonary artery pressures ≥ 60 mmHg. The average STS PROM for isolated aortic valve replacement for the cohort was $10.1\% \pm 6.4\%$. The average total predicted risk of mortality which includes incremental risk factors not accounted for in the Society of Thoracic Surgeons risk model was $14.6\% \pm 6.9\%$.

Postoperative morbidity is shown in Table 2. Overall operative mortality was 11.6%. Nineteen (44.2%) patients required prolonged ventilation, 10 (23.3%) patients had new renal failure with 6 (14.0%) patients requiring dialysis. Median time to postoperative extubation was 21.5 h (interquartile range 12 h – 141 h), median length of intensive care unit stay was 136.0 h (interquartile range 46 h – 586 h), and median length of hospital stay from day of surgery was 13 days (interquartile range 9 days - 24 days). Of the 38 patients who survived to discharge, 12 (31.6%) patients were discharged to home.

The mortality rate was 23% at six months, 33% at 1 year and 42% at 2 years (Fig. 1). There were no

Table 1 Pre-Operative Characteristics of the Patient Population

Pre-Operative Characteristics	Number (Percent) $n = 43$
Male	15 (34.88)
Body Mass Index	26.7 ± 7.1
Urgent Procedure	31 (72.09)
Re-Operation	19 (44.19)
Severe Chronic Obstructive Lung Disease	15 (34.88)
Creatinine	1.7 ± 1.2
Dialysis Dependent	5 (11.63)
Diabetes	17 (39.53)
Hypertension	39 (90.70)
Dyslipidemia	28 (65.12)
Cerebrovascular Disease	10 (23.26)
Peripheral Vascular Disease	7 (16.28)
Previous MI	7 (16.28)
Atrial Fibrillation/Flutter	17 (39.53)
Congestive Heart Failure	39 (90.70)
Age (years)	80 ± 6
Pulmonary Hypertension (≥60 mmHg)	14 (32.56)
Ejection Fraction	49.9 ± 13
STS PROM for isolated AVR	10.1 ± 6.4
Total Predicted Risk of Mortality for isolated AVR	14.6 ± 6.9

Table 2 Postoperative Complication Rates of the Patient Population

Postoperative Complications	Number (Percent)
Composite Morbidity	30 (69.77)
Operative Mortality	5 (11.63)
Re-Op Bleeding	1 (2.33)
Re-Op non Cardiac Cause	12 (27.91)
Deep Sternal Wound Infection	0 (0.00)
Sepsis	2 (4.65)
Stroke	1 (2.33)
Prolonged Ventilation	19 (44.19)
Pneumonia	1 (2.33)
Renal Failure	10 (23.26)
Dialysis Required	6 (13.95)
Cardiac Arrest	2 (4.65)

Table 3 Association between Preoperative Risk Factors and Survival

Categorical Factors	p-value
Urgency of Operation	0.1199
Re-operation	0.8097
Severe Chronic Lung Disease	0.4225
Dialysis	0.1915
Diabetes	0.5321
Age	0.4274
Ejection fraction	0.6072

associations between preoperative risk factors and survival (Table 3).

Discussion

High risk patients with concomitant aortic stenosis and mitral regurgitation are left with uncorrected mitral valve disease after their TAVR. As the presence of significant mitral regurgitation is associated with reduced survival for patients undergoing TAVR, it is unclear if such patients would be better served with surgical correction of both the aortic and mitral valves rather than TAVR alone. The purpose of this study was to determine the outcomes of high risk patients who would have been candidates for TAVR who underwent surgical aortic valve replacement and mitral valve surgery.

Prior studies have shown increased postoperative mortality and morbidity with concomitant aortic and mitral valve surgery [12–16]. Maleska et al. reports a 91% and

71% survival rates at 30 days and 1 year, respectively, for octogenarians undergoing simultaneous aortic and mitral valve replacement [17]. However, the mortality risk of double valve surgery in patients with concomitant aortic and mitral valve disease who may be considered for TAVR remains unclear. This study is the first to look at outcomes of high risk patients with severe aortic stenosis undergoing surgical aortic valve replacement and mitral valve surgery. Although the actual operative mortality rate of 11.6% in our study cohort was lower than the total predicated risk of mortality rate for AVR alone of 14.6%, the long term 1 year and 2 year survival rate was only 67% and 58%, respectively. Therefore, our study demonstrates that, despite reasonable operative survival rates, high risk patients with concomitant severe aortic stenosis and mitral valve disease have poor long term prognosis even after surgical correction of both valvular abnormalities.

Numerous studies have demonstrated increased mortality in patients with significant MR undergoing TAVR [6, 8, 18, 19]. A meta-analysis of eight studies including 8015 patients found increased overall 30-day and 1-year mortality with an odds ratio of 1.49 and 1.92,

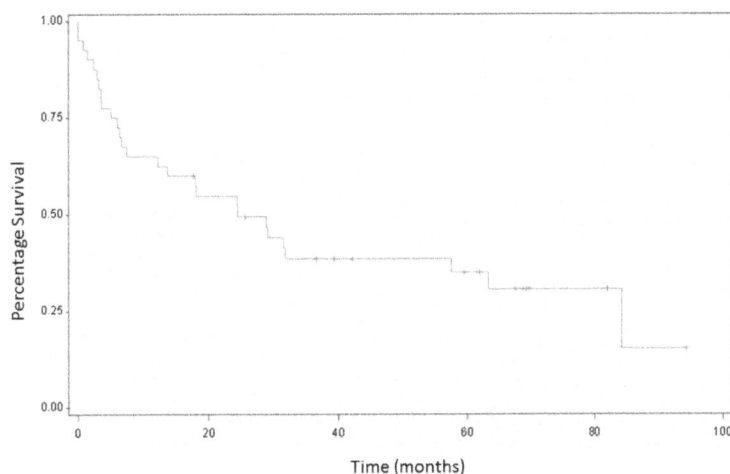

Fig. 1 Kaplan Meier Log Rank Survival Curve

respectively, in TAVR patients with significant MR as compared to those without [4]. Another meta-analysis of 16 studies and 13,672 patients demonstrated a similar increase in early and overall all-cause mortality in patients with significant MR as compared to patients without MR or with non-significant MR with an odds ratio of 2.17 and a hazard ratio of 1.81, respectively [5]. A large multicenter study of 1110 patients by Cortes et al. found that patients with significant pre-TAVR MR had a 3 fold increase in 6 month mortality as compared with patients without significant pre-TAVR MR (35.0% vs. 10.2%, $p < 0.001$) [2]. The same study found that although the degree of MR have been shown to improve in up to 60% of patients undergoing TAVR, improvement of baseline MR was not associated with improved cardiac mortality [2]. Mavromatis et al. reported a one year motality and heart failure rehospitalization rate of 28.0% and 23.4%, respectively, in patients who underwent TAVR with severe MR [9]. A study by Toggweiler et al. looked at the outcomes of patients undergoing TAVR with concomitant severe MR [6]. With 49% having previous open-heart surgery, 26% having chronic obstructive pulmonary disease, 35% having pulmonary hypertension, and an average STS risk score of 9.7%, the study population in their study was comparable to that of the current study. They report a survival of 84%, 65% and 59% at 30 days, 1 year and 2 years, respectively, which is comparable to the survival rate of 77%, 67% and 58% reported in our study [6].

Although significant MR is associated with increased short and long term mortality in patients undergoing TAVR, they are comparable to the mortality rates for our study cohort of similar patients undergoing concomitant aortic and mitral valve surgery. As such, surgical correction of both valves may not alter the long term outcomes in these high risk patients as compared to TAVR alone. Furthermore, the advent of percutaneous interventions for treating mitral valve disease may offer appropriate patients percutaneous alternatives for the management of residual MR after TAVR [20]. Percutanous edge to edge mitral valve repair with MitraClip (Abbott Vascular, Menlo Park, CA) has been the most widely used and studied for the treatment of significant MR after TAVR. Rudolph et al. reported a case series of 11 patients receiving both TAVR and MitraClip therapy with successful reduction of MR severity to <2+ in 10 patients [21]. Another case series of 12 patients who underwent MitraClip placement after TAVR by Kische et al. reported a 100% procedural success rate with MitraClip with no patients with greater than 1+ MR after MitraClip. All patients in that series also experienced functional improvement after MitraClip [22]. A contemporary series of 14 patients undergoing MitraClip after TAVR reported a 92.9% procedural success rate with 21.4% of patients with

recurrent 3+ MR at one year [23]. Interestingly, the reported one year survival rate of 66.5% in that series is similar to that of our study [23]. This may further support that correction of the mitral regurgitation may not offer survival benefit in this select high risk patient population.

There are several limitations to this study. First, as an STS score is unable to be calculated for double valve surgery, we used the STS score for isolated AVR as the basis for expected mortality risk for risk stratification. Although this inevitably underestimates the surgical risk for double valve surgery, its use is justified for the purpose of this study as the same score would be used for the risk stratification of patients with concomitant mitral and aortic valve disease being considered for TAVR. Secondly, as this study was limited to patients to high risk patients undergoing concomitant surgical aortic valve replacement and mitral valve surgery, the results of this study may not be applicable to intermediate and low risk patients undergoing similar surgeries. Lastly, as with all single center studies, the results of this study may not be generalizable to all institutions.

Conclusion

In conclusion, high-risk patients with severe aortic stenosis and mitral valve disease undergoing concomitant surgical aortic valve replacement and mitral valve surgery have similar long term survival as that described for such patients undergoing TAVR. Surgical correction of double valvular disease in this patient population may not confer mortality benefit compared to TAVR alone.

Abbreviations
LOS: length of stay; MR: mitral regurgitation; STS PROM: Society of Thoracic Surgery predicted risk of mortality; TAVR: transcatheter aortic valve replacement

Acknowledgements
Not applicable.

Funding
None.

Authors' contributions
PY designed the study, gathered and interpreted the data, and drafted the manuscript; AM gathered and interpreted the data; HC analyzed the data; RE analyzed the data; FM analyzed the data; NK did the statistical analysis; ARH interpreted the data. All authors read and approved the final manuscript.

Competing interests
The authors declare that they have no competing interests.

Author details

[1]Department of Cardiovascular and Thoracic Surgery, Hofstra Northwell School of Medicine, 300 Community Drive, 1DSU, Manhasset, NY 11030, USA.
[2]The Feinstein Institute for Medical Research, Manhasset, NY, USA.

References

1. Nombela-Franco L, Ribeiro HB, Urena M, et al. Significant mitral regurgitation left untreated at the time of aortic valve replacement: a comprehensive review of a frequent entity in the transcatheter aortic valve replacement era. J Am Coll Cardiol. 2014;63:2643–58.
2. Cortes C, Amat-Santos IJ, Nombela-Franco L, et al. Mitral regurgitation after transcatheter aortic valve replacement: prognosis, imaging predictors, and potential management. JACC Cardiovasc Interv. 2016;9:1603–14.
3. Khawaja MZ, Williams R, Hung J, et al. Impact of preprocedural mitral regurgitation upon mortality after transcatheter aortic valve implantation (tavi) for severe aortic stenosis. Heart. 2014;100:1799–803.
4. Nombela-Franco L, Eltchaninoff H, Zahn R, et al. Clinical impact and evolution of mitral regurgitation following transcatheter aortic valve replacement: a meta-analysis. Heart. 2015;101:1395–405.
5. Takagi H, Umemoto T. All-literature investigation of cardiovascular evidence G. Coexisting mitral regurgitation impairs survival after transcatheter aortic valve implantation. Ann Thorac Surg. 2015;100:2270–6.
6. Toggweiler S, Boone RH, Rodes-Cabau J, et al. Transcatheter aortic valve replacement: outcomes of patients with moderate or severe mitral regurgitation. J Am Coll Cardiol. 2012;59:2068–74.
7. Goncalves A, Solomon SD. Mitral regurgitation in transcatheter aortic valve replacement: the complexity of multivalvular disease. Circulation. 2013;128:2101–3.
8. Bedogni F, Latib A, De Marco F, et al. Interplay between mitral regurgitation and transcatheter aortic valve replacement with the corevalve revalving system: a multicenter registry. Circulation. 2013;128:2145–53.
9. Mavromatis K, Thourani VH, Stebbins A, et al. Transcatheter aortic valve replacement in patients with aortic stenosis and mitral regurgitation. Ann Thorac Surg. 2017;104:1977-985.
10. Adams DH, Popma JJ, Reardon MJ, et al. Transcatheter aortic-valve replacement with a self-expanding prosthesis. N Engl J Med. 2014;370:1790–8.
11. Reardon MJ, Kleiman NS, Adams DH, et al. Outcomes in the randomized corevalve us pivotal high risk trial in patients with a society of thoracic surgeons risk score of 7% or less. JAMA Cardiol. 2016;1:945–9.
12. Galloway AC, Grossi EA, Baumann FG, et al. Multiple valve operation for advanced valvular heart disease: results and risk factors in 513 patients. J Am Coll Cardiol. 1992;19:725–32.
13. Mueller XM, Tevaearai HT, Stumpe F, et al. Long-term results of mitral-aortic valve operations. J Thorac Cardiovasc Surg. 1998;115:1298–309.
14. Litmathe J, Boeken U, Kurt M, Feindt P, Gams E. Predictive risk factors in double-valve replacement (avr and mvr) compared to isolated aortic valve replacement. Thorac Cardiovasc Surg. 2006;54:459–63.
15. Connelly KA, Creati L, Lyon W, et al. Early and late results of combined mitral-aortic valve surgery. Heart Lung Circ. 2007;16:410–5.
16. Nicolini F, Agostinelli A, Fortuna D, et al. Outcomes of patients undergoing concomitant mitral and aortic valve surgery: results from an italian regional cardiac surgery registry. Interact Cardiovasc Thorac Surg. 2014;19:763–70.
17. Maleszka A, Kleikamp G, Zittermann A, Serrano MR, Koerfer R. Simultaneous aortic and mitral valve replacement in octogenarians: a viable option? Ann Thorac Surg. 2008;86:1804–8.
18. Rodes-Cabau J, Webb JG, Cheung A, et al. Transcatheter aortic valve implantation for the treatment of severe symptomatic aortic stenosis in patients at very high or prohibitive surgical risk: acute and late outcomes of the multicenter canadian experience. J Am Coll Cardiol. 2010;55:1080–90.
19. Zahn R, Gerckens U, Linke A, et al. Predictors of one-year mortality after transcatheter aortic valve implantation for severe symptomatic aortic stenosis. Am J Cardiol. 2013;112:272–9.
20. Ando T, Takagi H, Briasoulis A, et al. A systematic review of reported cases of combined transcatheter aortic and mitral valve interventions. Catheter Cardiovasc Interv. 2017. doi:10.1002/ccd.27256.
21. Rudolph V, Schirmer J, Franzen O, et al. Bivalvular transcatheter treatment of high-surgical-risk patients with coexisting severe aortic stenosis and significant mitral regurgitation. Int J Cardiol. 2013;167:716–20.
22. Kische S, D'Ancona G, Paranskaya L, et al. Staged total percutaneous treatment of aortic valve pathology and mitral regurgitation: institutional experience. Catheter Cardiovasc Interv. 2013;82:E552–63.
23. D'Ancona G, Paranskaya L, Oner A, Kische S, Ince H. Mitro-aortic pathology: a point of view for a fully transcatheter staged approach. Neth Heart J. 2017;25:605–8.

4

Identification of preoperative prediction factors of tumor subtypes for patients with solitary ground-glass opacity pulmonary nodules

Meishuang Li[1,2,3,4], Yanan Wang[1,2,3,4], Yulong Chen[1,2,3,4] and Zhenfa Zhang[1,2,3,4*]

Abstract

Background: Recent wide spread use of low-dose helical computed tomography for the screening of lung cancer have led to an increase in the detection rate of very faint and smaller lesions known as ground-glass opacity nodules. The purpose of this study was to investigate the clinical factors of lung cancer patients with solitary ground-glass opacity pulmonary nodules on computed tomography.

Methods: A total of 423 resected solitary ground-glass opacity nodules were retrospectively evaluated. We analyzed the clinical, imaging and pathological data and investigated the clinical differences in patient with adenocarcinoma in situ / minimally invasive adenocarcinoma and those with invasive adenocarcinoma.

Results: Three hundred and ninety-three adenocarcinomas (92.9%) and 30 benign nodules were diagnosed. Age, the history of family cancer, serum carcinoembryonic antigen level, tumor size, ground-glass opacity types, and bubble-like sign in chest CT differed significantly between adenocarcinoma in situ / minimally invasive adenocarcinoma and invasive adenocarcinoma (p:0.008, 0.046, 0.000, 0.000, 0.000 and 0.001). Receiver operating characteristic curves and univariate analysis revealed that patients with more than 58.5 years, a serum carcinoembryonic antigen level > 1.970 μg/L, a tumor size> 13.50 mm, mixed ground-glass opacity nodules and a bubble-like sign were more likely to be diagnosed as invasive adenocarcinoma. The combination of five factors above had an area under the curve of 0.91, with a sensitivity of 82% and a specificity of 87%.

Conclusion: The five-factor combination helps us to distinguish adenocarcinoma in situ / minimally invasive adenocarcinoma from invasive adenocarcinoma and to perform appropriate surgery for solitary ground-glass opacity nodules.

Keywords: Solitory ground-glass opacity pulmonary nodules, ROC curve, Clinical features, Five-factor combination, Pathology

Background

Recent widespread use of low-dose helical computed tomography (CT) for the screening of lung cancer have led to an increase in the detection rate of very faint and smaller lesions known as ground-glass opacity (GGO) nodules. GGO is a nonspecific finding that may be caused by various disorders, including inflammatory disease, hyperemia, focal fibrosis and neoplastic disease. The new interdisciplinary IASLC/ATS/ERS classification of lung adenocarcinoma has achieved a considerable impact since its publication in the year 2011. It puts forward that the preinvasive lesions atypical adenomatous hyperplasia (AAH) and adenocarcinoma in situ (AIS) together with minimally invasive adenocarcinoma (MIA) have an excellent prognosis after complete resection with 100% survival or approaches 100% survival. Several recent studies have demonstrated comparable

* Correspondence: zhangzhenfa1973@163.com
[1]Department of Lung Cancer, Tianjin Medical University Cancer Institute and Hospital, Huanhu West Road, Tianjin 300060, China
[2]National Clinical Research Center for Cancer, Key Laboratory of Cancer Prevention and Therapy, Tianjin 300060, China
Full list of author information is available at the end of the article

recurrence and survival rates for lobectomy and sublobar resection, even in good-risk patients with small stage I lung cancer [1–4]. A GGO appearance on chest CT has been reported to be associated with a favorable histology such as non-or minimally invasive adenocarcinoma in lung cancer [5]. These GGO lesions are also likely to be amenable to sublobar resection. Serum carcinoembryonic antigen (CEA) is a useful circulating biomarker and now well-known and validated serum biomarker for lung cancer. Maeda et al. [6] reported that CEA level was an important clinical predictor of tumor invasiveness in patients with clinical stage IA non-small cell lung cancer (NSCLC).

Although some studies have identified some clinical and imaging factors and used the combination of the selected parameters for the preoperative prediction of tumor subtypes in patients with T1 lung cancer, there is no report about solitary GGO nodules on chest CT. Therefore, the purpose of our study was to investigate parameters that preoperatively predicted histological subtypes in patients with solitary GGO nodules on chest CT.

Methods
Study population
This study was approved by the institutional review board of Tianjin Medical University Cancer Institute and Hospital, Tianjin, China. Between January 2013 and December 2016, 6317 patients with pulmonary nodules underwent surgical resection with curative intent at Cancer Institute and Hospital of Tianjin Medical University. Of these patients, 423 were selected according to inclusion criteria and exclusion criteria. Our inclusion criteria were as follows: (1) patients with solitary GGO nodules on chest CT scan, (2) patients who had their lesions surgically removed and had postoperative pathological diagnosis, (3) R0 resection. Our exclusion criteria included: (1) patients who had no CT scan, (2) pulmonary multiple GGO nodules, mixed GGO with consolidation to the maximum tumor diameter greater than 0.75 or pure solid tumors, (3) patients with history of lung cancer or who had a malignancy elsewhere. All patients underwent lobectomy or limited resection (segmentectomy or wedge resection) with hilar and mediastinal lymphadenectomy or lymph node sampling. There were no objective criteria for limited resection, and the indications depended on each surgeon's preference. A patient with a GGO > 5-8 mm may be subjected to surgical treatment and with a GGO less than 20 mm may be given the limited resection, including segmentectomy and wedge resection.

Clinical and pathological characteristics
For each patient, age, gender, smoking status, a family history of cancer, location of tumor, the serum tumor markers: carcinoembryonic antigen (CEA) and carbohydrate antigen 19–9 (CA19–9) and histological subtypes were extracted from patient medical records. Classification of lung adenocarcinoma was assessed by two pathologists in accordance with the new interdisciplinary IASLC/ATS/ERS classification of lung adenocarcinoma. We classified all patients into two groups: AIS /MIA group and invasive adenocarcinoma (IA) group.

CT imaging
Chest CT scans were performed before surgery by using one of three multi-detector CT systems: Somatom Sensation 64 (Siemens Medical Solutions, Forchheim, Germany), Light speed 16, and Discovery CT750 HD (GE Healthcare, Milwaukee, WI, USA) scanner. Scanning parameters were as follows: 120kVp with tube current adjusted automatically, 1.5 mm reconstructionthickness with 1.5 mm reconstruction interval for 64-detector scanner; and 120kVp, 150–200 mA, 1.25 mm reconstruction thickness with 1.25 mm reconstruction interval for the other two scanners. GGO was defined as a hazy increase in lung attenuation without obscuring the underlying vascular marking. Two observers who were unaware of pathologic staging viewed each CT scan of 423 solitary GGO nodules and assessed nodules morphology blindly. Morphology included density, size, air bronchogram, bubble-like sign, spicule sign, pleural tag or lobular. Based on the density via CT, GGO nodules were classified into two groups: pure GGO (pGGO) (a tumor without solid component), and mixed GGO (mGGO) (a tumor with both GGO and solid components).

Blood specimen collection and measurement
About 3 ml of peripheral blood was collected from each case in coagulated tube. The serum was separated by centrifuging at 3000×g for 5 min, and then transferred to a new Eppendorf tube, and stored at – 80 °C for further analysis. Tumor biomarkers, including CEA, CA19–9 were measured using electrochemiluminescence immunoassays according to standard procedure of Roche Company's kit and Roche E170 automatic immunity analyzer. The cut-off points for each tumor biomarker determined by the manufacturer, were as follows: CEA, 5 μg/l; CA19–9, 39 U/ml.

Statistical analysis
Statistical analysis performed by using SPSS 24.0 software. The T test, Mann-Whitney U test, χ^2 test or Fisher's exact test were used to test for difference in clinical factors and imaging characters between different pathology groups, asappropriate. T test was used for categorical variables fitted normal distribution and expressed by x ± s. Mann-Whitney U test was used for categorical variablesfitted non-normal distribution and expressed by

M (P25, P75). χ^2 test or Fisher's exact test was used for categorical variables. Receiver operating characteristics (ROC) curves were generated to evaluate the predictive potential of identified clinical and imaging signatures for IA, then combined all identified factors to predict histological types by adding all five factors to a bivariable-adjusted logistic regression model. Optimal cut-off values were calculated by ROC cures. Univariate logistic regression and binary logistic regression analysis were also performed to assess the diagnostic accuracy by using cut-off values. All statistical tests were two-sided, and a p value ≤ 0.05 was considered statistically significant.

Results

Patients demographics

There were total 423 patients with solitory GGO nodules. Among them, 393 had adenocarcinoma and 30 had benign nodules. The clinicopathologic characteristics of 393 (92.9%) patients with adenocarcinoma were summarized in Table 1. There were 117 male and 276 female patients (median age, 57 years; range: 27–78 years). Two hundred and ninety-six of 393 (75.3%) patients were never active smokers. Sixty-six patients had a family history of other cancers (such as liver cancer, gastric cancer, colorectal cancer and bone cancer) and 50 (43.1%) patients had a family history of lung cancer. Of 393 patients, preoperative serum CEA and CA19–9 were tested in 379 patients. The number of patients with elevated CEA and CA19–9 were 25 (6.6%) and 81 (21.4%), respectively. GGO nodules were often found in the superior lobe of right lung ($n = 163$), followed by the superior lobe of left lung ($n = 98$). The histological types according to IASLC/ATS/ERS classification were as follows: 269 (68.4%) patients with IA, 115 (29.3%) patients with MIA, 9 (2.3%) patients with AIS. Lobectomy, segmentectomy and wedge resection were performed in 349 (88.8%), 21 (5.3%) and 23 (5.9%) patients, respectively.

Clinical and imaging factors that predict histological subtypes

Age, family history of cancer, Serum CEA level, GGO size, type of GGO and bubble-like sign differed significantly between patients with AIS/MIA and those with IA (p: 0.008, 0.046, 0.000, 0.000, 0.000, and 0.001). (Table 2). By the bivariate logistic analysis, tumor size, mixed GGO and bubble-like sign were independent predictors of IA (p:0.000, 0.000 and 0.021, respectively). ROC curves were generated to assess the IA prediction accuracy of the six factors identified in univariate analysis. It showed that a family history of cancer had a poor accuracy ($p = 0.1148$). Therefore, this parameter was not brought into muti-factor combination. Figure 1 shows the true-positive ratios (sensitivity) and false-positive ratios (1 minus specificity) for age, CEA, tumor

Table 1 Characteristic of the patients with GGO

Variable	Number (%)
Gender	
Male	117 (29.8)
Female	276 (70.2)
Age	
≤ 60	233 (59.3)
> 60	160 (40.7)
Smoking	
Current/ever	97 (24.7)
Never	296 (75.3)
Family history of cancer	
Yes	116 (29.5)
No	277 (70.5)
Tumor marker	
CEA(+)	25 (6.6)
CA19–9(+)	4 (1.1)
Surgical method	
Lobectomy	349 (88.8)
Segmentectomy	21 (5.3)
Wedge resection	23 (5.9)
Pathological type	
AIS/MIA	9/115 (31.6)
IA	269 (68.4)
Pathological stage	
0	9 (2.3)
IA	370 (94.1)
IB	14 (3.6)
Lymphatic metastasis	0

Abbreviation: *CEA* carcinoembryonic antigen, *CA19–9* carbohydrate antigen 19-9, *AIS* adenocarcinoma in situ, *MIA* minimally invasive adenocarcinoma, *IA* invasive pulmonary adenocarcinoma

size, GGO type and bubble-like sign. The areas under curves (AUCs) for age, serum CEA level, tumor size, GGO type and bubble-like sign were 0.59, 0.62, 0.87, 0.72, and 0.58 (p: 0.0058, 0.0002, < 0.0001, < 0.0001, and 0.001, respectively), with sensitivities of 57%, 54%, 86%, 71%, 35% and specificities of 59%, 65%, 72%, 73%, 83%. We also assessed the IA prediction accuracy of these five factors in combination via bivariate logistic regression analysis. The AUC of the five-factor combination was 0.91, with a sensitivity of 82% and a specificity of 87% (p < 0.0001). (Table 3). To further distinguish the IA from AIS/MIA, we performed univariate and multivariate analyses using the optimal cut-off values calculated from the ROC curves (Table 4). According to the univariate analysis, patients were more likely to be diagnosed with IA if they had these factors: more than 58.5 years, a serum CEA level > 1.970 µg/L, a tumor size > 13.50 mm,

Table 2 Correlation between histological subtypes and clinical and CT imaging characteristics

Variable	AIS/MIA(124)	IA(269)	p value
Gender			0.984
Male	37	80	
Female	87	189	
Median age	55.85 ± 9.42	58.49 ± 9.00	0.008*
Smoking			0.246
Current/ever	98	198	
Never	26	71	
History of family cancer			0.046*
Yes	45	71	
No	79	198	
CEA	1.5 (1.0,2.4)	2.1 (1.3,3.1)	0.000*
CA19–9	11.0 (8.4,17.4)	9.4 (6.5,15.3)	0.081
Location of tumor			0.084
RUL	52	111	
RML	8	12	
RLL	15	50	
LUL	39	59	
LLL	10	37	
GGO size	1.2 (0.8,1.6)	2.0 (1.6,2.5)	0.000*
GGO type			0.000*
pGGO	90	77	
mGGO	34	192	
Air bronchogram	18	71	0.074
Bubble-like sign	22	92	0.001*
Spicule sign	32	79	0.140
Pleural tag	31	71	0.163
Pathological stage			0.000*
0/IA	124	255	
IB	0	14	
Lymphatic metastasis	–	–	–

*Statistically significant p value, CEA carcinoembryonic antigen, CA19–9 carbohydrate antigen 19–9, pGGO pure ground-glass opacity nodule, mGGN mixed ground-glass opacity nodule, RUL superior lobe of right lung, RML middle lobe of right lung, RLL inferior lobe of right lung, LUL superior lobe of left lung, LLL inferior lobe of left lung

mGGO and bubble-like sign (p: 0.005, 0.001, 0.000, 0.000, and 0.001, respectively). According to the bivariate analyses, the combination of these five factors was an independent diagnostic factor for IA (p:0.000).

Discussion

Limited resection including segmentectomy and wedge resection has been recently advocated for patients with AIS or MIA due to its preservation of lung function. But it is not suitable for patients with IA. Thus, it would be helpful to use preoperative factors to predict the histological type of GGO because many GGO nodules were AIS or MIA. Due to the low cellularity in GGO lesions, the diagnostic yield of percutaneous needle biopsy for GGO lesions was reported to be significantly lower than that of solid lesions [7]. Therefore, circulating tumor marker levels and CT imaging are attractive alternatives.

Numerous studies proved that the CT findings were useful for evaluating the histological nature of the tumors and correlated with the IASLC/ATS/ERS classification [8–10]. Our results showed that benign lesions only accounted for 7.1%, the reason may be the selection of candidate patients for surgery. Because we usually resected GGNs which were more likely to be malignant, such as larger tumor diameter (more than 8 mm), mGGO with solid contents, changing of diameter or contents of GGNs during follow-up. From a survey of 492 lung cancers of all pathological types and stages, Seki et al. [11] reported that GGO was found only in adenocarcinoma. In line with these findings, our results showed that all patients with pulmonary GGO nodules are confirmed to be lung adenocarcinoma. Generally, the larger the nodules are, the more likely they will be IA. Our study revealed that tumor size was an independent predictive factor for IA. We distinguished IA from AIS/ MIA when an optimal cut-off value of 13.50 mm was used. Lee et al. [12] reported that optimal cut-off values of 10 mm and 14 mm for distinguishing preinvasive lesions from invasive pulmonary lesions in cases of pGGO and mGGO, respectively. However, a study recommended that 11 mm was the tumor size cut-off value for differentiating IA from AIS and MIA in patients with T1 lung adenocarcinoma.

A study reported that lesions with GGO appearance were more likely to be "early" adenocarcinoma such as BAC, AIS, or MIA, whereas more advanced adenocarcinomas include a larger solid component within the GGO region [13, 14]. Our study revealed that a solid component was associated with IA.. In our study, the presence of mGGO nodule predicted IA with an AUC of 0.72. Although our study showed that CT findings were useful diagnostic factors of pathological types, other factors should be identified to improve sensitivity and specificity.

Serum biomarker as a diagnostic tool with less invasive and rapid detection was widely used for malignant tumor. Serum CEA is a useful circulating biomarker and now a well-known and validated serum biomarker for lung adenocarcinoma. However, the optimal cut-off value for serum CEA level varies in the literature [15]. Using the optimal cut-off value identified in our study (> 1.970 µg/L,), We found CEA was associated IA in patients with GGOs.

A significant difference was also noted in age, which could be explained by the hypothesis of sequential

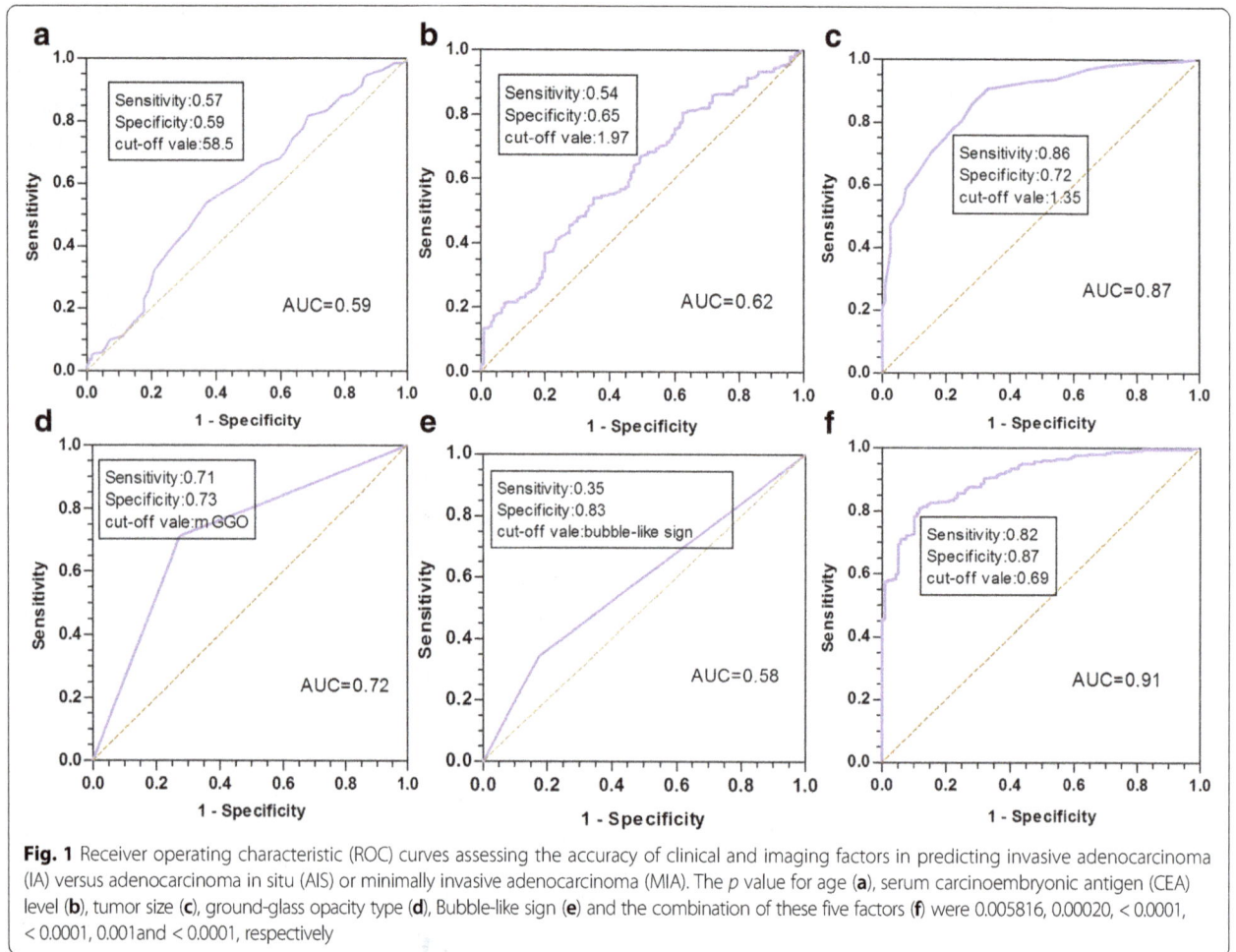

Fig. 1 Receiver operating characteristic (ROC) curves assessing the accuracy of clinical and imaging factors in predicting invasive adenocarcinoma (IA) versus adenocarcinoma in situ (AIS) or minimally invasive adenocarcinoma (MIA). The *p* value for age (**a**), serum carcinoembryonic antigen (CEA) level (**b**), tumor size (**c**), ground-glass opacity type (**d**), Bubble-like sign (**e**) and the combination of these five factors (**f**) were 0.005816, 0.00020, < 0.0001, < 0.0001, 0.001and < 0.0001, respectively

development of small AAH to adenocarcinoma. However, it was sometimes unreasonable to accurately predict the pathological types using only a single factor in patients with GGO nodules. To possibly improve accuracy, we combined the five factors (age, serum CEA level, GGO type, tumor size, and bubble-like sign) that distinguished AIS/MIA from IA preoperatively. Therefore, if patients have the following parameters: age ≤ 58.5 years, serum CEA level ≤ 1.970 µg/L, tumor size ≤13.5 mm, pGGO,

and without a bubble-like sign in chest CT scan, limited resection was suggested.

There are limitations of this study. First, this was a single institution retrospective analysis and the number of patients was small. Second, all patients in our study were resected within 4 years. We didn't make the survival analysis because patients with GGOs had excellent prognoses. Finally, variations in nodule measurement and characterization of lesions might be possible due to different observers.

Table 3 Results of ROC curves assessing the accuracy of clinical and imaging factors in predicting IA versus AIS / MIA

variable	Area	95% CI	Sensitivity	Specificity	Cut-off vale	*p* value
Tumor size	0.87	(0.83,0.91)	0.86	0.72	1.35	<0.0001
Age	0.59	(0.53,0.65)	0.57	0.59	58.50	0.005816
History of family cancer	0.55	(0.49,0.61)	0.74	0.36	0.66	0.1148
CEA	0.62	(0.56,0.68)	0.54	0.65	1.97	0.00020
GGO type	0.72	(0.66,0.77)	0.71	0.73	0.66	<0.0001
Bubble-like sign	0.58	(0.53,0.64)	0.35	0.83	0.63	0.00100
Five-factor combination	0.91	(0.88,0.94)	0.82	0.87	0.69	<0.0001

Five factors including tumor size, age, serum CEA level, GGO type and Bubble-like sign

Table 4 Univariate and bivariate analysis to predict pathological subtype using optimal cut-off values

Variable		Univariate			Bitivariate		
	Cut-off vale	OR	95%CI	p value	OR	95%CI	p value
GGO size	>13.50	15.944	(9.453,26.894)	0.000	2.413	(0.845,6.812)	0.093
Age	>58.50	1.860	(1.208,2.862)	0.005	1.650	(0.872,3.136)	0.106
CEA	>1.97	2.185	(1.396,3.419)	0.001	1.217	(0.638,2.305)	0.536
GGO type	mGGO	2.569	(2.026,3.258)	0.000	1.446	(0.917,2.283)	0.112
Imaging feature	Bubble-like sign	1.936	(1.258,4.263)	0.001	1.213	(0.645,2.134)	0.127
Five-factor combination	0.69	313.679	(107.5868.8)	0.000	58.238	(7.536,440.632)	0.000*

* Statistically significant p value

Conclusion

The results revealed that the persistent presence of a solitary GGO nodule may be lung adenocarcinoma. Our results successfully validated potential usefulness of serum CEA level, tumor size and GGO type and bubble-like sign in predicting pathological types in patients with solitary GGO pulmonary nodules. The five-factor combination helps us to distinguish AIS/MIA from IA in patients with GGO and to perform an appropriate surgical resection.

Abbreviations

AAH: Atypical adenomatous hyperplasia; AIS: Adenocarcinoma in situ; AUCs: Area under curves; CA-19-9: Carbohydrate antigen 19–9; CEA: Carcinoembryonic antigen; GGO: Ground-glass opacity; IA: Invasive adenocarcinoma; mGGO: Mixed GGO; MIA: Minimally invasive adenocarcinoma; NSCLC: Non-small cell lung cancer; pGGO: Pure GGO; ROC: Receiver operating characteristics

Acknowledgements
No applicable

Funding
No applicable

Authors' contributions
ML carried out the data collection, statistical analysis and drafted the manuscript. YW, YC helped draft the manuscript. ZZ participated in the design and coordination of the study. All authors read and approved the final manuscript.

Competing interests
The authors declare that they have no competing interests.

Author details
[1]Department of Lung Cancer, Tianjin Medical University Cancer Institute and Hospital, Huanhu West Road, Tianjin 300060, China. [2]National Clinical Research Center for Cancer, Key Laboratory of Cancer Prevention and Therapy, Tianjin 300060, China. [3]Tianjin's Clinical Research Center for Cancer, Tianjin 300060, China. [4]Tianjin Lung Cancer Center, Tianjin 300060, China.

References
1. Kodama K, Doi O, Higashiyama M, Yokouchi H. Intentional limited resection for selected patients with T1 N0 M0 non-small-cell lung cancer: a single-institution study. J Thorac Cardiovasc Surg. 1997;114:347–53.
2. Koike T, Yamato Y, Yoshiya K, Shimoyama T, Intentional SR. Limited pulmonary resection for peripheral T1 N0 M0 small-sized lung cancer. J Thorac Cardiovasc Surg. 2003;125:924–8.
3. Okada M, Koike T, Higashiyama M, Yamato Y, Kodama K, Tsubota N. Radical Sublobar resection for small-sized non-small cell lung cancer: a multicenter study. J Thorac Cardiovasc Surg. 2006;132:769–75.
4. Watanabe A, Ohori S, Nakashima S, et al. Feasibility of video-assisted thoracoscopic surgery segmentectomy for selected peripheral lung carcinomas. Eur J Cardiothorac Surg. 2009;35:775–80. discussion 780
5. Sakurai H, Dobashi Y, Mizutani E, et al. Bronchioloalveolar carcinoma of the lung 3 centimeters or less in diameter: a prognostic assessment. Ann Thorac Surg. 2004;78:1728–33.
6. Maeda R, Suda T, Hachimaru A, Tochii D, Tochii S, Takagi Y. Clinical significance of preoperative carcinoembryonic antigen level in patients with clinical stage IA non-small cell lung cancer. J Thorac Dis. 2017;9:176–86.
7. Shimizu K, Ikeda N, Tsuboi M, Hirano T, Kato H. Percutaneous CT-guided fine needle aspiration for lung cancer smaller than 2 cm and revealed by ground-glass opacity at CT. Lung Cancer. 2006;51:173–9.
8. Kudo Y, Matsuhayashi J, Saji H, et al. Association between high-resolution computed tomography findings and the IASLC/ATS/ERS classification of small lung adenocarcinomas in Japanese patients. Lung Cancer. 2015;90:47–54.
9. Lederlin M, Puderbach M, Muley T, et al. Correlation of radio- and histomorphological pattern of pulmonary adenocarcinoma. Eur Respir J. 2013;41:943–51.
10. Qiu ZX, Cheng Y, Liu D, et al. Clinical, pathological, and radiological characteristics of solitary ground-glass opacity lung nodules on high-resolution computed tomography. Ther Clin Risk Manag. 2016;12:1445–53.
11. Seki N, Sawada S, Nakata M, et al. Lung cancer with localized ground-glass attenuation represents early-stage adenocarcinoma in nonsmokers. J Thorac Oncol. 2008;3:483–90.
12. Lee SM, Park CM, Goo JM, Lee HJ, Wi JY, Kang CH. Invasive pulmonary adenocarcinomas versus preinvasive lesions appearing as ground-glass nodules: differentiation by using CT features. Radiology. 2013;268:265–73.
13. Kodama K, Higashiyama M, Yokouchi H, et al. Prognostic value of ground-glass opacity found in small lung adenocarcinoma on high-resolution CT scanning. Lung Cancer. 2001;33:17–25.
14. Aoki T, Tomoda Y, Watanabe H, et al. Peripheral lung adenocarcinoma: correlation of thin-section CT findings with histologic prognostic factors and survival. Radiology. 2001;220:803–9.
15. Lee HJ, Goo JM, Lee CH, et al. Predictive CT findings of malignancy in ground-glass nodules on thin-section chest CT: the effects on radiologist performance. Eur Radiol. 2009;19:552–60.

5

Influence of coronary territory on flow profiles of saphenous vein grafts

Sanaz Amin[1,2*], Raphael S. Werner[3], Per Lav Madsen[4], George Krasopoulos[1,2] and David P. Taggart[1,2]

Abstract

Background: Differing perfusion of the left and right ventricular coronary territory may influence flow-profiles of saphenous vein grafts (SVGs). We compared flow parameters, measured by transit-time flowmetry (TTFM), in left- and right-sided SVGs during coronary artery by-pass grafting (CABG).

Methods: Routine TTFM measurements were obtained in 167 SVGs to the left territory (55%) and 134 SVGs to the right territory (total of 301 SVGs in 207 patients). The four standard TTFM parameters, [mean graft flow (MGF), pulsatility index (PI), percentage diastolic filling (%DF), and percentage backward flow (%BF)] were compared. Differences in flow parameters were also examined according to surgical technique (on- vs. off-pump).

Results: No significant difference between coronary territories was found for MGF, PI and %BF. However, a higher %DF was noted in left-sided SVGs in the overall cohort as well as in the on-pump (both $p < 0.001$) and the off-pump cohorts ($p = 0.07$). Further, a significantly higher %BF was found in SVGs performed off-pump to the left territory (1.2 ± 2.5 vs. 2.3 ± 3.0, $p = 0.023$). In a multivariate regression analysis, anastomosing a SVG to the left territory was weakly associated with higher PI ($OR = 0.36$, $p = 0.026$) and strongly associated with higher %DF ($OR = 5.1$, $p < 0.001$). No significant association was found for MGF, PI, %DF or %BF in either the on-pump nor the off-pump cohorts.

Conclusions: Although statistically significant, the established differences in TTFM parameters between left- and right-sided vein grafts were small and unlikely to be of clinical relevance.

Keywords: Transit time flowmetry, TTFM, Coronary artery by-pass surgery, CABG, Intraoperative graft patency assessment, Saphenous vein graft

Background

Coronary artery by-pass surgery (CABG) remains the optimal treatment for complex coronary artery disease [1], but despite the survival benefit of CABG, long-term graft patency remains a concern. Current European guidelines on CABG recommend intraoperative graft assessment with specific cut-off values for mean graft flow (MGF) and pulsatility index (PI) by transit-time flowmetry (TTFM) technique [2]. However, a limitation of current guideline recommendations is that they do not take into account the known differences in physiological pattern of flow between the right and left coronary artery territories [2].

The transmyocardial pressure is higher on the left side of the heart compared to the right, as the left ventricle provides circulatory support for the high-pressure systemic circulation, and hence a larger fraction of the myocardial blood flow in the left coronary territory takes place during ventricular diastole [3–5]. These differences in coronary blood flow of the left and right coronary territory might therefore be expected to influence flow in by-pass grafts. Few studies, however, have specifically addressed flow in left- vs. right-sided grafts, and have included cohorts of both arterial and venous conduits. Hence, current evidence for any potentially clinically relevant difference is scarce and contradictory [6–8].

The aim of this study was to compare all TTFM parameters MGF, PI, percentage of diastolic filling (%DF), and percentage of backward flow (%BF) in saphenous vein grafts (SVGs) supplying the left and right coronary territories in a larger cohort of CABG patients. Results

* Correspondence: sanaz.amin@nds.ox.ac.uk
[1]University of Oxford, Oxford, UK
[2]Department of Cardiovascular Surgery, Oxford University Hospitals Trust, Oxford, UK
Full list of author information is available at the end of the article

were then analysed according to on-pump (ONCABG) vs. off-pump (OPCABG). We hypothesized that the higher pressure on the left side would particularly influence diastolic run off in SVGs.

Methods

Study design and population

This study was designed as a comparative, non-interventional study, in which data was collected retrospectively. The population consisted of 268 consecutive CABG patients (total of 659 by-pass grafts) undergoing standard elective or urgent isolated OPCABG or ONCABG. After exclusion of arterial conduits, the study population included 207 CABG patients with a total of 301 SVGs operated in one Centre (John Radcliffe Hospital, Oxford, UK) from July 2015 to April 2017. The study group breakdown is depicted in Fig. 1. TTFM parameters, mean arterial pressure (MAP), demographic data, and risk profile were prospectively collected.

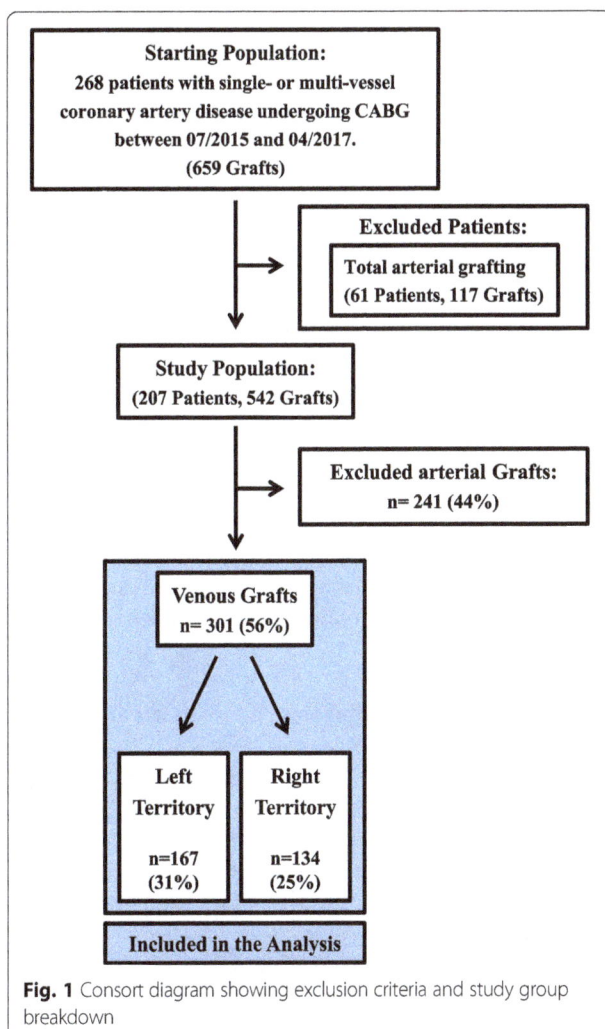

Fig. 1 Consort diagram showing exclusion criteria and study group breakdown

The degree of proximal stenosis in the coronary arteries was assessed by one blinded operator (SA) using quantitative coronary angiography (Horizon Cardiology version 12.2, McKesson, Israel). All TTFM measurements were performed with the VeriQC device (Medistim ASA, Oslo, Norway).

Procedure

General

All patients underwent CABG via a median sternotomy. SVGs were endoscopically harvested as skeletonized conduits and stored in heparinized blood prior to performing the anastomosis. The vast majority of SVGs were used as single grafts to graft the obtuse marginal (OM), the right coronary artery (RCA), or the posterior descending arteries (PDA). However, most grafts anastomosed to the right territory were anastomosed to the PDA. Two surgeons (DPT and GK) performed all CABGs. The routine practice of one surgeon (DPT) was OPCABG, and the routine practice of the other surgeon (GK) was ONCABG.

The average vessel diameter and the extent of native coronary artery vessel disease was assessed by one blinded operator (SA) using quantitative coronary angiography (QCA) (Horizon Cardiology version 12.2, McKesson, Israel).

Principle of TTFM measurement

Prior to TTFM measurement, the surgeon selected an appropriately sized TTFM probe according to a visual estimation of the external conduit diameter. Mainly probe size 4 or 5 mm was used. Ultrasound gel was applied to the lumen of the probe so that the graft occupied a minimum of 75% of the lumen. During TTFM measurement, the ultrasound probe was placed as close as possible to the distal anastomosis *for the most accurate reading of the flow dynamics across the anastomosis, as previous studies have demonstrated slightly lower %DF and higher PI in the proximal compared to the distal segment of a by-pass graft* [9]. TTFM measurements are routinely measured at a mean systemic blood pressure of 75–85 mmHg to exclude the effects on flow of excessively low or high blood pressure. Traction on the pericardium was released, and the stabilizer was removed from the pericardial surface to allow the heart to return to its natural anatomic position. *All TTFM parameters and MAPs were measured after protamine administration. The rational for measuring TTFM after reversal of heparin was to ascertain that the TTFM reading reflected the most accurate interpretation of the graft quality prior to sending the patient out of the operating room.*

OPCABG

Complete anticoagulation with heparin was achieved as in the ONCABG group. The lateral and inferior walls were exposed by means of a combination of a deep pericardial stay suture, Trendelenburg and right decubitus position, and opening of the right side of the pericardium to the inferior vena cava. Regional myocardial immobilization was achieved with a suction stabilizer (Octopus Evolution AS, Tissue Stabilizer TS2500, Medtronic Inc.). The target coronary vessels were snared proximally with silastic slings. An intracoronary shunt (Clearview 31,175, Medtronic Inc.) was used during construction of the anastomosis. Shunts were used routinely in all OPCABG cases. A surgical blower-mister device was used to enhance visualization (Clearview 22,150, Medtronic Inc). Proximal anastomoses were made to the ascending aorta at a controlled systolic pressure of between 70 and 80 mmHg and a side-biting vascular clamp.

ONCABG

Cardiopulmonary bypass was instituted by ascending aorta cannulation and a two-stage venous cannula in the right atrium. A standard cardiopulmonary by-pass circuit incorporated a roller pump (Jostra HL 20) and a hollow-fiber membrane oxygenator (Inspire Sorin, Fusion Medtronic). The extracorporeal circuit was primed with 1000 mL of Hartmann solution, 500 ml Gelespan, 100 ml mannitol (20% Baxter solution), and 2500 IU of heparin. Non-pulsatile flow was maintained with a flow rate of 2.4 l/min/m^2. The extra-corporeal circuit was without arterial filtration, and cardiotomy suction was used routinely. Acid-base balance was managed with alpha-stat control. During construction of anastomoses, the patient temperature was allowed to drift to 34 °C before rewarming. Myocardial protection was achieved with intermittent antegrade cold blood-based cardioplegia solution (a mixture of patient's blood and Harefield cardioplegia solution at ratio of 4:1 during induction and 8:1 for maintenance doses). On completion of all distal anastomoses, the aortic cross-clamp was removed, and the proximal anastomosis was performed with partial clamping.

Statistical analysis

Continuous variables are reported as mean ± standard deviation. Normality was assessed with the Kolmogorov-Smirnov test. Comparisons were made with the unpaired t-test for normal distributions and the Mann-Whitney U-test for non-normal distributions. Categorical variables are expressed as frequencies and percentages and were compared using the Chi^2-Pearson test. A multivariable linear regression model was applied to investigate the effect of the grafted territory (left or right) on TTFM parameters whilst controlling for potential confounding variables. Variables were incorporated into the multivariable analysis if associated with the dependent variables

in a univariable analysis ($p < 0.1$). Significance of the multivariable regression model was assessed using the F-test. Results of the regression model are presented as regression coefficients (B) with 95% confidence intervals (95% CI) and the corresponding p-values. A p-value < 0.05 (two-sided) was considered statistically significant. Data analysis was performed in IBM SPSS Statistics Version 22 (SPSS Inc., Chicago, IL).

Statistical power calculations were based on pilot data on MGF from our group and the assumption that for any territory-related difference to be of clinical importance, it should change a normal value by > 10% [10]. With a double-sided alpha-value of 0.05 and a beta-value of 0.80, changing MGF from 48 ml/min by at least 5 ml/min (estimated sigma of 10 ml/min) requires 63 patients in each group. To provide the possibility of further exploration of data including multivariate analysis, we aimed for at least 130 SVGs in each group.

Results
Patient baseline characteristics including target vessel disease

Two hundred seven patients receiving a total of 301 SVGs were included in the final analysis (Table 1). 167 SVGs (55%) were grafted to the left territory, and 134 SVGs were grafted to the right territory (Fig. 1). One hundred twenty one patients were operated ONCABG (184 SVGs, 61%), and 86 patients were operated OPCABG (117 SVGs). Patient demographics and their pre-operative risk profile are presented in Table 1. The distribution of the target vessels grafted is shown in Table 2.

The extent of native coronary artery vessel disease is shown in Table 3. Target vessel stenosis severity, as judged by QCA, was significant lower in the left coronary territory compared to the right coronary territory both in the overall cohort (86.1 ± 11.8% vs. 90.6 ± 9.8%, $p < 0.001$) and in the OPCABG cohorts (84.5 ± 13 vs. 91.7 ± 9.4%, $p < 0.04$) and ONCABG (87.2 ± 10.4% vs. 90.4 ± 10.1%, $p = 0.002$) cohorts. Non-obstructed target coronary artery diameter, average lumen diameter, and lesion length were comparable between coronary territories.

Comparison of TTFM parameters between left and right coronary territory

TTFM measurements, MAP at the time of measurement, and by-pass times are presented in Fig. 2 and Table 4. As intended, MAP at the time of TTFM measurement was similar between grafts anastomosed to the left and the right territories. No significant differences between SVGs supplying the two coronary territories were found for MGF, PI, and %BF. However, a higher %DF was noted in left-sided SVGs in comparison to right-sided SVGs in the overall (63.3 ± 12.0% vs. 58.1 ±

Table 1 Patient demographics and preoperative risk profile for both groups

Variable	Study population
Total patients	207 (100%)
Age (yrs)	67 ± 8
Male	176 (85%)
Body Mass Index (kg/m^2)	28.7 ± 4.0
Diabetes mellitus	
Insulin dependent	9 (4%)
Noninsulin dependent	61 (29%)
No history of diabetes	137 (66%)
Chronic obstructive pulmonary disease	24 (12%)
Peripheral vascular disease	22 (11%)
New York Heart Association class	
0	2 (1%)
I	48 (23%)
II	115 (56%)
III	40 (19%)
IV	2 (1%)
Canadian Cardiovascular Society class	
0	13 (6%)
I	19 (9%)
II	132 (64%)
III	32 (15%)
IV	11 (5%)
Left ventricular ejection fraction (%)	58 ± 7
By-pass time (min)	96.1 ± 26.0
Cross-clamp time (min)	66.8 ± 20.8
Surgeon	
"DT"	176 (85%)
"GK"	31 (15%)
Total grafts and territory	542 (100%)
Venous	301 (56%)
Left territory	167 (31%)
Right territory	134 (25%)

10.5%, $p < 0.001$), OPCABG (63.1 ± 12.1% vs. 59.5 ± 10.4%, $p = 0.07$) and ONCABG (63.5 ± 12.0% vs. 57.3 ± 10.5%, $p < 0.001$) cohorts.

Impact of OPCABG vs. ONCABG on TTFM parameters in the left and right territory

No significant territory-related difference was found for MGF, PI, and %DF between OPCABG and ONCABG

Table 2 Distribution of target vessels grafted using saphenous vein grafts (SVGs)

Conduit (No.)	LAD	DIAG	IM	OM	RCA	PDA
SVG (301)	5	35	12	115	38	96

SVG saphenous vein graft, *LAD* left anterior descending artery, *DIAG* diagonal artery, *IM* intermediate artery, *OM* obtuse marginal branch of circumflex artery, *RCA* right coronary artery, *PDA* posterior descending artery

cohorts. However, for the left territory, a significantly higher %BF was found in OPCABG SVGs compared to ONCABG SVGs (2.3 ± 3.0% vs. 1.2 ± 2.5%, $p = 0.023$) (Table 4).

Multivariable linear regression model

The variables MGF, PI, %DF, %BF, mean arterial pressure at TTFM, age, sex, diabetes, surgeon, ONCABG and OPCABG, grafted territory, native coronary artery stenosis and minimal luminal diameter were incorporated into the multivariable analysis based on their association in the univariable analysis ($p < 0.1$). The grafted coronary territory did not have a significant influence on MGF. However, the coronary territory had a significant influence on PI and %DF: Thus, grafting to the left territory led to higher PI and %DF of SVGs ($B = 0.36$, 95% CI 0.04–0.67, $p = 0.026$ and $B = 5.1$, 95% CI 2.86–7.34, $p < 0.001$, respectively). No significant influence of grafted territory was found for %BF. Moreover, no significant association was found between TTFM parameters and OPCABG *or* ONCABG technique.

Some of the covariates used to adjust for the effect of the grafted territory were also independently associated with the TTFM parameters: older age was associated with higher MGF ($p = 0.034$) and lower %DF ($p < 0.05$), and male gender was associated with higher %DF ($p = 0.025$). Furthermore, higher MGF was associated with lower %BF ($p = 0.012$) and greater %DF ($p = 0.009$), while higher PI was associated with greater %BF ($p < 0.001$) and lower %DF ($p < 0.001$). Moreover, higher %DF itself was associated with lower %BF ($p = 0.004$).

Discussion

As demonstrated by Transit-time flowmetry in patients undergoing CABG, our study has shown that saphenous vein grafts (SVGs) anastomosed to the left and right coronary territory have comparable mean graft flow (MGF), pulsatility index (PI), and percentage of backward flow (%BF) irrespective of surgical technique (OPCABG *or* ONCABG). However, SVGs anastomosed to the left territory have a significantly higher diastolic filling (%DF) than SVGs anastomosed to the right territory both during OPCABG and ONCABG. Moreover, compared to ONCABG, a significantly higher %BF was found in OPCABG SVGs supplying the left coronary territory (Table 4). In a multi-regression analysis, grafting to the left territory was weakly associated with higher PI and strongly associated with higher %DF of SVGs.

In keeping with our finding of no significant difference between territories with respect to MGF, the study by Tokuda et al. [6], including a mixture of arterial and venous grafts, found no statistically significant difference in MGF between grafts anastomosed to the left or the right coronary territory [6]. On the other hand, the study

Table 3 Native vessel disease: quantitative coronary angiography data

Variable	Host coronary artery diameter (mm)	Average lumen stenosis diameter (mm)	Host coronary artery stenosis (% area)	Lesion length (mm)
Venous grafts				
Overall (n = 301)				
Left territory (n = 167)	2.0 ± 0.7	0.69 ± 0.37	86.1 ± 11.8	9.4 ± 4.7
Right territory (n = 134)	2.0 ± 0.8	0.67 ± 0.40	90.6 ± 9.8	9.3 ± 4.3
p-value	0.9	0.8	< 0.001	0.9
On-pump CABG (n = 184)				
Left territory (n = 99)	2.0 ± 0.7	0.67 ± 0.36	87.2 ± 10.4	9.6 ± 4.4
Right territory (n = 85)	2.0 ± 0.9	0.69 ± 0.44	90.4 ± 10.1	9.0 ± 4.2
p-value	0.5	0.4	0.002	0.5
Off-pump CABG (n = 117)				
Left territory (n = 68)	2.0 ± 0.7	0.71 ± 0.38	84.5 ± 13.5	9.2 ± 5.1
Right territory (n = 49)	1.9 ± 0.5	0.65 ± 0.33	91.7 ± 9.4	9.9 ± 4.5
p-value	0.6	0.4	0.040	0.4
p-value*	0.8	0.5	0.1	0.6
p-value**	0.5	0.6	0.5	0.3

*; comparing on- and off-pump CABG to the left territoty
**; comparing on- and off-pump CABG to the right territory

by Kim et al. [7], including a total of 117 arterial conduits (all operated as OPCABG), found a higher MGF in grafts anastomosed to the left than to the right territory. However, as only arterial grafts were assessed, the structural and physiological differences between arterial and venous conduits [11, 12] may explain these conflicting results, and further research is thus warranted to address this topic.

In further concordance with our results of no significant territory-related difference in PI, the study by Tokuda et al. [6] also found no statistically significant difference between grafts anastomosed to the left or the right territory with respect to PI [6]. In contrast to this finding, the study by Kim et al. [7] found a higher PI in grafts anastomosed to the right coronary territory. Again, since the study by Kim et al. [7] only included arterial conduits, this may well explain these conflicting results. Another explanation for why a higher PI may be found in right-sided grafts may be due to the position of the TTFM probe during measurement. Repositioning of the heart into anatomical position at the end of surgery will obscure the distal end of the graft. Consequently, TTFM measurement is often performed proximally on right-sided grafts, where PI is usually higher, *as the high pressured forward flow from the aorta results in higher systolic peak flows in the proximal segment of a by-pass graft and hence in a bigger difference between maximum flow and minimum flow* [9], *as further explained in the*

following. In theory, a slightly higher PI may well be expected in grafts anastomosed to the left territory, as the PI is obtained by dividing the difference between maximum and minimum flow by the mean flow: $\frac{(Q_{Max} - Q_{Min})}{Q_{Mean}}$. Therefore, a larger difference between maximum and minimum flow, resulting in a higher PI value, may be expected on the left side of the heart where the higher transmyocardial pressure results in a higher pressure amplitude between systole and diastole [13]. Indeed, the multi-regression analysis suggested that grafting to the left territory was weakly associated with higher PI in SVGs.

In agreement with our study suggesting Tokuda et al. [6] and Kim et al. [7] both demonstrated a higher %DF in grafts anastomosed to the left compared to the right coronary territory compared. As previously noted, a higher %DF is indeed expected on the left side of the heart due to the higher transmyocardial pressure, which lowers systolic coronary flow, irrespective of conduit type (arterial or venous) or surgical technique. However, it is important to acknowledge that the established differences in %DF found in our study is of a mere 5%-points. Although this may reach statistical significance, the established difference is in most situations clinically insignificant.

Tokuda et al. [6] also found no significant difference in %BF in left vs. right-sided by-pass grafts. In contrast, however, Kim et al. [7] found a higher %BF in grafts anastomosed to the left coronary territory. Notably, all grafts were performed by OPCABG technique, which is consistent with our results showing higher %BF only in OPCABG SVGs anastomosed to the left coronary territory (Table 4). A higher %BF is indeed expected on the left side due to the higher transmyocardial pressure, which forces blood backward during isovolumetric contraction. However, these differences were also too small to be of any clinical relevance.

No other parameters were significantly different in grafts anastomosed in OPCABG vs. ONCABG surgery. Notwithstanding this however, previously published papers on TTFM parameters in OPCABG vs. ONCABG found a higher MGF in grafts performed with the latter technique [14–16]. In a prospective study [14] including a total of 266 grafts (203 OPCABG vs. 63 ONCABG) in 100 patients, Taggart and colleagues reported a lower MGF in SVGs performed by OPCABG technique despite a higher mean arterial pressure when compared to ONCABG ($p < 0.05$) [14]. The authors suggested that these findings might be related to vasodilatation following a period of myocardial ischaemia. Indeed, it has been well documented that despite the use of cardioplegia, cross-clamping in ONCABG leads to global myocardial

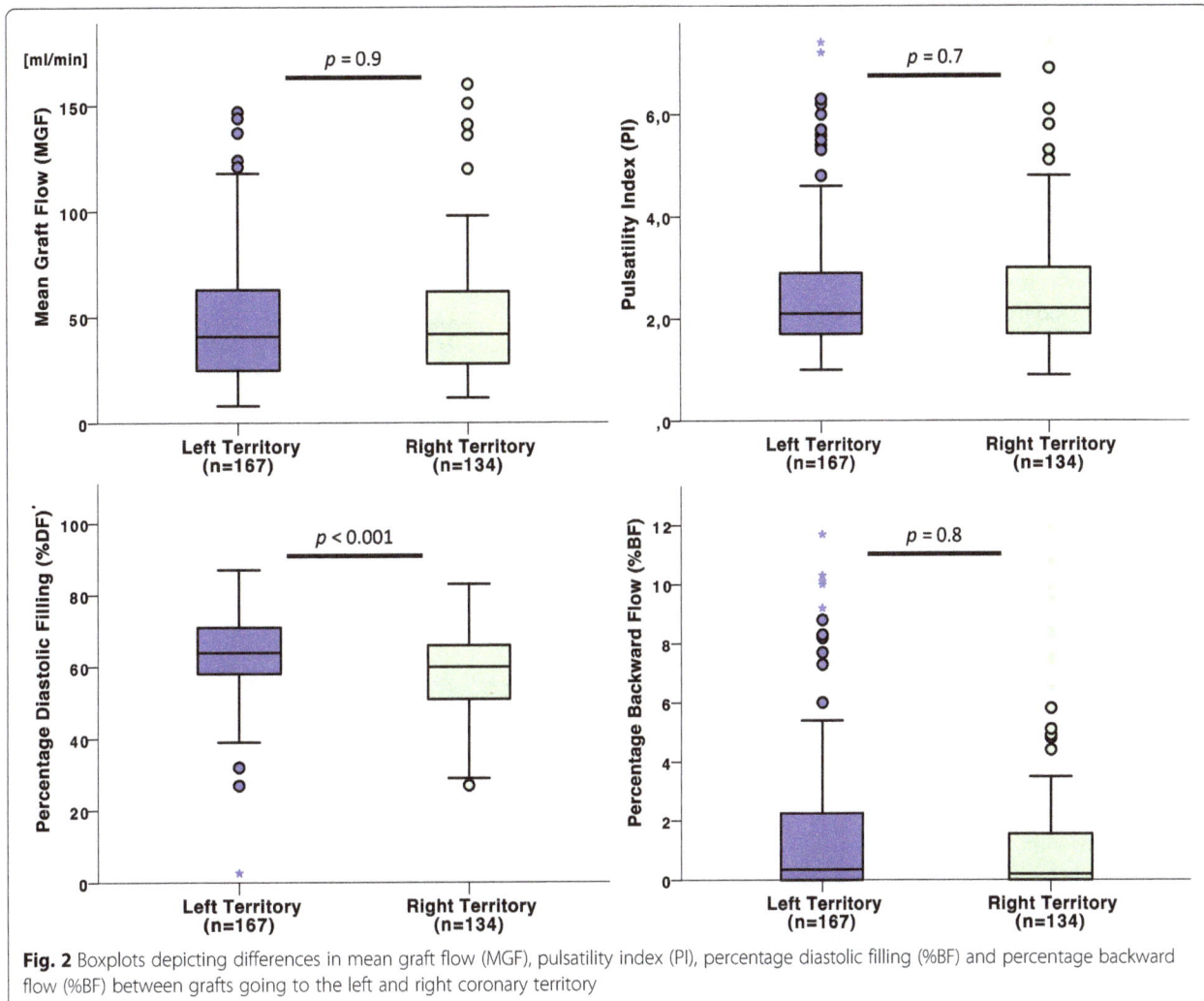

Fig. 2 Boxplots depicting differences in mean graft flow (MGF), pulsatility index (PI), percentage diastolic filling (%BF) and percentage backward flow (%BF) between grafts going to the left and right coronary territory

Table 4 Comparison of intraoperative TTFM parameters between venous grafts going to the left and to the right territory

Variable	Mean graft flow (ml/min)	Pulsatility Index	Diastolic filling (%)	Backward flow (%)	By-pass time (min)	Mean arterial pressure at TTFM (mmHg)
Saphenous vein grafts						
Overall (n = 301)						
Left territory (n = 167)	48.3 ± 33.8	2.6 ± 1.7	63.3 ± 12.0	1.8 ± 3.2	94.5 ± 23.4	80.9 ± 8.1
Right territory (n = 134)	48.3 ± 29.1	2.5 ± 1.2	58.1 ± 10.5	1.6 ± 3.0	98.8 ± 28.4	80.7 ± 6.2
p-value	0.9	0.7	< 0.001	0.8	0.3	0.9
On-pump CABG (n = 184)						
Left territory (n = 99)	51.7 ± 28.1	2.5 ± 1.9	63.5 ± 12.0	1.2 ± 2.5	94.5 ± 23.4	80.8 ± 5.8
Right territory (n = 85)	49.0 ± 30.1	2.5 ± 1.3	57.3 ± 10.5	1.6 ± 3.2	98.8 ± 28.4	80.1 ± 5.4
p-value	0.5	0.9	< 0.001	0.4	0.3	0.3
Off-pump CABG (n = 117)						
Left territory (n = 68)	43.5 ± 40.4	2.7 ± 1.4	63.1 ± 12.1	2.3 ± 3.0	–	81.0 ± 10.6
Right territory (n = 49)	47.0 ± 27.5	2.6 ± 1.2	59.5 ± 10.4	1.6 ± 2.6	–	82.0 ± 7.3
p-value	0.6	0.5	0.071	0.2	–	0.6
p-value*	0.1	0.3	0.8	0.023	–	0.9
p-value**	0.7	0.7	0.3	0.9	–	0.095

*comparing on- and off-pump CABG to the left territoty
**comparing on- and off-pump CABG to the right territory

ischaemia and subsequent acidosis with resultant dilatation of coronary arteries [17]. Thus, a higher MGF may be expected in ONCABG vs. OPCABG by-pass grafts. Although our results did demonstrate a numerically higher MGF in the ONCABG SVG cohort, this difference did not reach clinical or statistical significance.

Of note, the multi-regression analysis of this study showed significant associations between the four TTFM parameters, which suggests that these parameters should thus be considered complementary rather than in isolation when assessing quality of SVGs intraoperatively [4, 5, 10]. This is supported by studies demonstrating that high quality grafts, as determined by angiographic graft patency assessment, have high MGF due to good run-off with concomitant low PI, predominant %DF, and little %BF [6, 18–22].

Conclusions

Saphenous vein grafts supplying the left coronary artery territory have a higher diastolic flow (%DF) when compared to right-sided SVGs, irrespective of whether the procedure is performed ONCABG or OPCABG. Furthermore, multi-regression analysis suggests that SVGs grafted to the left coronary territory are weakly associated with higher PI. The magnitude of differences are numerically small and unlikely to be of clinical significance.

Limitations

Our study was observational and confounding cannot be excluded due to lack of randomisation. Further, while the statistical power-analysis allowed for clinically significant changes to be excluded, we cannot exclude if smaller changes may be of importance for long-term patency. Furthermore, the extent of host coronary artery stenosis was statistically higher in the right coronary territory (Table 3). However, the mean host coronary artery stenosis was over 80% in both territories, which should make the difference between the two territories clinically irrelevant and results thus comparable [23]. Notably, this study only describes perioperative flow-profiles of SVGs; hence these results may not necessarily reflect the long-term flow-profile in either group.

Abbreviations

BF: Backward flow; CABG: Coronary artery bypass grafting; DF: Diastollic filling; MGF: Mean graft flow; OM : Obtuse marginal artery; ONCABG: On-pump coronary artery bypass grafting; OPCABG: Off-pump coronary artery bypass grafting; PDA: Posterior descending artery; PI: Pulsatility index; RCA: Right coronary artery; SVG: Saphenous vein graft; TTFM: Tansit time flowmetry

Acknowledgements
Not applicable.

Funding
Not applicable.

Authors' contributions
All authors meet ICMJE guidelines for contribution: made substantial contributions to conception and design, or acquisition of data, or analysis and interpretation of data; been involved in drafting the manuscript or revising it critically for important intellectual content; given final approval of the version to be published. Each author should have participated sufficiently in the work to take public responsibility for appropriate portions of the content; and agreed to be accountable for all aspects of the work in ensuring that questions related to the accuracy or integrity of any part of the work are appropriately investigated and resolved. All authors read and approved the final manuscript.

Competing interests
The senior author of this manuscript (DP Taggart) discloses a competing interest, as he has received research funding from Medistim as well as traveling fees and speaking honoraria. David Taggart is an Editor-in-Chief for the Journal of Cardiothoracic Surgery.

Author details
[1]University of Oxford, Oxford, UK. [2]Department of Cardiovascular Surgery, Oxford University Hospitals Trust, Oxford, UK. [3]Department of thoracic surgery, Faculty of Medicine, University of Zurich, Zurich, Switzerland. [4]Department of Cardiology, Copenhagen University Hospital, Herlev, Denmark.

References
1. Benedetto U, et al. Coronary surgery is superior to drug eluting stents in multivessel disease. Systematic review and meta-analysis of contemporary randomized controlled trials. Int J Cardiol. 2016;210:19–24.
2. Kolh P, et al. ESC/EACTS guidelines on myocardial revascularization: the task force on myocardial revascularization of the European Society of Cardiology (ESC) and the European Association for Cardio-Thoracic Surgery (EACTS). Developed with the special contribution of the European Association of Percutaneous Cardiovascular Interventions (EAPCI). Eur J Cardiothorac Surg. 2014;46(4):517–92.
3. Pijls NH, et al. Experimental basis of determining maximum coronary, myocardial, and collateral blood flow by pressure measurements for assessing functional stenosis severity before and after percutaneous transluminal coronary angioplasty. Circulation. 1993;87(4):1354–67.
4. D'Ancona G, et al. Graft patency verification in coronary artery bypass grafting: principles and clinical applications of transit time flow measurement. Angiology. 2000;51(9):725–31.
5. D'Ancona G, et al. Intraoperative graft patency verification in coronary artery surgery: modern diagnostic tools. J Cardiothorac Vasc Anesth. 2009;23(2):232–8.
6. Tokuda Y, et al. Predicting early coronary artery bypass graft failure by intraoperative transit time flow measurement. Ann Thorac Surg. 2007; 84(6):1928–33.
7. Kim KB, Kang CH, Lim C. Prediction of graft flow impairment by intraoperative transit time flow measurement in off-pump coronary artery bypass using arterial grafts. Ann Thorac Surg. 2005;80(2):594–8.
8. Nordgaard H, Vitale N, Haaverstad R. Transit-time blood flow measurements in sequential saphenous coronary artery bypass grafts. Ann Thorac Surg. 2009;87(5):1409–15.
9. Jelenc M, et al. Understanding coronary artery bypass transit time flow curves: role of bypass graft compliance. Interact Cardiovasc Thorac Surg. 2014;18(2):164–8.
10. Amin S, Pinho-Gomes AC, Taggart DP. Relationship of Intraoperative transit time Flowmetry findings to angiographic graft patency at follow-up. Ann Thorac Surg. 2016;101(5):1996–2006.
11. Singh RN, Beg RA, Kay EB. Physiological adaptability: the secret of success of the internal mammary artery grafts. Ann Thorac Surg. 1986;41(3):247–50.
12. Desai ND, et al. A randomized comparison of radial-artery and saphenous-vein coronary bypass grafts. N Engl J Med. 2004;351(22):2302–9.
13. Ofili EO, Labovitz AJ, Kern MJ. Coronary flow velocity dynamics in normal and diseased arteries. Am J Cardiol. 1993;71(14):3D–9D.

14. Balacumaraswami L, et al. The effects of on-pump and off-pump coronary artery bypass grafting on intraoperative graft flow in arterial and venous conduits defined by a flow/pressure ratio. J Thorac Cardiovasc Surg. 2008;135(3):533–9.

15. Schmitz C, et al. Transit time flow measurement in on-pump and off-pump coronary artery surgery. J Thorac Cardiovasc Surg. 2003;126(3):645–50.

16. Hassanein W, et al. Intraoperative transit time flow measurement: off-pump versus on-pump coronary artery bypass. Ann Thorac Surg. 2005;80(6):2155–61.

17. Graffigna AC, et al. Continuous monitoring of myocardial acid-base status during intermittent warm blood cardioplegia. Eur J Cardiothorac Surg. 2002;21(6):995–1001.

18. Tokuda Y, et al. Predicting midterm coronary artery bypass graft failure by intraoperative transit time flow measurement. Ann Thorac Surg. 2008;86(2):532–6.

19. Une D, et al. Cut-off values for transit time flowmetry: are the revision criteria appropriate? J Card Surg. 2013;28(1):3–7.

20. Kieser TM, et al. Transit-time flow predicts outcomes in coronary artery bypass graft patients: a series of 1000 consecutive arterial grafts. Eur J Cardiothorac Surg. 2010;38(2):155–62.

21. Di Giammarco G, et al. Predictive value of intraoperative transit-time flow measurement for short-term graft patency in coronary surgery. J Thorac Cardiovasc Surg. 2006;132(3):468–74.

22. Lehnert P, et al. Transit-time flow measurement as a predictor of coronary bypass graft failure at one year angiographic follow-up. J Card Surg. 2015; 30(1):47–52.

23. Honda K, et al. Graft flow assessment using a transit time flow meter in fractional flow reserve-guided coronary artery bypass surgery. J Thorac Cardiovasc Surg. 2015;149(6):1622–8.

6

Primary and metastatic cardiac tumors: echocardiographic diagnosis, treatment and prognosis in a 15-years single center study

Natsumi Nomoto[1], Tomoko Tani[2*], Toshiko Konda[1], Kitae Kim[3], Takeshi Kitai[3], Mitsuhiko Ota[3], Shuichiro Kaji[3], Yukihiro Imai[4], Yukikatsu Okada[5] and Yutaka Furukawa[3]

Abstract

Background: The frequency of primary cardiac tumors is rare at about 0.3% by autopsy. Our objective was to investigate the characteristics and locations of cardiac tumors and to provide a prognostic analysis in our hospital.

Methods: We collected data on 95 patients with echocardiographic diagnosis or detection of cardiac tumors in a prospective analysis from 1999 to 2014. The median follow-up period was 43 months (0.5–183 months).

Results: The subjects included 56 men and 39 women with a mean age of 65 years. Clinical diagnosis revealed primary tumors in 61 patients (64%) and secondary metastatic tumors in 34 patients (36%). In the 61 patients, 41 patients (67%) underwent surgery and tissue samples were obtained. Of these 41 patients, benign tumors were found in 30 cases (73%). One patient (2%) was diagnosed with thrombus. Among the benign tumors, myxoma (67%) was the most common type followed by papillary fibroelastoma (23%). The most common site was the left atrium (35%) followed by the right atrium (25%). Primary malignant tumors were diagnosed in 10 cases (24%), including 6 angiosarcomas, 3 lymphomas, and 1 leiomyosarcoma. The diagnostic accuracy of echocardiography was 80%. The patients with benign tumors were all alive at the end of the follow-up period. In contrast, 7 patients with malignant tumors died (70%) ($p < 0.0001$).

Conclusions: Our data is in line with previous literature. Our study also suggests the necessity of extending our knowledge of the characteristics of cardiac tumors for diagnosis.

Keywords: Cardiac tumor, Echocardiography, Diagnosis, Prognosis

Background

Cardiac tumors are classified into primary tumors that arise from part of the heart or metastatic tumors that involve the heart. Primary cardiac tumors include benign and malignant tumors. Primary cardiac tumors are rare and the incidence is from 0.001 to 0.3% by autopsy [1, 2]. There have only been a few published studies about cardiac tumors and their management in the past half century. The majority of papers about cardiac tumors report only on a limited number of primary cardiac tumors, especially benign tumors. Cardiac tumors present various clinical situations. The most common primary cardiac tumor is cardiac myxoma, and it was reported that 50–70% of all primary cardiac tumors were myxomas [2, 3].

We have been able to detect and accurately diagnose cardiac tumors with clinically useful imaging techniques, especially echocardiography. We investigated prospectively the characteristics of cardiac tumors that have been diagnosed by transthoracic echocardiography (TTE) or transesophageal echocardiography (TEE) at our hospital. We performed a comparison of the tumors with the pathological data from patients who underwent surgery.

* Correspondence: tomokot@tr.kobe-ccn.ac.jp
[2]Basic Medical Science, Kobe City College of Nursing, 3-4 Gakuennishi-machi, Nishi-ku, Kobe 651-2103, Japan
Full list of author information is available at the end of the article

Moreover, we studied the clinical course of each case with a cardiac tumor in a single center.

Methods

We prospectively identified 95 patients who had complete echocardiographic records and who were diagnosed or detected with cardiac tumors from August 1999 to December 2014.

We confirm that our study complied with the principles of the declaration of Helsinki. Approval to conduct this study was obtained from the Institutional Review Board in our hospital. All participants gave their informed consent to participate in the study.

The medical records of all the cardiac tumor patients were reviewed and details regarding diagnosis, treatment, and follow-up were obtained after echocardiographic examination. We calculated overall survival times from the date of surgery to the date of death or to the date when we were able to confirm the patient's survival.

Echocardiography

Two-dimensional transthoracic echocardiography (TTE) was performed by experienced sonographers according to a standardized echocardiographic protocol using commercially available equipment (ARTIDA/Aplio SSA-770A Toshiba, Tochigi, Japan; HDI 5000/iE33/EPIQ7c Philips Medical Systems, Andover, MA, USA; ACUSON SC2000 Siemens, Munchen, DEU). Images were obtained using standard views. Transesophageal echocardiography (TEE) was performed using commercially available equipment and standard imaging planes for patients who needed a more detailed examination. Some patients were not able to undergo TEE because of their physical condition.

Diagnosis of tumor type

The tumor type was diagnosed based on location, site of attachment, shape, size, mobility and other morphologic characteristics on echocardiography. For the diagnosis of malignant tumors, the localization and growth of the tumor lesions, permeation to the great vessels, and the presence of malignancy characteristics were evaluated as follows; about localization: intracardiac, extracardiac,; about growth: invasion, infiltration, compression; about surface/border: smooth, filiform, rough. Other characteristics associated with malignancy were defined as pericardial effusion and direct invasion into the myocardium. Metastatic tumors were easily diagnosed if the tumors showed direct invasion in addition to the above characteristics. However, cases of metastatic tumors often underwent an echocardiographic examination for the purpose of determining whether cardiac metastasis might exist. All tumors were evaluated independently by two experienced investigators blinded to the patient's clinical diagnosis. All pathology records were reviewed and confirmed by a single pathologist. We collected the pathological data from the medical records. As for the cases in the non-surgery group, the results of other imaging methods after echocardiography were confirmed.

Statistical analysis

The Kaplan–Meier method was used to analyze survival, and the log-rank test was used for all survival differences. All statistical analyses were performed with the commercially available software package SPSS for Windows, version 23 (IBM Corporation, Chicago, IL, USA).

Results

Patient characteristics

There were 56 men and 39 women with a mean age of 65 years (age 65 ± 14 years). The median follow-up period was 43 months (0.5–183 months).

Tumor characteristics

Of the 95 cardiac tumor cases, 61 (64%) were diagnosed as primary cardiac tumors by echocardiography. All primary cardiac tumors were diagnosed without information about the history of cardiac tumors from echocardiographic order. Thirty-four cases (36%) were detected as secondary metastatic cardiac tumors and 5 of 34 cases (15%) were accidentally diagnosed by echocardiography with no information about primary disease and other imaging data. Among the 61 patients with primary tumors, 41 patients (67%) underwent partial or complete tumor resection and had a histologic diagnosis. Twenty patients (33%) refused surgery. The majority of the surgical cases ($n = 30$, 73%) were diagnosed with benign tumors. One case was diagnosed with thrombus, not a tumor (Fig. 1). Tumors were detected in all cardiac chambers and extracardiac sites. Locations of the tumors are listed in Table 1. One case was diagnosed with thrombus, not a tumor. In 4 cases, tumors were detected at two sites in each. The most frequent tumor sites were the atrium: 35% in the left atrium and 25% in the right atrium. The tumor types are listed in Table 2. Figure 2 shows the distribution of 40 cases diagnosed pathologically by surgery. One case was excluded because of a thrombus diagnosis. The most common type of all cardiac tumors was myxoma ($n = 20$, 50%). The second-most common tumor was papillary fibroelastoma ($n = 7$, 18%). Among cases with malignant tumors ($n = 10$, 25%), angiosarcoma ($n = 6$, 15%) was the most common pathological type. Other malignant tumors were malignant lymphoma ($n = 3$, 7.5%) and leiomyosarcoma (n = 1, 2.5%).

As for the cases with primary cardiac tumors in the non-surgery group, benign cardiac tumors were diagnosed in all 20 cases. We diagnosed myxoma in 13 cases, papillary fibroelastoma in 6 cases and lipoma in one case. After echocardiography, we confirmed other imaging data.

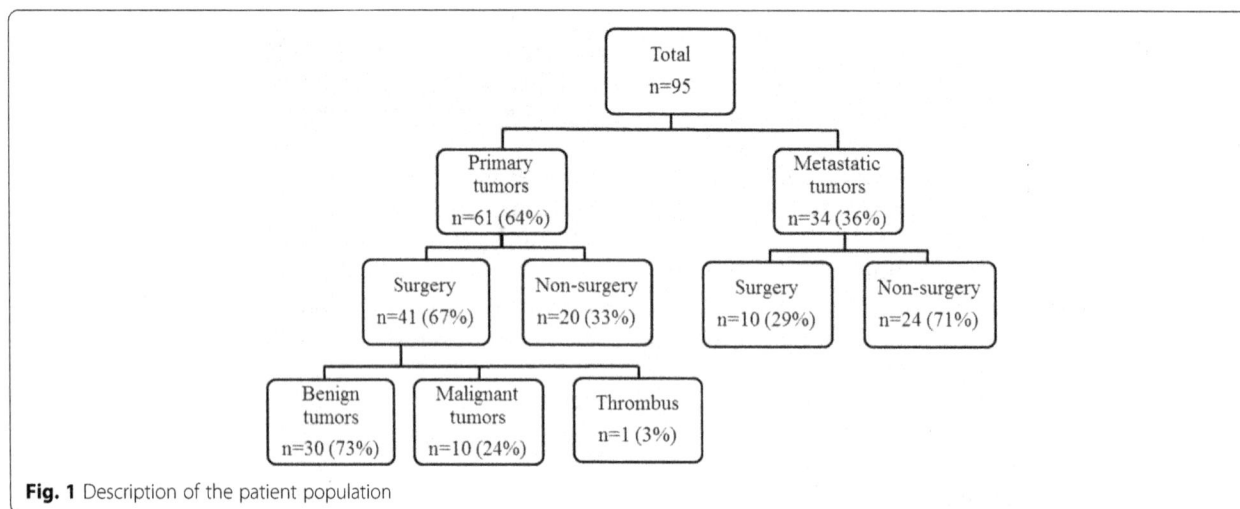

Fig. 1 Description of the patient population

These cases were highly suspected primary benign tumors, but no definitive diagnosis could be obtained.

Diagnosis of cardiac tumor

Table 3 shows the comparison of the echocardiographic diagnosis with the pathological diagnosis. By echocardiography, 41 cases were diagnosed with primary cardiac tumors. TEE was performed in 27 (66%) of the operated 41 patients. Four cases (10%) could only be diagnosed by TEE, not by TTE. Tumor types diagnosed by TEE were myxoma in 1 case and angiosarcoma in 3 cases. The patients diagnosed with papillary fibroelastoma and the patients diagnosed with angiosarcoma by echocardiography were all concordant with pathological results.

Otherwise, in 6 cases with angiosarcoma diagnosed by pathology, 3 cases (50%) could not be diagnosed by TTE but were diagnosed by TEE. Two cases (33%) could be diagnosed as an angiosarcoma by TTE. One case of angiosarcoma (17%) could not have the tumor type diagnosed by echocardiography. One case was diagnosed with myxoma by echocardiography, but was found to be a thrombus on pathology. One case could not determine the tumor type by echocardiography, but was a clear hemangioma by pathology. In summary, we could not diagnose the tumor types in 7 cases (17%) by echocardiography. These tumors were

Table 1 The location of cardiac tumors in 94 cases included 4 overlapping sites

Location	Total $n = 95$ (99 sites[a])	Primary cardiac tumors $n = 60$ (61 sites)				Metastatic cardiac tumors $n = 34$ (37 sites)	
		Surgery Group $n = 40$ (41 sites)		Non-surgery Group $n = 20$ (20 sites)		Surgery Group $n = 10$ (12 sites)	Non-surgery Group $n = 24$ (25 sites)
		Benign tumor $n = 31$ (31 sites)	Malignant tumor $n = 10$ (11 sites)				
Left Atrium	34 (34%)	22 (71%)	0	5 (25%)		1 (8%)	6 (24%)
Right Atrium	25 (26%)	2 (6%)	8 (73%)	4 (20%)		4 (34%)	7 (28%)
Left Ventricle	6 (6%)	1 (3%)	0	4 (20%)		0	1 (4%)
Right Ventricle	7 (7%)	0	2 (18%)	1 (5%)		1 (8%)	3 (12%)
Aortic Valve	10 (10%)	5 (16%)	0	5 (25%)		0	0
Mitral Valve	1 (1%)	0	0	1 (5%)		0	0
Pulmonary Valve	1 (1%)	1 (3%)	0	0		0	0
Inferior vena cava	6 (6%)	0	0	0		4 (34%)	2 (8%)
Aorta	4 (4%)	0	0	0		1 (8%)	3 (12%)
Pulmonary Artery	2 (2%)	0	1 (9%)	0		0	1 (4%)
Pericardium	3 (3%)	0	0	0		1 (8%)	2 (8%)

[a]In 4 cases, tumors were detected at two sites in each

Table 2 Histopathology of primary cardiac tumors

Pathology	No. of patients
Benign tumors	30
Myxoma	20 (67%)
Papillary fibroelastoma	7 (23%)
Hemangioma	1 (3%)
Bronchogenic cyst	1 (3%)
Calcified tumor	1 (3%)
Malignant tumors	10
Angiosarcoma	6 (60%)
Malignant lymphoma	3 (30%)
Leiomyosarcoma	1 (10%)
Thrombus	1

malignant lymphoma in 3 patients (7.3%), and 1 case each of angiosarcoma (2.4%), leiomyosarcoma (2.4%), hemangioma (2.4%) and bronchogenic cyst (2.4%). Figure 3a shows the case with thrombus that was misdiagnosed as a right atrial myxoma by echocardiography. Figure 3b shows the case with leiomyosarcoma that could not be diagnosed by echocardiography. The diagnostic accuracy of cardiac tumors by echocardiography was 80% (33/41).

The characteristics of secondary metastatic cardiac tumors

Thirty-four of 95 cases (36%) were detected or diagnosed as metastatic cardiac tumors by echocardiography. From the echocardiographic images, these were diagnosed as metastatic cardiac tumors for the following reasons: direct invasion to the heart, a massive pericardial effusion, or an irregular mass. We performed echocardiography in 6

cases without the information about primary disease and other imaging data from the echocardiographic order. The metastatic cardiac tumors were initially diagnosed by echocardiography in 5 of 6 cases. However, one case could not be distinguished from a pericardial cyst. The diagnostic rate was 15% of all metastatic tumors. The information about the primary disease or other imaging data from echocardiographic order was obtained in 28 cases before examination.

From the echocardiographic characteristics, a definite diagnose of the metastatic tumors could be made in 30 of all 34 cases, with or without information about the tumor in echocardiographic order. With echocardiographic diagnosis, a diagnosis could be made because of the specific characteristics. Concretely, the echocardiographic characteristics that allowed us to make a metastatic tumor diagnosis were direct invasion of the aorta in 4 cases, a mass of inferior vena cava (IVC) in 10 cases, direct invasion of the right ventricle (RV) in 3 cases, direct invasion of the left atrium (LA) in 3 cases, direct invasion of the right atrium (RA) in 2 cases, penetration of interatrial septum in one case, tumors that continued into the left atrium from the pulmonary vein (PV) in 2 cases and a tumor that continued into the right atrium from the supra vena cava in one case. One case diagnosed as lymphoma was detected as a metastatic tumor at the tricuspid annulus, which is a specific metastatic site for lymphoma. The metastatic tumors at the pericardium and pericardial effusion found in 3 cases were diagnosed accurately because of primary disease from echocardiographic order. Otherwise, the irregular mass in the chambers could be suspected as malignant tumors in 3 cases. However, we unable to diagnose whether

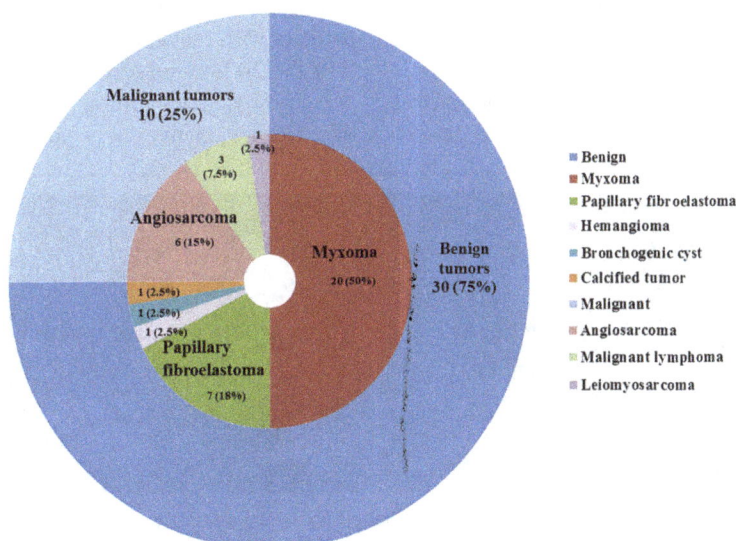

Fig. 2 Distribution of cardiac tumors diagnosed and treated at our hospital. We excluded one case that was diagnosed as thrombus by pathological data

Table 3 The diagnostic accuracy of echocardiography

Pathology	Echocardiographic diagnosis	Accuracy
Myxoma (n = 20)	Myxoma (n = 20)	100%
Thrombus (n = 1)	Myxoma	0%
Papillary fibroelastoma (n = 7)	Papillary fibroelastoma (n = 7)	100%
Angiosarcoma (n = 6)	Angiosarcoma (n = 5)	83%
	No definite diagnosis (n = 1)	
Malignant lymphoma (n = 3)	No definite diagnosis	0%
Leiomyosarcoma (n = 1)	No definite diagnosis	0%
Bronchogenic cyst (n = 1)	No definite diagnosis	0%
Hemangioma (n = 1)	No definite diagnosis	0%
Calcified amorphous tumor (n = 1)	Calcified amorphous tumor	100%

these were metastatic tumors or not only by echocardiography. The most frequent tumor sites were the atrium: 30% in the right atrium and 19% in the left atrium. The second-most common tumor site was the inferior vena cava (16%). Primary diseases of metastatic cardiac tumors are shown in Fig. 4. The most common primary disease was lung cancer followed by renal cell carcinoma and thymoma. Ten of the 34 cases (29%) underwent surgery for their cardiac tumors.

Operative data

All benign tumors were completely resected without major complications. The patient with a bronchogenic cyst was implanted a permanent epicardium pacemaker for atrioventricular block.

In ten patients with primary malignant tumors, one patient underwent surgery twice for recurrence.

Two patients with sarcoma underwent complete resections.

Seven of 10 patients (70%) required reconstructions of RA with autologous or bovine pericardium. One patient required tricuspid annuloplasty and aortocoronary bypass to right coronary artery.

One patient with direct invasion of the ascending aorta underwent concomitant ascending aorta replacement.

Ten patients with secondary metastatic tumors underwent surgery. All IVC tumors were completely resected. The IVC wall was directly incised in 3 patients. In one patient, the free wall of the RA was incised and then an IVC tumor was resected. The patient with direct tumor invasion of the aorta received a replacement of the descending aorta with an artificial blood vessel. In the patient whose tumor was a continuous invasion from the PV into LA, the tumor with the partial portion of the LA wall and PV was resected. Thereafter, the posterior wall of the LA was repaired with self pericardium. In the patient whose tumor was directly invading the RA wall, the tumor with the anterior wall of the RA was resected and the defect portion was recreated with equine pericardium.

Mortality

The median follow-up period was 43 months (0.5–183 months). The patients diagnosed with benign tumors were all alive at the end of the follow-up period ($p < 0.0001$; Fig. 5). The mean survival of the patients with malignant tumors was 113.5 ± 34.1 months. Seven patients with malignant tumors died (70%). Five of these 7 patients were diagnosed with angiosarcoma and the other two were each diagnosed with leiomyosarcoma or malignant lymphoma. All of the patients with malignant tumors received adjuvant chemotherapy after resection. The median survival for the patients with angiosarcoma was 42.2 months (10–113 months). Median survival for the patients with other malignant tumors was 21.8 months (0.8–64 months). The 1-month mortality of patients with malignant cardiac tumors was 30% (Fig. 5).

In the 20 non-surgery patients with primary tumors, a primary malignant tumor was found in only one patient. Seventeen patients were followed up. Three patients

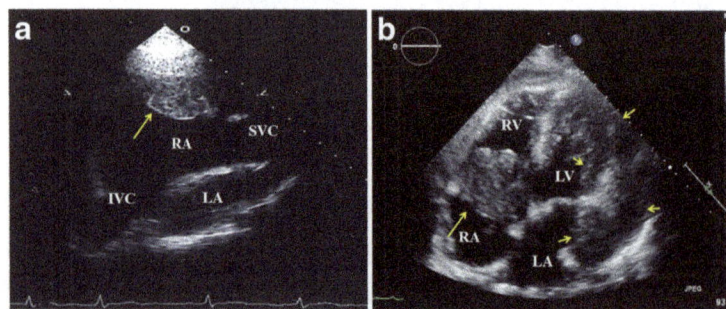

Fig. 3 Representative cases incorrectly diagnosed by transthoracic echocardiography. **a**. Horizontal section of a right parasternal view. Thrombus attached to RA appendage (arrow). We misdiagnosed this as an RA myxoma. **b**. Left parasternal four-chamber view. We could not diagnose the tumor type before surgery. A leiomyosarcoma arose from the coronary sinus and was detected around the LV (arrows). RA = right atrium, LA = left atrium, IVC = inferior vena cava, SVC = superior vena cava, LV = left ventricle, RV = right ventricle

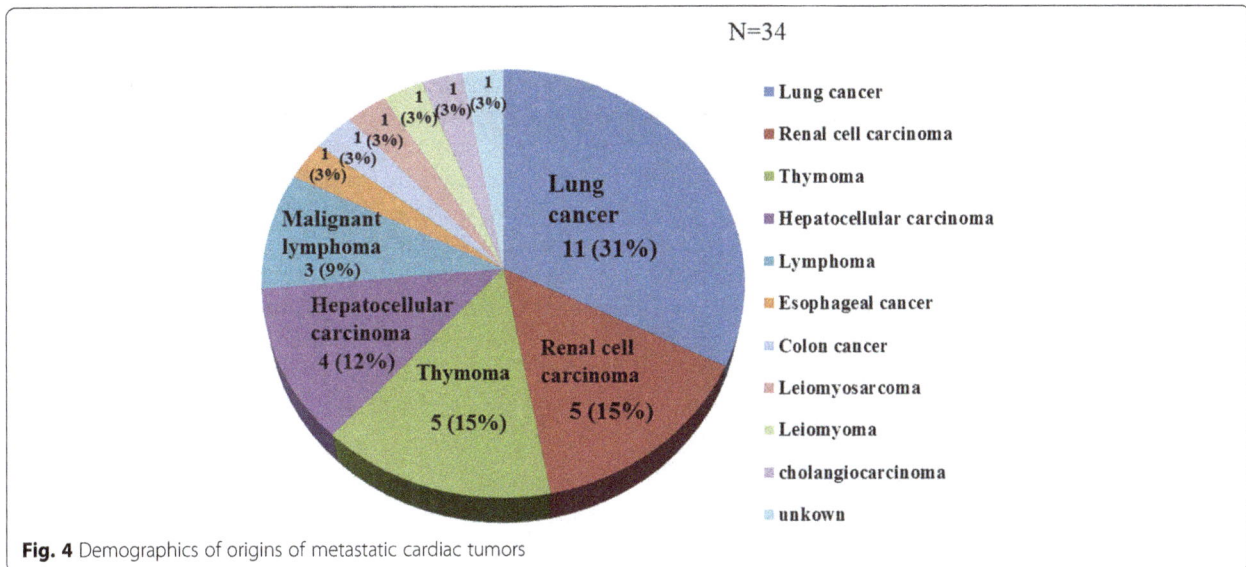

Fig. 4 Demographics of origins of metastatic cardiac tumors

died. The patient diagnosed with angiosarcoma died 47 days after the diagnosis. The other 2 patients diagnosed with benign tumor died because of non-cardiac diseases. The maximum survival was 6-years.

In the 24 non-surgery patients with metastatic malignant tumors, 20 patients could be followed up. Eighteen patients died. The maximum survival for these 18 patients was 7-years in the patient diagnosed with lymphoma. The minimum survival was 2 days in the patient with colon cancer. The maximum survival for all patients with metastatic malignant tumors was 11.5-years.

Discussion

Indeed, there might be few new information, however, some clinically important information has been found in our study. Firstly, our study reconfirmed previous

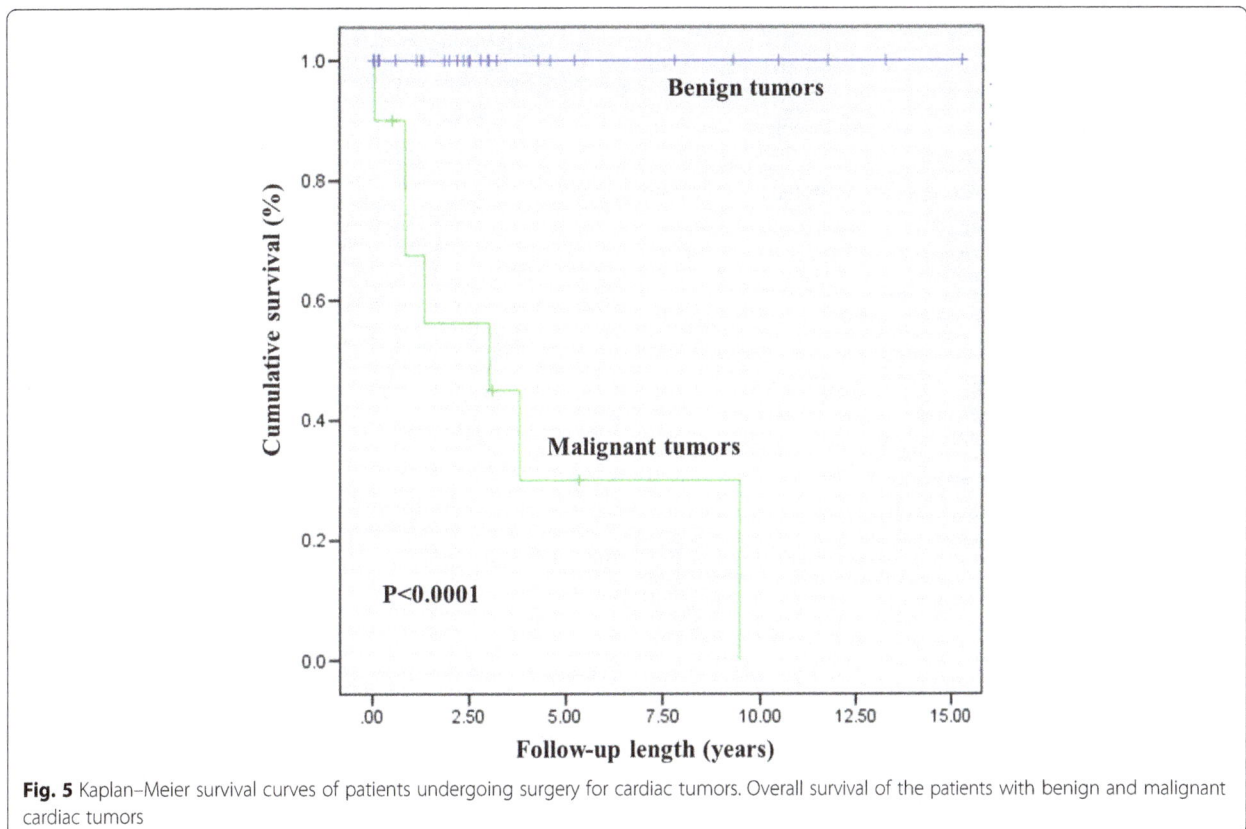

Fig. 5 Kaplan–Meier survival curves of patients undergoing surgery for cardiac tumors. Overall survival of the patients with benign and malignant cardiac tumors

reports about cardiac tumors. Previously, echocardiography had been shown to be a useful technique for detecting cardiac masses [4]. Secondly, the present study reconfirmed the echocardiographic characteristics of cardiac tumors and histological diagnoses. Moreover, this study also confirmed the utility of echocardiography in the diagnosis of uncommon cardiac tumors in a single center. This study had a clinical importance to address the characteristics of cardiac tumors and to reconfirm the usefulness and problems of echocardiography.

Characteristics of cardiac tumors

Primary cardiac tumors are rare and the incidence is 0.001–0.3% by autopsy, while metastatic tumors to the heart are reported to be 20 to 40 times more common by an autopsy report [5]. The reported clinical incidence of primary cardiac tumors has varied between 0.001% -0.03% in most studies, with cardiac tumors as the cause of only 0.3%–0.85% of all open-heart surgeries [1, 6]. Approximately 75% of all primary cardiac tumors are benign, with myxoma accounting for at least half of the reported cases [1, 7, 8]. 25% of primary cardiac tumors are malignant with sarcoma accounting for a majority of the reported cases [9]. Kumar et al. reported that 184 of 188 cases (98%) had primary cardiac tumors, with 170 cases (92%) of benign cardiac tumors and 14 cases (8%) of primary malignant cardiac tumors. Only 4 of 188 cases (2%) were secondary metastatic tumors [9]. Other studies reported that only 3.3% of all cardiac tumors were metastases [10]. In our study, 64% (61/95) of all cardiac tumors were primary cardiac tumors and metastatic tumors were detected in 36% of cases (34/95). Compared with previous reports, the numbers of metastatic tumor cases in our hospital was higher. The main reason is that many cancer patients were referred to our hospital for higher-level treatment. Therefore, the proportion of metastatic cardiac tumors was higher.

Our study confirms the results from previous studies in that the majority of primary cardiac tumors are benign (≥ 75%) and most benign cardiac tumors are atrial myxomas. Although significantly less common, papillary fibroelastoma is the second-most common benign cardiac tumor. One unusual case in our study was diagnosed with a very rare bronchogenic cyst. A calcified tumor was detected in only a single case. The premortem diagnosis of primary malignant cardiac tumors is rare. In previous studies, malignant cardiac tumors were even more rare, representing 5.1–28.7% of all cardiac tumors [11]. In our study, 25% of the primary cardiac tumors (10/40) were malignant, with angiosarcoma representing 15% of all primary cardiac tumors and 60% of primary malignant tumors. The differences in the percentage of malignant cardiac tumors across studies may be explained by characteristics of the hospital. If the

hospital is famous for the treatment of malignant diseases, the number of cases with primary or secondary malignant cardiac tumors may increase. Mortality in cases of primary benign tumor is low [12–14]. However, < 50% of patients with primary malignant cardiac tumors were alive by the end of the first year after diagnosis, with a sharp decrease in survival for sarcoma patients [15]. In our study, 70% of patients with primary malignant cardiac tumors were alive at the end of the first year. However, after one year, the survival rate decreased sharply. Metastatic cardiac tumors make up 0.7–3.5% of cardiac tumors. The major primary lesion was lung cancer in our study, consistent with a prior study [16].

Echocardiographic diagnosis

Echocardiography and cardiac magnetic resonance imaging (MRI) are also useful to identify cardiac tumors and malignant masses [17]. However, TTE is now the principle imaging technique for cardiac tumor detection. It can usually provide adequate diagnostic information, such as a cardiac site, size, and shape of a tumor. Thereafter, the mass can be checked in detail by computed tomography (CT) or MRI. In our practice, we can accurately diagnose the masses that have characteristic images by echocardiography. The diagnostic accuracy of echocardiography is good (80%). The diagnosable tumors include myxoma, papillary fibroelastoma, and angiosarcoma [18, 19]. The most common tumor type is myxoma, and second is papillary fibroelastoma. These tumors can be diagnosed easily by echocardiography because of specific characters, and we think that this is the reason for the high diagnostic accuracy of echocardiography for cardiac tumors. Therefore, echocardiography is very useful for the diagnosis of benign cardiac tumors. Otherwise, it is difficult to diagnose the rarer tumors. For these cases, TEE is a useful method of imaging cardiac masses. In our study, we could not diagnose the tumor type using TTE in 4 patients, but were able to diagnose them using TEE. Recently, 3-dimensional TEE can provide a clearer view of the characteristics of cardiac mass. However, TEE is more invasive than TTE. Therefore, the necessity of TEE must be considered individually. Further effort needs to be taken to understand the tumor characteristics on echocardiography. However, it is difficult to diagnose cases with rare types of tumors using echocardiography.

Clinical implications

Primary cardiac tumor is very rare, however, cardiac tumors are sometimes found at the time of echocardiographic examination. Therefore, we should recognize the echocardiographic characteristics of cardiac tumors and make an effort to diagnose them accurately. As for benign tumors, the specific echocardiographic characteristics and locations are very important for diagnosis.

We canreconfirm the importance of echocardiographic characteristics.

When we suspect malignant tumors, the extent of tumor invasion must be examined attentively to decide the patient's operative status. Furthermore, surgeons need information regarding how much of the tumor can be removed The extent of resection is an important factor contributing to the prognosis. Many cases of metastatic cardiac tumors could be diagnosed by other imaging modalities. Malignant diseases generally undergo follow-up examination, especially using computed tomography. Therefore, the importance of echocardiography may be the diagnostic tool for the progression degree, rather than the diagnosis itself. However, in fact, the small number of cases could be initially diagnosed by echocardiography. We recommend that the chief physician follow up by not only CT but also echocardiography when the patients with malignancy arefollowed up. We also must understand the limitations of echocardiography.

Limitations

First, this study was performed in a single center. Therefore, the number of cases was very small. We need to perform a multicenter study that includes more patients with cardiac tumors. Second, we only evaluated biopsy-proved masses, and therefore, no conservatively managed masses were included. Third, the follow-up period varied by the kind of tumor, especially in primary malignant tumors. Fourth, we only investigated the diagnostic accuracy and importance of echocardiography. We also need to study the diagnostic accuracy and importance of computed tomography and magnetic resonance imaging. Finally, our data may be biased because many patients with malignant tumors visited our hospital for advanced treatment. This point can be addressed by performing a multicenter study.

Conclusion

Cardiac tumor is a rare and important disease of the heart. Our results are consistent with previous reports in regards to the incidence, tumor characteristics and prognosis of cardiac tumors. Echocardiography offers advantages in early identification of cardiac masses noninvasively and in providing clinically important information about the characteristics of the masses. Our study also suggests the necessity of extending our knowledge of the characteristics of cardiac tumors.

Abbreviations

CT: Computed tomography; MRI: Magnetic resonance imaging; TEE: Transesophageal echocardiography; TTE: Transthoracic echocardiography

Acknowledgements
Not applicable.

Funding
None.

Authors' contributions
NN is the primary investigator, including data collection. NN and TT were responsible for study design, analysis and interpretation of data and manuscript drafting. TK collected data. TK, KK, TK, MO and SK were responsible for study design and interpretation of data. YI contributed to pathological examination. YO carried out the operation. YF have supervised and commented the manuscript. All authors read and approved the final manuscript.

Competing interests
The authors declare that they have no competing interests.

Author details
[1]Department of Clinical Technology, Kobe City Medical Center General Hospital, 2-1-1 Minatojima-Minamimachi, Chuo-ku, Kobe 650-0047, Japan. [2]Basic Medical Science, Kobe City College of Nursing, 3-4 Gakuennishi-machi, Nishi-ku, Kobe 651-2103, Japan. [3]Department of Cardiovascular Medicine, Kobe City Medical Center General Hospital, 2-1-1 Minatojima-Minamimachi, Chuo-ku, Kobe 650-0047, Japan. [4]Department of Pathology, Kobe City Medical Center General Hospital, 2-1-1 Minatojima-Minamimachi, Chuo-ku, Kobe 650-0047, Japan. [5]Department of Cardiovascular Surgery, Kobe City Medical Center General Hospital, 2-1-1 Minatojima-Minamimachi, Chuo-ku, Kobe 650-0047, Japan.

References
1. Patel J, Sheppard MN. Pathological study of primary cardiac and pericardial tumours in a specialist UK Centre: surgical and autopsy series. Cardiovasc Pathol. 2010;19:343–52.
2. Reynen K. Frequency of primary tumors of the heart. Am J Cardiol. 1996;77(1):107.
3. Centofanti P, Di Rosa E, Deorsola L, Dato GM, Patane F, La Torre M, et al. Primary cardiac tumors: early and late results of surgical treatment in 91 patients. Ann Thorac Surg. 1999;68:1236–41.
4. Peters PJ, Reinhardt S. The echocardiographic evaluation of intracardiac masses: a review. J Am Soc Echocardiogr. 2006;19:230–40.
5. Al-Mamgani A, Baartman L, Baaijiens M, de Pree I, Incrocci L, Levendag PC. Cardiac metastases. Int J Clin Oncol. 2008;13:369–72.
6. Strecker T, Rosch J, Weyand M, Agaimy A. Primary and metastatic cardiac tumors: imaging characteristics, surgical treatment, and histopathological spectrum: a 10-year-experience at a German heart center. Cardiovasc Pathol. 2012;21:436–43.
7. Habertheuer A, Laufer G, Wiedemann D, Andreas M, Ehrlich M, Rath C, et al. Primary cardiac tumors on the verge of oblivion: a European experience over 15 years. J Cardiothorac Surg. 2015;10:56.
8. Kuroczynski W, Peivandi AA, Ewald P, Pruefer D, Heinemann M, Vahl CF. Cardiac myxomas: short- and long-term follow-up. Cardiol J. 2009;16:447–54.
9. Kumar N, Agarwal S, Ahuja A, Das P, Airon B, Ray R. Spectrum of cardiac tumors excluding myxoma: experience of a tertiary center with review of the literature. Pathol Res Pract. 2011;207:769–74.
10. Yu K, Liu Y, Wang H, Hu S, Long C. Epidemiological pathological characteristics of cardiac tumors: a clinical study of 242 cases. Interact Cardiovasc Thorac Surg. 2007;6(5):636–9.
11. Burazor I, Aviel-Ronen S, Imazio M, Markel G, Grossman Y, Yosepovich A, et al. Primary malignancies of the heart and pericardium. Clin Cardiol. 2014;37(9):582–8.
12. Kamiya H, Yasuda T, Nagamine H, Sakakibara N, Nishida S, Kawasuji M, et al. Surgical treatment of primary cardiac tumors: 28 years' experience in Kanazawa university hospital. Jpn Circ J. 2001;65:315–9.
13. Elbardissi AW, Dearani JA, Daly RC, Mullany CJ, Orszulak TA, Puga FJ, et al.

Survival after resection of primary cardiac tumors: a 48-year experience. Circulation. 2008;118(14 suppl):S7–15.

14. Pacini D, Careddu L, Pantaleo A, Berretta P, Leone O, Marinelli G, et al. Primary benign cardiac tumours: long-term results. Eur J Cardiothorac Surg. 2012;41(4):812–9.

15. Guilherme HO, Al-Kindi SG, Hoimes C, Park SJ. Characteristics and survival of malignant cardiac tumors. A 40-year analysis of > 500 patients. Circulation. 2015;132:2395–402.

16. Goldberg AD, Blankstein R, Padera RF. Tumors metastatic to heart. Circulation. 2013;128:1790–4.

17. Patel R, Lim RP, Saric M, Nayar A, Babb J, Ettel M, et al. Diagnostic performance of cardiac magnetic resonance imaging and echocardiography in evaluation of cardiac and paracardiac masses. Am J Cardiol. 2016;117:135–40.

18. Cianciulli TF, Soumoulou JB, Lax JA, Saccheri MC, Cozzarin A, Beck MA, et al. Papillary fibroelastoma: clinical and echocardiographic features and initial approach in 54 cases. Echocardiography. 2016;33:1811–7.

19. Kupsky DF, Newman DB, Kumar G, Maleszewski JJ, Edwards WD, Klarich KW. Echocardiographic features of cardiac angiosarcomas: the Mayo Clinic experience (1976-2013). Echocardiography. 2016;33:186–92.

7

Short-term outcomes of robot-assisted minimally invasive esophagectomy for esophageal cancer: a propensity score matched analysis

Haiqi He, Qifei Wu, Zhe Wang, Yong Zhang, Nanzheng Chen, Junke Fu and Guangjian Zhang[*]

Abstract

Background: Minimally invasive esophagectomy (MIE) was shown to be effective in reducing the morbidity and was adopted increasingly. The robot-assisted minimally invasive esophagectomy (RAMIE) remains in the initial stage of application. This study evaluated its safety and feasibility by comparing short-term outcomes of RAMIE and video-assisted minimally invasive esophagectomy (VAMIE).

Methods: Between March 2016 and December 2017, 115 consecutive patients underwent RAMIE or VAMIE at our institute. The baseline characteristics, pathological data and short-term outcomes of these two group patients were collected and compared. RAMIE patients were propensity score matched with VAMIE patients for a more accurate comparison.

Results: Matching based on propensity scores produced 27 patients in each group. After propensity score matching (PSM), the baseline characteristics between the two groups were comparable. The operation time in RAMIE group was significantly longer than that in VAMIE group (349 and 294 min, respectively; $P < 0.001$). The blood loss volume in RAMIE group was less than that in VAMIE group (119 and 158 ml, respectively), but with no statistically significant difference ($P = 0.062$). There was no significant difference between the two groups with respect to the mean number of dissected lymph nodes (20 and 19, respectively; $P = 0.420$), postoperative hospital stay (13.8 and 12.7 days, respectively; $P = 0.548$), the rate of overall complications (37.0 and 33.3%, respectively; $P = 0.776$) and the rates of detailed complications between the two groups.

Conclusions: The short-term outcomes of RAMIE is comparable to VAMIE, demonstrating safety and feasibility of RAMIE.

Keywords: Esophageal cancer, Esophagectomy, Minimally invasive esophagectomy, Robot-assisted, Video-assisted

Background

Esophageal cancer is one of the most commonly diagnosed cancers around the world. At present, esophageal cancer is the sixth and ninth leading causes of cancer-related mortality among men and women, respectively [1]. In China, it is estimated that there are approximately 477,900 new esophageal cancer cases and 375,000 deaths in 2015 [2]. For esophageal cancer, surgical resection with radical lymphadenectomy remains a critical element in the multimodality management [3], and transthoracic esophagectomy is the preferred surgical procedure worldwide, which is conducive to en bloc resection of the tumor along with the mediastinal lymph nodes [4]. However, the open transthoracic approach is associated with high rates of postoperative complications due to the surgical trauma [5]. Therefore, to reduce the morbidity as a result of surgical trauma from open procedures, minimally invasive esophagectomy (MIE) was adopted. The role of MIE has been well established in the last few years [6–9]. Nevertheless, the MIE is not routinely applied worldwide for its high technical complexity and steep learning curve [10].

As an alternative, robotic surgery may provide the minimally invasive option for more surgeons and

* Correspondence: michael8039@163.com
Department of thoracic surgery, The First Affiliated Hospital of Xi'an Jiaotong University, 277 West Yanta Road, Xi'an, Shaanxi 710061, China

patients, because the robotic platform provides improved visualization with a magnified three-dimensional view and improved articulation of instruments with seven degrees of freedom, and thereby allows for precise manipulation and dissection. Although the robot-assisted esophagectomy was completed as early as 2003 [11, 12], it remains in the initial stage of application [13]. At present, there were few reports comparing RAMIE with VAMIE.

Thus, the aim of this study was to determine the safety and feasibility by comparing the short-term outcomes between RAMIE and VAMIE in patients with esophageal cancer.

Methods

Patient selection

We retrospectively reviewed the medical records of consecutive 115 patients who underwent McKeown minimally invasive esophagectomy in our institution for esophageal cancer without any previous neoadjuvant

therapy from March 2016 to December 2017. Preoperatively, all patients underwent upper gastrointestinal endoscopy, contrast-enhanced computed tomography (CT) scan of the chest and upper abdomen, pulmonary function routinely, and were evaluated as resectable esophageal cancer. This study was approved by the ethics committee of Xi'an Jiaotong University. Each patient gave consent before the operation.

Operation method

All patients underwent RAMIE or VAMIE with two-field lymph node dissection. RAMIE was completed using da Vinci surgical system (Intuitive Surgical, Inc., Sunnyvale, CA, USA). All patients were intubated with a double-lumen tube. During the thoracic phase, the patients were placed in the left lateral decubitus position. The trocars for thoracic part of RAMIE were placed as shown in Fig. 1a. An 8-mm robotic trocar was placed in the 3rd or 4th intercostal space (ICS) on the anterior axillary line, and another 8-mm robotic trocar

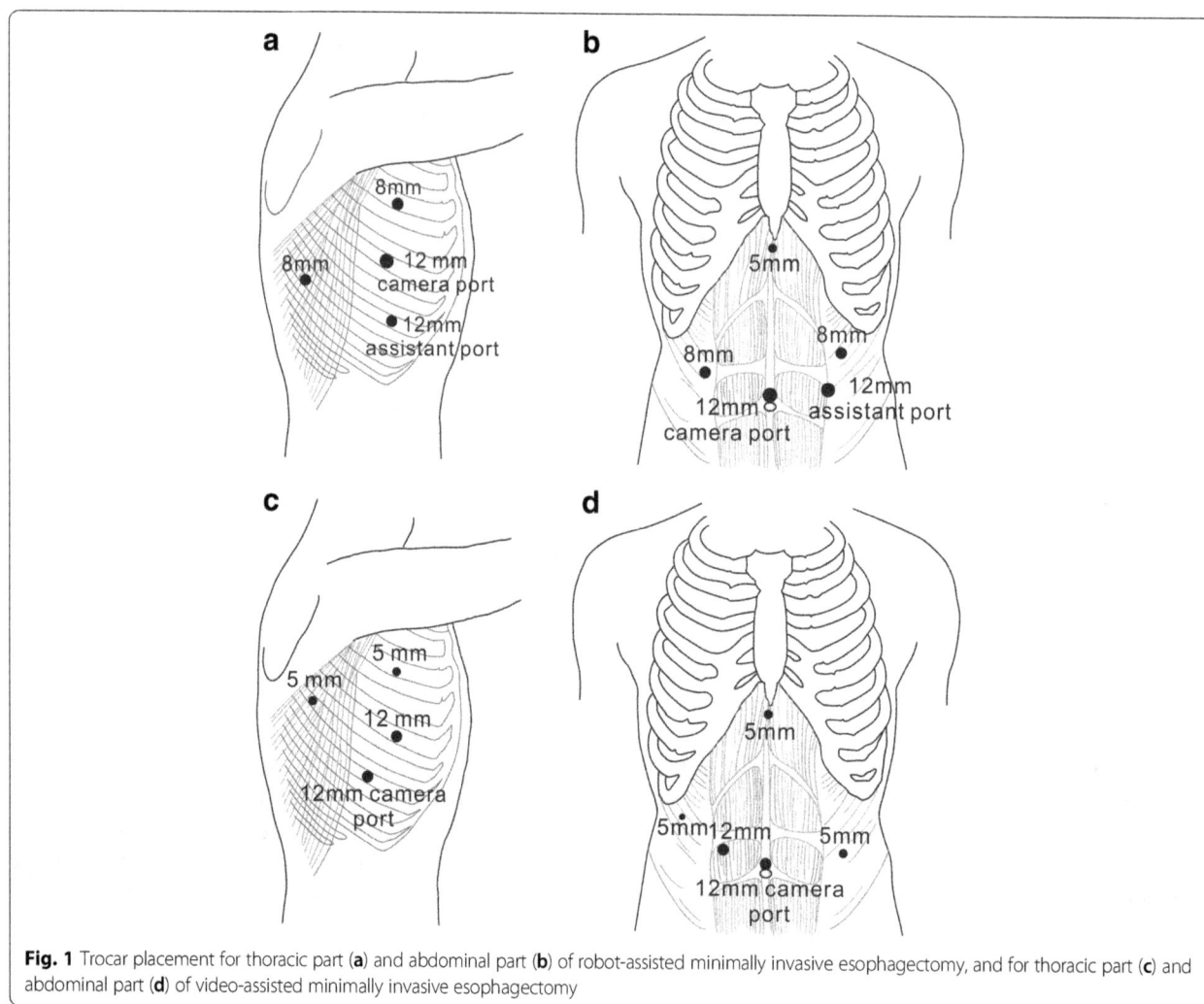

Fig. 1 Trocar placement for thoracic part (**a**) and abdominal part (**b**) of robot-assisted minimally invasive esophagectomy, and for thoracic part (**c**) and abdominal part (**d**) of video-assisted minimally invasive esophagectomy

was placed in the 8th ICS between the posterior axillary line to scapular line. A 12-mm camera trocar was placed in the 5th or 6th ICS on the middle axillary line. A 12-mm assistant trocar was placed in the 7th ICS on the anterior axillary line. The trocars for thoracic part of VAMIE were placed as follows: a 5-mm and a 12-mm working trocar were placed in the 4th and 6th ICS on the anterior axillary line, respectively; a 12-mm camera trocar was placed in the 7th ICS on the middle axillary line; a 5-mm assistant trocar was placed in the 6th ICS between the posterior axillary line to scapular line. Insufflation with CO_2 at a pressure of 7–10 mmHg was used for both RAMIE and VAMIE during thoracic part. The esophagus was mobilized along with all periesophageal lymph nodes. The azygous vein was routinely ligated with Hem-o-lock clips and divided. The lymph nodes along bilateral recurrent laryngeal nerve were dissected carefully.

Trocar placement for abdominal part of RAMIE and VAMIE were shown in Fig. 1b and d. A 5-mm trocar under the xiphoid process was used in both RAMIE and VAMIE to retract the liver. When the mobilized stomach was taken out through the upper abdominal small incision, a 4-cm-wide gastric conduit was constructed with the linear tissue staplers. Then the gastric tube was pulled up to the neck through the mediastinum and a cervical end-to-side anastomosis was performed with a circular stapler.

Data collection

The baseline characteristics, pathological data and short-term outcomes were retrospectively collected, including gender, age, body mass index (BMI), Charlson comorbidity index, forced expiratory volume in 1 s (FEV1%), tumor location, tumor grade, operation time, blood loss, the number of retrieved lymph nodes, pathological stage, postoperative hospital stay and postoperative complications. All patients were staged using the American Joint Committee on Cancer (AJCC) 7th edition TNM staging system. The postoperative complications were diagnosed and categorized based on clinical symptoms, combined with laboratory tests and radiological imaging findings. Pulmonary complications were defined as pneumonia, atelectasis requiring sputum suction bronchoscopy, acute respiratory failure, acute respiratory distress syndrome (ARDS). Recurrent laryngeal nerve injury was diagnosed at any sign of voice change or aspiration. The diagnosis of anastomotic leakage was based on definite clinical features, confirmed by esophagography and gastroscopy. Other complications were also recorded, including chylothorax, delayed gastric emptying, hemorrhage, pleural effusion and wound infection. Postoperative death was defined as death within 90 days after surgery.

Statistical analysis

SPSS software version 22.0 was used for statistical analysis. In order to overcome the data heterogeneity, the RAMIE cases were propensity scored matched to VAMIE cases according to gender, age, BMI, Charlson comorbidity index, forced expiratory volume in 1 s (FEV1%), tumor location, pathologic T stage, and pathologic N stage. The operation time, blood loss, the number of dissected lymph nodes and postoperative complications were compared between the RAMIE and the VAMIE groups. Data were expressed as the mean ± standard deviation for continuous variables or number (%) for categorical data. Continuous variables were analyzed using Student's test or Mann-Whitney U test, depending on normality of distribution; while categorical data were analyzed using chi-square or Fisher's exact test. $P < 0.05$ was considered statistically significant.

Results

A total of 115 patients with esophageal cancer met the inclusion criteria between March 2016 and December 2017. Twenty-seven patients underwent RAMIE, and 88 patients received VAMIE. The baseline characteristics were shown in Table 1. There were significant differences between the two groups in FEV1% predicted and pathologic T stage. The average pulmonary function represented by FEV1% predicted was higher in RAMIE group than VAMIE group ($P = 0.012$). Patients in the VAMIE group presented more frequently with advanced T stage ($P = 0.042$). Other characteristics were similar between the two groups.

The operation time in RAMIE group was significantly longer than that in VAMIE group (349 and 294 min, respectively; $P < 0.001$). However, the blood loss in RAMIE was less than that in VAMIE group (118 and 165 ml, respectively; $P = 0.030$). The mean number of dissected lymph nodes in RAMIE group was similar to that in VAMIE group (20 and 18, respectively; $P = 0.214$). Within 90 days after surgery, there were two patients died in VAMIE group; whereas there was no patient died in RAMIE group ($P = 1.000$). There were no differences between the two groups with respect to postoperative hospital stay (13.8 and 14.1 days, respectively; $P = 0.548$) as well as the rates of overall postoperative complications (37.0 and 42.0%, respectively; $P = 0.643$) and detailed complications (Table 2).

To reduce the bias arising from baseline characteristics such as FEV1% predicted and pathologic T stage, a 1:1 propensity score matching analysis was performed. Propensity score matching analysis produced 27 patients in each group. After PSM, patient characteristics were well balanced between the two matched groups (Table 1). The operation time was still significantly longer in RAMIE group (349 and 285 min, respectively; $P < 0.001$). Although

Table 1 Patients' characteristics before and after propensity score matching

Variables	Before matching			After matching		
	RAMIE (n = 27)	VAMIE (n = 88)	P value	RAMIE (n = 27)	VAMIE (n = 27)	P value
Gender			0.636			1.000
Male	20 (74.1)	61 (69.3)		20 (74.1)	20 (74.1)	
Female	7 (25.9)	27 (30.7)		7 (25.9)	7 (25.9)	
Age	61.0 ± 8.0	62.9 ± 8.3	0.310	61.0 ± 8.0	61.6 ± 9.8	0.621*
BMI (kg/m²)	21.5 ± 2.7	21.4 ± 2.7	0.935	21.5 ± 2.7	21.9 ± 2.8	0.578
FEV1% predicted	94.5 ± 13.8	84.2 ± 19.6	0.012	94.6 ± 13.8	92.9 ± 23.0	0.747
Charlson comorbidity index			0.198			0.506
1	1 (3.7)	6 (6.8)		1 (3.7)	4 (14.8)	
2	10 (37.0)	20 (22.7)		10 (37.0)	8 (29.6)	
3	13 (48.1)	37 (42.0)		13 (48.1)	11 (40.7)	
4	3 (11.1)	25 (28.4)		3 (11.1)	4 (14.8)	
Tumor location			0.457			0.514
Proximal	1 (3.7)	8 (9.1)		1 (3.7)	3 (11.1)	
Middle	18 (66.6)	48 (54.5)		18 (66.6)	15 (55.6)	
Distal/EGJ	8 (29.6)	32 (36.4)		8 (29.6)	9 (33.3)	
Histological type			0.395			0.334†
Squamous cell carcinoma	23 (85.2)	80 (90.9)		23 (85.2)	25 (92.6)	
other	4 (14.8)	8 (9.1)		4 (14.8)	2 (7.4)	
Pathologic T stage			0.042			0.334
T1	4 (14.8)	13 (14.8)		4 (14.8)	1 (3.7)	
T2	13 (48.1)	21 (23.9)		13 (48.1)	13 (48.1)	
T3	10 (37.0)	54 (61.4)		10 (37.0)	13 (48.1)	
Pathologic N stage			0.260			0.387
N0	13 (48.1)	58 (65.9)		13 (48.1)	18 (66.6)	
N1	10 (37.0)	17 (19.3)		10 (37.0)	8 (29.6)	
N2	3 (11.1)	11 (12.5)		3 (11.1)	1 (3.7)	
N3	1 (3.7)	2 (2.3)		1 (3.7)	0	
Tumor grade			0.399			0.285
Well differentiated	2 (7.4)	13 (14.8)		2 (7.4)	6 (22.2)	
Moderate differentiated	19 (70.4)	63 (71.6)		19 (70.4)	17 (63.0)	
Poorly differentiated	6 (22.2)	12 (13.6)		6 (22.2)	4 (14.8)	

Data were presented as mean ± standard deviation for continuous variables or number (%) for categorical data
*Mann-Whitney U test; †Fisher's exact test
RAMIE robot-assisted minimally invasive esophagectomy, *VAMIE* video-assisted minimally invasive esophagectomy, *BMI* Body mass index, *FEV1* forced expiratory volume in 1 s, *GEJ* gastroesophageal junction

the mean blood loss volume in RAMIE group was still less than that in VAMIE group, this difference was no longer statistically significant (119 and 158 ml, respectively; P = 0.062). There was no significant difference between the two groups with respect to the mean number of dissected lymph nodes (20 and 19, respectively; P = 0.420), postoperative hospital stay (13.8 and 12.8 days, respectively; P = 0.128) as well as the rates of overall postoperative complications (37.0 and 33.3%, respectively; P = 0.776) and detailed complications.

Discussion

In the recent years, multiple reports have demonstrated that MIE could decrease blood loss, the length of stay, and surgical complications [6–9]. This encourages the surgeon to use and develop the minimally invasive techniques. As a novel minimally invasive technique, the robot-assisted approach has been successfully used for esophagectomy. However, the safety and feasibility of RAMIE have not been completely determined. Therefore, the present study compared the short-term outcomes of

Table 2 Postoperative outcomes of propensity score-unmatched and matched patients

Postoperative outcomes	Before matching			After matching		
	RAMIE (n = 27)	VAMIE (n = 88)	P value	RAMIE (n = 27)	VAMIE (n = 27)	P value
Operation time (minutes)	349 ± 45	294 ± 52	< 0.001	349 ± 45	285 ± 66	< 0.001
Blood loss (mL)	118 ± 71	165 ± 107	0.030*	119 ± 72	158 ± 82	0.062*
Number of harvested LNs	20 ± 7	18 ± 6	0.214*	20 ± 7	19 ± 5	0.420*
Postoperative hospital stay (day)	13.8 ± 2.0	14.1 ± 4.2	0.548*	13.8 ± 2.0	12.8 ± 2.7	0.128
Overall complication (at least one) [n (%)]	10 (37.0)	37 (42.0)	0.643	10 (37.0)	9 (33.3)	0.776
RLN injury [n (%)]	4 (14.8)	14 (15.9)	0.891	4 (14.8)	3 (11.1)	1.000†
Pulmonary complication [n (%)]	5 (18.5)	16 (18.2)	0.968	5 (18.5)	2 (7.4)	0.224
Arrhythmia [n (%)]	1 (3.7)	8 (9.1)	0.362	1 (3.7)	0	1.000†
Anastomotic leak [n (%)]	3 (11.1)	9 (10.2)	0.763	3 (11.1)	1 (3.7)	0.351†
Chylothorax [n (%)]	0	1 (1.1)	1.000†	0	1 (3.7)	1.000†
Bleeding [n (%)]	1 (3.7)	2 (2.3)	0.556†	1 (3.7)	1 (3.7)	1.000†
Delayed gastric emptying [n (%)]	1 (3.7)	7 (8.0)	0.448	1 (3.7)	0	1.000†
90-day mortality [n (%)]	0	2 (2.3)	1.000†	0	1 (3.7)	1.000†

Data were presented as mean ± standard deviation for continuous variables or number (%) for categorical data
*Mann-Whitney U test; †Fisher's exact test
RAMIE robot-assisted minimally invasive esophagectomy, *VAMIE* video-assisted minimally invasive esophagectomy, *RLN* recurrent laryngeal nerve

RAMIE with that of VAMIE. We found that there were no significant differences in blood loss, the number of dissected lymph nodes, postoperative hospital stay, and rates of postoperative complications, although RAMIE took longer operation time than VAMIE, mainly attributing to the docking and undocking. These results suggested that RAMIE is a safe and feasible technique, comparable to VAMIE.

Because of the high technical complexity and steep learning curve, the conventional VAMIE is not routinely applied worldwide [10]. Theoretically, the magnified three-dimensional view combined with seven degrees of freedom of the articulating surgical instruments facilitates meticulous dissection and thereby can accelerate the learning curve of RAMIE and decrease the operation time [14]. Narula et al. [15] evaluated technical enhancement of robotic and laparoscopic instrumentation in the task performance, using a computerized assessment system, and they found that the tasks were performed faster and more precisely with the robotic technology than standard laparoscopy. Further study by Chandra et al. [16] compared robotic and laparoscopic-assisted suturing performance for experts and novices. For laparoscopic novices, robotic technology significantly improves performance and accuracy. For laparoscopic experts, robotic technology significantly decreases the total instrument path length. Therefore, the robot is particularly useful for performing precise dissection in limited spaces, such as the mediastinal lymphadenectomy.

Actually, the advantages of RAMIE over VAMIE have not been well confirmed so far, even though RAMIE was completed as early as 2003 [11, 12]. During the past

decade, several groups have reported their results describing the safety and feasibility of the technique [13, 17–23]. Weksler et al., [24] compared 11 patients who underwent RAMIE and 26 patients who underwent VAMIE. They found that RAMIE was equivalent to VAMIE in terms of operation time, blood loss, the number of dissected lymph nodes, postoperative complications and length of stay. Yerokun et al. [7] reached the same conclusion by comparing the short-term outcomes of 117 cases with RAMIE and 117 cases with VAMIE. In terms of postoperative complications, most previous studies [24–27] together with our present study suggested that the rates of complications were comparable between RAMIE and VAMIE, although a higher rate of anastomotic leakage was found in the RAMIE in the study by Suda et al. [28].

The lymphadenectomy is a key step in radical esophagectomy for esophageal cancer. Lymph node dissection along bilateral recurrent laryngeal nerves (RLN) has always been a challenge in MIE due to frequent recurrent laryngeal nerve injury. The robot-assisted lymphadenectomy along bilateral RLNs was demonstrated to be technically feasible and safe [29]. The study by Park et al. [25] included 62 RAMIE and 43 VAMIE. They found that RAMIE yielded more number of dissected lymph nodes than VAMIE. The same conclusion was drawn by Deng et al. [27] in a recent study, which included 42 patients in both RAMIE and VAMIE groups. Suda et al. [28] showed that RAMIE reduced the incidence of RLN injury, although it did not increase the number of harvest lymph nodes. Chao et al. [26] found that RAMIE yielded more lymph nodes along the left RLN than VAMIE. However, other previous studies [7, 24] together with our study suggested that the number of dissected lymph nodes of RAMIE was comparable to that of VAMIE. These results varied from series to series may be due to their different experience.

Anyway, this study combined with previous studies suggested that RAMIE is a safe and feasible technique, and its efficacy is comparable to VAMIE in terms of short-term outcomes. However, the limitation of our study is that it has a small sample size and it is a non-randomized controlled study. At present, there aren't large-scale studies comparing these two minimally invasive technologies for esophagectomy. Interestingly, an ongoing randomized controlled trial by van der Sluis et al. [30] are now comparing robot-assisted with conventional open transthoracic esophagectomy. The result of ROBOT trial will provide more conclusive data.

Conclusions

RAMIE is technically safe and feasible. The short-term outcomes of RAMIE are comparable to VAMIE. The advantages of robotic system may allow precise dissection of lymph nodes in the mediastinum and help us to decrease blood loss.

Abbreviations

BMI: Body mass index; CT: Computed tomography; FEV1: Forced expiratory volume in 1 s; GEJ: Gastroesophageal junction; ICS: Intercostal space; MIE: Minimally invasive esophagectomy; PSM: Propensity score matching; RAMIE: Robot-assisted minimally invasive esophagectomy; RLN: Recurrent laryngeal nerve; VAMIE: Video-assisted minimally invasive esophagectomy

Authors' contributions

HH collected the data, wrote the manuscript. QW and NC collected and analyzed the data. GZ carried out the study design, made the main correction and participate in surgery. JF performed the surgeries and approved the final manuscript. YZ and ZW participate in surgery. All authors read and approved the final manuscript.

Competing interests

The authors declare that they have no competing interests.

References

1. Torre LA, Bray F, Siegel RL, Ferlay J, Lortet-Tieulent J, Jemal A. Global cancer statistics, 2012. CA Cancer J Clin. 2015;65(2):87–108.
2. Chen W, Zheng R, Baade PD, Zhang S, Zeng H, Bray F, Jemal A, Yu XQ, He J. Cancer statistics in China, 2015. CA Cancer J Clin. 2016;66(2):115–32.
3. Mariette C, Piessen G, Triboulet JP. Therapeutic strategies in oesophageal carcinoma: role of surgery and other modalities. Lancet Oncol. 2007;8(6): 545–53.
4. Boone J, Livestro DP, Elias SG, Borel Rinkes IH, van Hillegersberg R. International survey on esophageal cancer: part I surgical techniques. Dis Esophagus. 2009;22(3):195–202.
5. Hulscher JB, van Sandick JW, de Boer AG, Wijnhoven BP, Tijssen JG, Fockens P, Stalmeier PF, ten Kate FJ, van Dekken H, Obertop H, et al. Extended transthoracic resection compared with limited transhiatal resection for adenocarcinoma of the esophagus. New Engl J Med. 2002;347(21):1662–9.
6. Biere SS, van Berge Henegouwen MI, Maas KW, Bonavina L, Rosman C, Garcia JR, Gisbertz SS, Klinkenbijl JH, Hollmann MW, de Lange ES, et al. Minimally invasive versus open oesophagectomy for patients with oesophageal cancer: a multicentre, open-label, randomised controlled trial. Lancet. 2012;379(9829):1887–92.
7. Yerokun BA, Sun Z, Jeffrey Yang CF, Gulack BC, Speicher PJ, Adam MA, D'Amico TA, Onaitis MW, Harpole DH, Berry MF, et al. Minimally invasive versus open Esophagectomy for esophageal Cancer: a population-based analysis. Ann Thorac Surg. 2016;102(2):416–23.
8. Luketich JD, Pennathur A, Awais O, Levy RM, Keeley S, Shende M, Christie NA, Weksler B, Landreneau RJ, Abbas G, et al. Outcomes after minimally invasive esophagectomy: review of over 1000 patients. Ann Surg. 2012; 256(1):95–103.
9. Zhou C, Zhang L, Wang H, Ma X, Shi B, Chen W, He J, Wang K, Liu P, Ren Y. Superiority of minimally invasive Oesophagectomy in reducing in-hospital mortality of patients with Resectable Oesophageal Cancer: a meta-analysis. PLoS One. 2015;10(7):e0132889.
10. Mamidanna R, Bottle A, Aylin P, Faiz O, Hanna GB. Short-term outcomes following open versus minimally invasive esophagectomy for cancer in England: a population-based national study. Ann Surg. 2012;255(2):197–203.
11. van Hillegersberg R, Boone J, Draaisma WA, Broeders IA, Giezeman MJ, Borel Rinkes IH. First experience with robot-assisted thoracoscopic esophagolymphadenectomy for esophageal cancer. Surg Endosc. 2006; 20(9):1435–9.
12. Kernstine KH, DeArmond DT, Karimi M, Van Natta TL, Campos JH, Yoder MR, Everett JE. The robotic, 2-stage, 3-field esophagolymphadenectomy. J Thorac Cardiovasc Surg. 2004;127(6):1847–9.
13. Ruurda JP, van der Sluis PC, van der Horst S, van Hillegersberg R. Robot-assisted minimally invasive esophagectomy for esophageal cancer: a systematic review. J Surg Oncol. 2015;112(3):257–65.
14. Finley DS, Nguyen NT. Surgical robotics. Curr Surg. 2005;62(2):262–72.
15. Narula VK, Watson WC, Davis SS, Hinshaw K, Needleman BJ, Mikami DJ, Hazey JW, Winston JH, Muscarella P, Rubin M, et al. A computerized analysis of robotic versus laparoscopic task performance. Surg Endosc. 2007;21(12): 2258–61.
16. Chandra V, Nehra D, Parent R, Woo R, Reyes R, Hernandez-Boussard T, Dutta S. A comparison of laparoscopic and robotic assisted suturing performance by experts and novices. Surgery. 2010;147(6):830–9.
17. Kernstine KH, DeArmond DT, Shamoun DM, Campos JH. The first series of completely robotic esophagectomies with three-field lymphadenectomy: initial experience. Surg Endosc. 2007;21(12):2285–92.
18. Puntambekar S, Kenawadekar R, Kumar S, Joshi S, Agarwal G, Reddy S, Mallik J. Robotic transthoracic esophagectomy. BMC Surg. 2015;15:47.
19. Sarkaria IS, Rizk NP, Finley DJ, Bains MS, Adusumilli PS, Huang J, Rusch VW. Combined thoracoscopic and laparoscopic robotic-assisted minimally invasive esophagectomy using a four-arm platform: experience, technique and cautions during early procedure development. Eur J Cardiothorac Surg. 2013;43(5):e107–15.
20. de la Fuente SG, Weber J, Hoffe SE, Shridhar R, Karl R, Meredith KL. Initial experience from a large referral center with robotic-assisted Ivor Lewis esophagogastrectomy for oncologic purposes. Surg Endosc. 2013;27(9): 3339–47.
21. Cerfolio RJ, Wei B, Hawn MT, Minnich DJ. Robotic Esophagectomy for Cancer: early results and lessons learned. Semin Thorac Cardiovasc Surg. 2016;28(1):160–9.
22. Park SY, Kim DJ, Yu WS, Jung HS. Robot-assisted thoracoscopic esophagectomy with extensive mediastinal lymphadenectomy: experience with 114 consecutive patients with intrathoracic esophageal cancer. Dis Esophagus. 2016;29(4):326–32.

Short-term outcomes of robot-assisted minimally invasive esophagectomy for esophageal cancer...

47

23. van der Sluis PC, Ruurda JP, Verhage RJ, van der Horst S, Haverkamp L, Siersema PD, Borel Rinkes IH, Ten Kate FJ, van Hillegersberg R. Oncologic long-term results of robot-assisted minimally invasive Thoraco-laparoscopic Esophagectomy with two-field lymphadenectomy for esophageal Cancer. Ann Surg Oncol. 2015;22(Suppl 3):S1350–6.

24. Weksler B, Sharma P, Moudgill N, Chojnacki KA, Rosato EL. Robot-assisted minimally invasive esophagectomy is equivalent to thoracoscopic minimally invasive esophagectomy. Dis Esophagus. 2012;25(5):403–9.

25. Park S, Hwang Y, Lee HJ, Park IK, Kim YT, Kang CH. Comparison of robot-assisted esophagectomy and thoracoscopic esophagectomy in esophageal squamous cell carcinoma. J Thorac Dis. 2016;8(10):2853–61.

26. Chao YK, Hsieh MJ, Liu YH, Liu HP. Lymph node evaluation in robot-assisted versus video-assisted Thoracoscopic Esophagectomy for esophageal squamous cell carcinoma: a propensity-matched analysis. World J Surg. 2018;42(2):590–8.

27. Deng HY, Huang WX, Li G, Li SX, Luo J, Alai G, Wang Y, Liu LX, Lin YD. Comparison of short-term outcomes between robot-assisted minimally invasive esophagectomy and video-assisted minimally invasive esophagectomy in treating middle thoracic *esophageal* cancer. Dis Esophagus. 2018; https://doi.org/10.1093/dote/doy012.

28. Suda K, Ishida Y, Kawamura Y, Inaba K, Kanaya S, Teramukai S, Satoh S, Uyama I. Robot-assisted thoracoscopic lymphadenectomy along the left recurrent laryngeal nerve for esophageal squamous cell carcinoma in the prone position: technical report and short-term outcomes. World J Surg. 2012;36(7):1608–16.

29. Kim DJ, Park SY, Lee S, Kim HI, Hyung WJ. Feasibility of a robot-assisted thoracoscopic lymphadenectomy along the recurrent laryngeal nerves in radical esophagectomy for esophageal squamous carcinoma. Surg Endosc. 2014;28(6):1866–73.

30. van der Sluis PC, Ruurda JP, van der Horst S, Verhage RJ, Besselink MG, Prins MJ, Haverkamp L, Schippers C, Rinkes IH, Joore HC, et al. Robot-assisted minimally invasive thoraco-laparoscopic esophagectomy versus open transthoracic esophagectomy for resectable esophageal cancer, a randomized controlled trial (ROBOT trial). Trials. 2012;13:230.

8

Near-infrared dye marking for thoracoscopic resection of small-sized pulmonary nodules: comparison of percutaneous and bronchoscopic injection techniques

Takashi Anayama[1]*[iD], Kentaro Hirohashi[1], Ryohei Miyazaki[1], Hironobu Okada[1], Nobutaka Kawamoto[1], Marino Yamamoto[1], Takayuki Sato[2] and Kazumasa Orihashi[1]

Abstract

Background: Minimally invasive video-assisted thoracoscopic surgery for small-sized pulmonary nodules is challenging, and image-guided preoperative localisation is required. Near-infrared indocyanine green fluorescence is capable of deep tissue penetration and can be distinguished regardless of the background colour of the lung; thus, indocyanine green has great potential for use as a near-infrared fluorescent marker in video-assisted thoracoscopic surgery.

Methods: Thirty-seven patients with small-sized pulmonary nodules, who were scheduled to undergo video-assisted thoracoscopic wedge resection, were enrolled in this study. A mixture of diluted indocyanine green and iopamidol was injected into the lung parenchyma as a marker, using either computed tomography-guided percutaneous or bronchoscopic injection techniques. Indications and limitations of the percutaneous and bronchoscopic injection techniques for marking nodules with indocyanine green fluorescence were examined and compared.

Results: In the computed tomography-guided percutaneous injection group ($n = 15$), indocyanine green fluorescence was detected in 15/15 (100%) patients by near-infrared thoracoscopy. A small pneumothorax occurred in 3/15 (20.0%) patients, and subsequent marking was unsuccessful after a pneumothorax occurred. In the bronchoscopic injection group ($n = 22$), indocyanine green fluorescence was detected in 21/22 (95.5%) patients. In 6 patients who underwent injection marking at 2 different lesion sites, 5/6 (83.3%) markers were successfully detected.

Conclusion: Either computed tomography-guided percutaneous or bronchoscopic injection techniques can be used to mark pulmonary nodules with indocyanine green fluorescence. Indocyanine green is a safe and easily detectable fluorescent marker for video-assisted thoracoscopic surgery. Furthermore, the bronchoscopic injection approach enables surgeons to mark multiple lesion areas with less risk of causing a pneumothorax.

Keywords: Indocyanine green fluorescence, Near-infrared spectroscopy, Small-sized pulmonary nodules, Video-assisted thoracoscopic surgery

* Correspondence: anayamat@kochi-u.ac.jp
Meeting presentation: The concept and a portion of data from the pilot study of this clinical trial were presented at the World Conference for Lung Cancer, 2015 (WCLC2015/IASLC) held in Denver, Colorado, U.S.A.
[1]Division of Thoracic Surgery, Department of Surgery II, Kochi Medical School, Kochi University, Kohasu Oko Nankoku Kochi 783-8505, Japan
Full list of author information is available at the end of the article

Background

Lung cancer is the leading cause of death worldwide. Computed tomography (CT) is currently the most effective screening method for detecting lung cancer and reducing lung cancer mortality [1, 2]. Bronchoscopy and percutaneous needle biopsy are performed for pulmonary lesions with a strong suspicion of malignancy based on CT findings. However, in cases where lung lesions are small in size, present in the periphery of the lung, or close to the visceral pleura, thoracoscopic biopsy may be performed [3]. Therefore, there is an increasing need for wedge resection of small-sized pulmonary nodules by means of video-assisted thoracic surgery (VATS) for both the diagnosis and treatment of lung cancer.

Nevertheless, localisation of small-sized pulmonary nodules is challenging. In particular, ground-glass nodule (GGN) lesions do not alter the surface of the visceral pleura, and the elevation of tumours cannot be perceived in the deflated lung during VATS; thus, GGNs are difficult to localise. Small-sized pulmonary nodules are often marked prior to VATS by using a VATS marker such as a hook-thread [4], spiral wire needle [5], microcoil [6], fiducial marker [7], or colour dyes such as methylene blue [8]; each of these is injected into the lung near the target using a CT-guided percutaneous injection approach. Alternatively, barium [9] or lipiodol [10] can be injected with CT guidance, and the labelled nodules can be intraoperatively detected by fluoroscopy. Radiotracer-guided localisation can also be used with gamma-emitting radioisotopes (technetium 99, Tc99m) for localising nodules with CT-guided injection [11, 12]. Gamma-ray emission signals can be detected intraoperatively using a gamma probe.

Bronchoscopic markers are an alternative to VATS markers. With a bronchoscopic approach, multiple markers can be placed in the lung without injuring the visceral pleura or causing a pneumothorax. Various materials, such as methylene blue [13], indigo carmine [14], and fiducial markers [15], as well as methods such as radiofrequency identification (RFID) have been used [16]. Navigation bronchoscopy technology, such as virtual bronchoscopy and electromagnetic navigation bronchoscopy (ENB) [17, 18], are used to guide the tip of the bronchoscope to the target lesion area. We have previously reported the concept of ENB-guided bronchoscopic injection of indocyanine green (ICG) and localisation of infrared ICG-fluorescence (ICG-FL) to localise small-sized pulmonary nodules using a porcine model [19]. In that study, we determined the optimal dose, concentration, and volume of ICG to produce a small ICG-FL spot in the lung parenchyma that could be visualised using a near-infrared (NIR) thoracoscope.

In the current study, we translated this basic research into a clinical investigation of the feasibility and the efficacy of ICG-FL marking to localise small-sized pulmonary nodules in human patients. We compared CT-guided percutaneous marking and bronchoscopic marking to clarify the benefits and detectability of these two techniques.

Methods

Patient enrolment

Thirty-seven patients who were scheduled for VATS wedge resection of a non-solid, partly solid, or solid pulmonary nodule with a maximum nodule diameter < 20 mm located in the peripheral part of the lung, were included in this study. The study period was from January 2013 to December 2014 for CT-guided percutaneous marking, and from January 2015 to December 2016 for bronchoscopic marking.

Ethics, consent, and permissions

Patients provided written informed consent to participate in the study and for individual patient data to be published. This study was approved by the Institutional Review Board of Kochi Medical School, Kochi University.

VATS marking procedures

An ICG/iopamidol mixture was prepared by diluting ICG 100-fold (2.5 mg/ml, 10 ml; Daiichi-Sankyo, Tokyo, Japan) with iopamidol (Lopamiron 370, Bayer, Leverkusen, Germany). A 1 ml syringe was filled with the ICG/iopamidol mixture and connected to either a CT-guided percutaneous needle or a bronchoscopic needle, and the needle lumen was filled with the marking solution prior to the marking procedure.

The CT-guided percutaneous marking procedure was performed as follows (Fig. 1). The patient was placed in either the prone, supine, or lateral position, depending on the location of the lesion. After a preliminary scan, the CT scanner was focused on the area of the pulmonary nodule. After providing local anaesthesia with lidocaine, a 23-gauge needle filled with marking solution was injected near the pulmonary nodule. Fifty microlitres of ICG/iopamidol marking solution was injected under real-time imaging using CT fluoroscopy. CT scans were performed repeatedly for 30 min after the injection to monitor for the occurrence of pneumothorax or air embolism. The total duration of the procedure was within 90 min, including observation time. In consideration of the possibility of late-onset pneumothorax, the marking procedure was performed in the morning, and surgery was performed on the same afternoon.

The bronchoscopic marking procedure was performed as follows (Fig. 2). Virtual bronchoscopy navigation images were generated from the CT DICOM data using the Synapse Vincent (Fuji Film, Tokyo, Japan) volume analyser. Bronchoscopy was performed according to

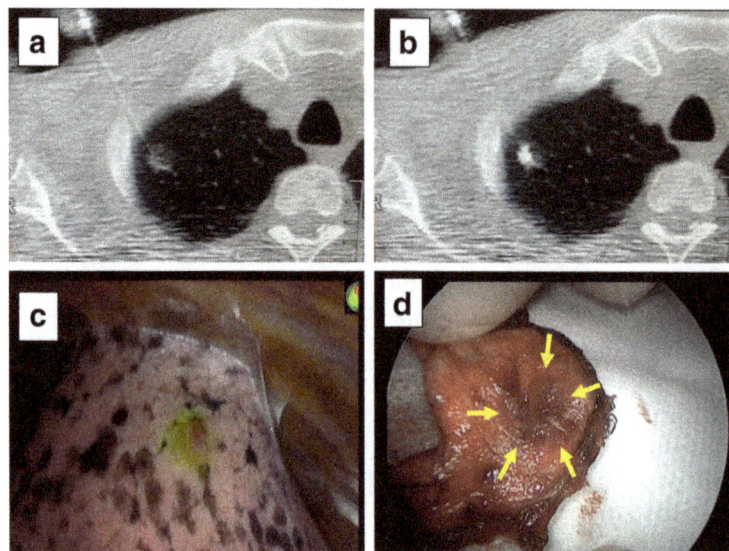

Fig. 1 Computed tomography (CT)-guided percutaneous marking, near-infrared (NIR) fluorescence detection, and wedge resection. **a**: A 23-gauge needle was inserted into the lung near a ground-glass nodule under CT guidance. **b**: A mixture (0.1 ml) of 100-fold diluted indocyanine green and iopamidol was injected into the lung parenchyma. **c**: The indocyanine green fluorescence was detected using NIR thoracoscopy (PINPOINT®, Novadaq). **d**: A resected lung specimen from the surgical field. The target pulmonary nodule is indicated by yellow arrows

conventional procedures. The upper airway (nasal passage, oropharynx, vocal cords, and trachea) was topically anesthetised using aerosolised 2% lidocaine and 1% lidocaine gel. After topical anaesthesia, moderate sedation was induced by administrating 2–3 mg of midazolam intravenously. A thin, flexible bronchoscope (P290, Olympus, Tokyo, Japan) was inserted nasally into the tracheobronchial tree. While viewing the virtual bronchoscopy navigation images, the tip of the bronchoscope was guided to the peripheral bronchus near the target lung tumour. A sheath containing a transbronchial aspiration cytology (TBAC) needle was inserted through the accessory channel of the bronchoscope to the peripheral end of the bronchus immediately below the visceral pleura under X-ray fluoroscopy. The sheath was retracted 3 cm from that position, the TBAC needle was exposed 1 cm from the sheath, and then the sheath and needle were advanced together 1 cm to puncture the lung parenchyma. Fifty microliters of ICG/iopamidol marking solution was injected into the lung parenchyma under X-ray fluoroscopy. The duration of bronchoscopic marking procedures was no more than 30 min. A chest CT image was then acquired and the marking point was confirmed. The surgical procedure was performed one day after the bronchoscopic marking.

Thoracoscopic NIR fluorescence detection and video-assisted thoracoscopic wedge resection

Two- and three-dimensional CT images of the marking point and the pulmonary nodule were prepared prior to surgery in order to clarify the positional relationship between the marker and the tumour (Fig. 3a, b). During thoracoscopic surgery, ICG-FL was visualised using the PINPOINT® endoscopic fluorescence imaging system (Novadaq, Mississauga, Canada) (Fig. 3c). The part of the lung believed to contain the tumour was partially excised using an automatic suturing device. Successful removal was confirmed using rapid pathological diagnosis.

Statistical analysis

Any significant differences among the categorized groups were compared using either the two-sided chi-squared test or Fisher's exact test, and 0.05 was the threshold for statistical significance. All analyses were performed using SPSS version 17.0 (SPSS Inc., Chicago, IL, USA) for Windows (Microsoft Corporation, Redmond, WA, USA).

Results

In total, 37 patients participated in this clinical trial. Percutaneous marking was performed in 15 patients and bronchoscopic marking in 22 patients. There was no difference in the clinical background data between the two patient groups (Table 1). Sub-centimetre nodules were found in 4 patients in the CT-guided percutaneous needle injection group, and in 13 patients in the bronchoscopic injection group. All pulmonary nodules were located at the 1/3 peripheral side of the lung. Each group included one patient with two pulmonary nodules in the ipsilateral side of lung.

In the CT-guided ICG-FL marking group, ICG fluorescence was detected using NIR thoracoscopy in all 15

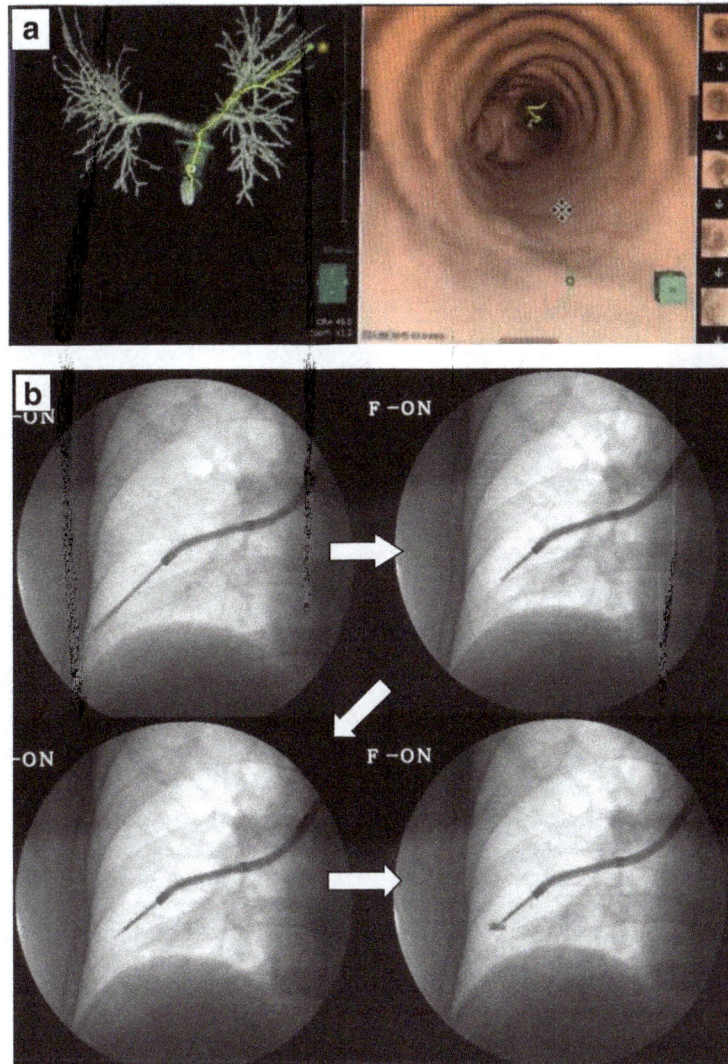

Fig. 2 Virtual bronchoscopy-guided bronchoscopic marking. **a**: Virtual bronchoscopy image created by Synapse Vincent (Fuji Film, Tokyo, Japan) to visualize the best path to reach the target pulmonary nodule. **b**: A thin bronchoscope was inserted into the peripheral bronchus based on the virtual bronchoscopy images. A transbronchial aspiration cytology (TBAC) needle enclosed within an outer sheath was advanced to the peripheral end of the bronchus until the operator could feel resistance. The outer sheath was retracted 3 cm, and 1 cm of the TBAC needle tip was exposed from the outer sheath. The TBAC needle and the outer sheath were advanced 1 cm to penetrate the lung parenchyma through the bronchial wall. The indocyanine green/iopamidol marking dye was injected through the TBAC needle into the lung parenchyma

(100%) patients, who all successfully underwent VATS wedge resection. A small pneumothorax occurred in 3/15 (20.0%) patients, none of whom required chest tube drainage. For one patient, a second marking procedure was attempted but was unsuccessful because the pneumothorax disrupted the lung anatomy and the localisation of the lesion (Fig. 4).

Bronchoscopic ICG-FL marking was successful in 20/22 (90.9%) patients (Table 2). In the 16 patients in whom an ICG-FL marker was placed, ICG-FL was detected by NIR thoracoscopy in 15 (93.8%) patients. In the patient in whom the ICG-FL marker could not be detected by NIR thoracoscopy, the ICG-FL marker was injected at a depth of 28 mm from the visceral pleura. In the 6 patients in whom the ICG-FL marker was placed at two different positions in the lung, both markers were detected in 5 (83.3%) patients (Fig. 5). One marker, which was injected at a depth of 30 mm from the visceral pleura, was not detected in a patient who had two markers placed.

For the 2 patients in whom the ICG marker was not detectable, the access portal was extended by approximately 3 cm and the surgeon was able to localise the pulmonary nodules by palpation. Ultimately, the target pulmonary nodules were successfully resected with a negative surgical margin in all patients.

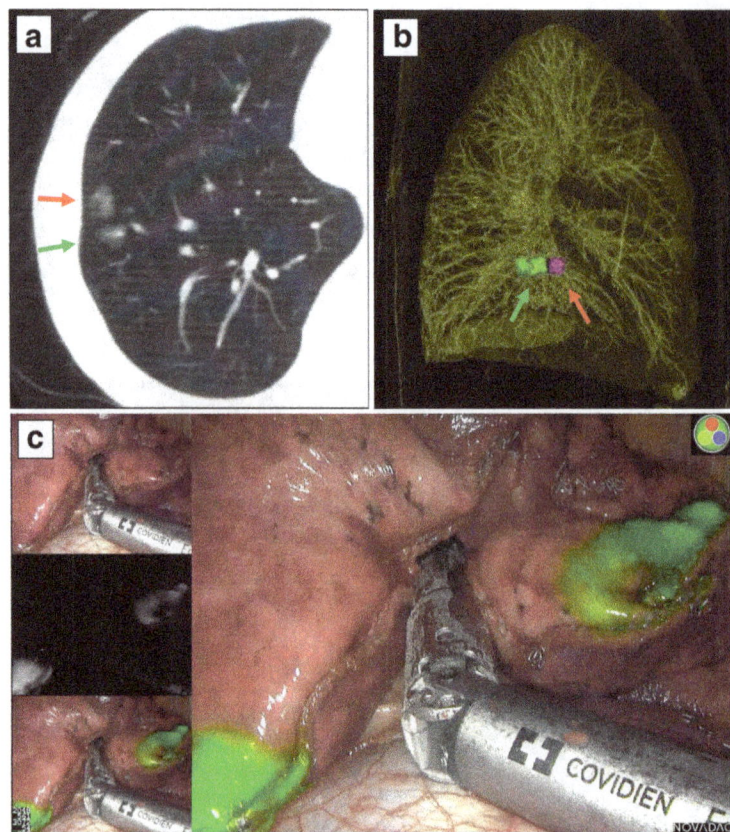

Fig. 3 Near-infrared fluorescence marked VATS wedge resection. **a**: computed tomography (CT) scan was performed after a bronchoscopic marking procedure to confirm the marked position. The indocyanine green (ICG)/iopamidol marking dye (green arrow) was injected into a 3 cm dorsal point of the target nodule (red arrow) in the same axial slice of the CT image. **b**: A three-dimensional CT image was constructed to assess the position of both the target pulmonary nodule (red arrow) and the ICG/iopamidol marker (green arrow) in the right anterior basal segment. **c**: During the surgery, ICG fluorescence was detected by the PINPOINT® (Novadaq) endoscopic fluorescence imaging system, and the pulmonary nodule was excised by cutting between the ICG-fluorescence marker and the anterior edge of the basal segment. PINPOINT® visualises white light images without infrared (on the left top), infrared signal only (on the left middle), and a hybrid mode with both the infrared signal and the white light image together (on the bottom left and right)

Other than a small pneumothorax in 3 patients, no complications were observed throughout the study period.

Discussion

Marking of a pulmonary mass using ICG-FL was confirmed to be a safe and reliable procedure using both percutaneous and bronchoscopic injection techniques. One of the advantages of NIR fluorescence marking is that NIR fluorescence can be detected using spectroscopy, regardless of the background colour of the lung; this can be especially valuable in patients with a smoking history whose lungs have black deposits. Another advantage of NIR fluorescence is its good tissue transparency properties [20–22]. As we previously demonstrated in an animal study, NIR dye is not necessarily present on the surface of the lung, but the NIR fluorescence of a marker injected into the lung at a depth of 20 mm can be detected by NIR thoracoscopy [19]. In the current

study, we injected a small amount of NIR marker (50 μl) into an area close to the tumour based on imaging studies and showed that it could be detected using NIR fluorescence thoracoscopy. Because the volume of ICG/iopamidol marker was as small as 50 μl, and it was injected near the tumour rather than within the tumour, the risk for spreading tumour cells was minimized.

Both percutaneous marking and bronchoscopic marking have benefits. Since percutaneous marking is not dependent on bronchial branching, it can easily be performed by interventional radiologists, using the same technique as CT-guided biopsy. The success rate of a single marking using the CT-guided percutaneous approach was 15/15 (100%). However, CT-guided percutaneous injection can injure the visceral pleura, potentially causing a pneumothorax. In the current study, the authors used a small-sized (23-gauge) needle to minimise damage to the visceral pleura. In our study, only 3/15 (20%) patients who underwent CT-guided percutaneous ICG-FL marking developed a pneumothorax,

Table 1 Patient characteristics

		CT-guided percutaneous needle injection group	Bronchoscopic injection group	p Value
Study period		Jan 2013 - Dec 2014	Jan 2015 - Dec 2016	
Patients (n)		15	22	
Age, years		61.5 ± 12.6	64.4 ± 10.0	N.S.
Sex	Male	10	13	N.S.
	Female	5	9	
Tumour	size (mm) size range (mm)	10 ± 3.4 (4.0–17.1)	9.2 ± 3.6 (3.5–16.0)	N.S.
	GGN (n) Solid (n)	12 4	10 13	
	Depth from visceral pleura	9.9 ± 7.7	9.8 ± 8.1	N.S.
	Localization			
	Right superior lobe (S1, S2, S3)	7 (1, 4, 2)	6 (4, 1, 1)	
	Right middle lobe (S4, S5) Right inferior lobe (S6, S7, S8, S9, S10) Left superior lobe (S1 + 2, S3, S4, S5) Left inferior lobe (S6, S8, S9, S10)	1 (0, 1) 4 (0, 0, 1, 2, 1) 3 (2, 1, 0, 0) 1 (0, 0, 1, 0)	1 (1, 0) 8 (0, 1, 2, 3, 2) 4 (3, 0, 1, 0) 4 (0, 1, 2, 1)	

Data presented as median ± standard deviation; GGN: ground-glass nodule; Jan: January; Dec: December; S1: apical segment; S2: posterior segment; S3: anterior segment; right S4: lateral segment; right S5: medial segment; S6: superior segment; right S7: medial-basal segment; right S8: anterior-basal segment; S9: lateral segment; S10: posterior-basal segment; S1 + 2: apico-posterior segment; left S4: superior lingular segment; left S5: inferior lingular segment; left S8: anteriomedial basal segment; N.S.: not significant

none of whom required chest tube drainage. However, these small pneumothoraces prevented repeated VATS marking procedures. Thus, the CT-guided percutaneous approach is not suitable for marking multiple lung regions.

Bronchoscopic marking enables the injection of ICG-FL markers into multiple lung sections without injuring the visceral pleura. In addition, the bronchoscopic approach can access regions of the lung that are difficult to reach using a percutaneous approach, such as the mediastinal side and the craniodorsal part that is obscured by the scapula. By referring to guidelines on lung biopsy, the bronchoscopic approach is chosen in preference to the percutaneous approach when accessible by bronchoscopy [23].

The success rate of the bronchoscopic approach was 20/22 (91.0%), which was lower than that of the CT-guided percutaneous approach. Furthermore, the

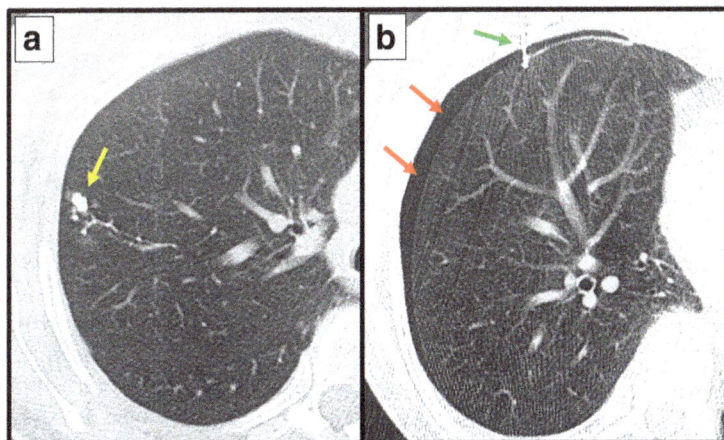

Fig. 4 Limitations of the percutaneous needle dye injection approach. **a**: indocyanine green/iopamidol marking dye was injected percutaneously (yellow arrow). **b**: A pneumothorax (red arrow) developed after the first injection, after which the lung was not stably fixed, even when breathing was stopped during the second attempt at percutaneous injection (green arrow)

Table 2 The success rates and complications of VATS marking

No. of markers	CT-guided percutaneous needle injection	Bronchoscopic injection
No. of patients	15	22
Single marking	14/14 (100%)	15/16 (86.0%)
Double marking	0/1 (0%)	5/6 (83.3%)
Complication		
Pneumothorax	3/15 (20%)	0/22 (0%)
Other	0 (0%)	0 (0%)

VATS video-assisted thoracic surgery

accuracy of virtual bronchoscopy navigation combined with X-ray fluoroscopy guidance was not as accurate as CT-guidance. In fact, we experienced two failed marking procedures. One case was a GGN located in the right apical segment, to which the ICG-iopamidol marker was injected into an area of lung deeper than 20 mm from the visceral pleura. In this case, only posterior-anterior projection X-ray fluoroscopy was used for image-guidance. Lateral projection X-ray fluoroscopy may have increased bronchoscopic marking accuracy. The other case involved GGNs located in the right medial basal segment. Because the segment overlapped with the cardiac shadow, it was technically difficult to inject ICG-iopamidol marker at the

correct point. In such a case, CT fluoroscopy is useful for confirming the position of the bronchoscopic needle. Additionally, electromagnetic navigation bronchoscopy may be more accurate than virtual bronchoscopy navigation, and should be evaluated in further studies.

In terms of cost, the CT-guided percutaneous approach involves only the expense of using the CT scanner unless complications, such as severe pneumothorax, occur. On the other hand, the bronchoscopic approach involves the costs of both the bronchoscopy and the CT imaging after the marking procedure.

When the target pulmonary nodule was not located near the bronchial tree, the VATS marker was injected in the vicinity of the pulmonary nodule. It was easy to determine the location of the nodule from the positional relationship between the marker and the tumour. Unlike metal markers, liquid markers do not necessarily have to be removed with the pulmonary nodules because they are absorbed by the body. The currently available devices, such as PINPOINT® and D-light P, have almost equivalent capabilities for detecting ICG NIR fluorescence, and either of these devices can be used for the method described in this study [19].

The use of ICG-FL as a thoracoscopic marker does have some disadvantages. In cases of severe pulmonary emphysema, there is concern that liquid markers do not form a distinct spot but rather diffuse into pulmonary cysts; therefore, ICG may not be ideal in such cases. Moreover, the equipment required to thoracoscopically visualise ICG-FL is expensive and is available only in a limited number of institutions.

Conclusions

ICG-FL is a VATS marker with good detectability and is capable of deep tissue penetration; ICG-FL can also be distinguished regardless of the tissue background colour. Pulmonary nodules can be marked with ICG-FL using either a CT-guided percutaneous or a bronchoscopic injection technique. Using the bronchoscopic approach, multiple VATS markers can be placed without causing a pneumothorax. ICG-FL using the bronchoscopic injection technique can be especially useful for marking multiple small-sized pulmonary nodules for minimally invasive resection.

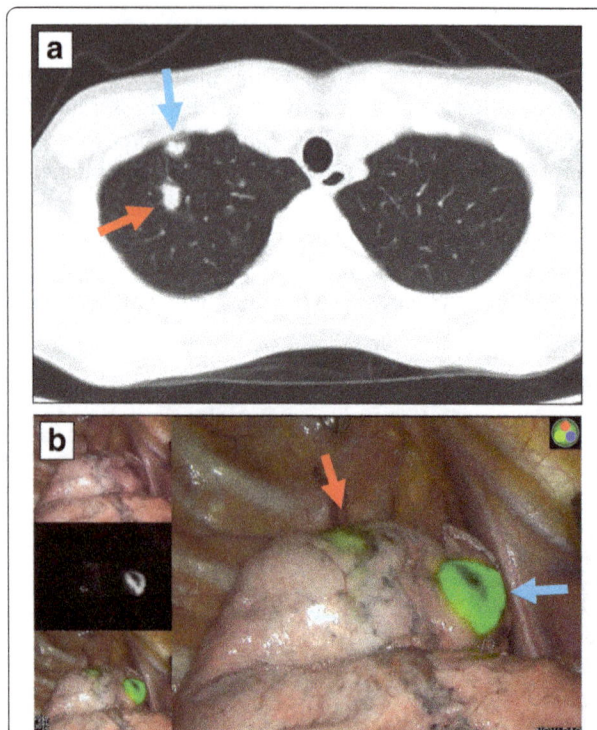

Fig. 5 CT (**a**) and near-infrared thoracoscopic (**b**) findings of a case with multiple bronchoscopic indocyanine green fluorescence markings. Two indocyanine green fluorescence markers were injected in both the median (red arrow) and anterior part (blue arrow) of the right apical segment. Both markers were visualised using a near-infrared thoracoscope

Abbreviations
CT: Computed tomography; ENB: Electromagnetic navigation bronchoscope; GGN: Ground-glass nodule; ICG: Indocyanine green; ICG-FL: Indocyanine green fluorescence; NIR: Near-infrared; TBAC: Transbronchial aspiration cytology; VATS: Video-assisted thoracic surgery

Acknowledgements
Not applicable.

Funding
This work was supported by JSPS KAKENHI Grant Number JP 15 K01294.

Authors' contributions
TA conceived and designed the study. TA, KH, HO, NK, and MY performed all bronchoscopic examinations and surgical procedures. TS advised on the settings for ICG-FL visualisation. TA analysed and interpreted the patient data and was a major contributor in writing the manuscript. OK supervised the entire study. All authors read and approved the final manuscript.

Competing interests
The authors declare that they have no competing interests.

Author details
[1]Division of Thoracic Surgery, Department of Surgery II, Kochi Medical School, Kochi University, Kohasu Oko Nankoku Kochi 783-8505, Japan. [2]Department of Circulation Control, Kochi Medical School, Kochi University, Kohasu Oko Nankoku Kochi 783-8505, Japan.

References
1. Aberle DR, Berg CD, Black WC, Church TR, Fagerstrom RM, Galen B, et al. The National Lung Screening Trial: overview and study design. Radiology. 2011;258:243–53.
2. Moyer VA. Screening for lung cancer U.S. preventive services task force recommendation statement. Ann Intern Med. 2014;160:330–8.
3. Hazelrigg SR, Nunchuck SK, LoCicero J. Video assisted thoracic surgery study group data. Ann Thorac Surg. 1993;56:1039–43.
4. Gossot D, Miaux Y, Guermazi A, Celerier M, Friga J. The hook-wire technique for localization of pulmonary nodules during thoracoscopic resection. Chest. 1994;105:1467–9.
5. Torre M, Ferraroli GM, Vanzulli A, Fieschi S. A new safe and stable spiral wire needle for thoracoscopic resection of lung nodules. Chest. 2004; 125:2289–93.
6. Lizza N, Eucher P, Haxhe JP, De Wispelaere JF, Johnson PM, Delaunois L. Thoracoscopic resection of pulmonary nodules after computed tomographic-guided coil labeling. Ann Thorac Surg. 2001;71:986–8.
7. Sancheti MS, Lee R, Ahmed SU, Pickens A, Fernandez FG, Small WC, et al. Percutaneous fiducial localization for thoracoscopic wedge resection of small pulmonary nodules. Ann Thorac Surg. 2014;97:1914–8.
8. Lenglinger FX, Schwarz CD, Artmann W. Localization of pulmonary nodules before thoracoscopic surgery: value of percutaneous staining with methylene blue. AJR Am J Roentgenol. 1994;163:297–300.
9. Moon SW, Wang YP, Jo KH, Kwack MS, Kim SW, Kwon OK, et al. Fluoroscopy-aided thoracoscopic resection of pulmonary nodule localized with contrast media. Ann Thorac Surg. 1999;68:1815–20.
10. Watanabe K, Nomori H, Ohtsuka T, Kaji M, Naruke T, Suemasu K. Usefulness and complications of computed tomography-guided lipiodol marking for fluoroscopy-assisted thoracoscopic resection of small pulmonary nodules: experience with 174 nodules. J Thorac Cardiovasc Surg. 2006;132:320–4.
11. Chella A, Lucchi M, Ambrogi MC, Menconi G, Melfi FM, Gonfiotti A, et al. A pilot study of the role of TC-99 radionuclide in localization of pulmonary nodular lesions for thoracoscopic resection. Eur J Cardiothorac Surg. 2000; 18:17–21.
12. Galetta D, Bellomi M, Grana C, Spaggiari L. Radio-guided localization and resection of small or ill-defined pulmonary lesions. Ann Thorac Surg. 2015; 100:1175–80.
13. Bolton WD, Howe H, Stephenson JE. The utility of electromagnetic navigational bronchoscopy as a localization tool for robotic resection of small pulmonary nodules. Ann Thorac Surg. 2014;98:471–5.
14. Sato M, Omasa M, Chen F, Sato T, Sonobe M, Bando T, et al. Use of virtual assisted lung mapping (VAL-MAP), a bronchoscopic multispot dye-marking technique using virtual images, for precise navigation of thoracoscopic sublobar lung resection. J Thorac Cardiovasc Surg. 2014;147:1813–9.
15. Anantham D, Feller-Kopman D, Shanmugham LN, Berman SM, MM DC, Gangadharan SP, et al. Electromagnetic navigation bronchoscopy-guided fiducial placement for robotic stereotactic radiosurgery of lung tumors. Chest. 2007;132:930–5.
16. Kojima F, Sato T, Takahata H, Okada M, Sugiura T, Oshiro O, et al. A novel surgical marking system for small peripheral lung nodules based on radio frequency identification technology: feasibility study in a canine model. J Thorac Cardiovasc Surg. 2014;147:1384–9.
17. Gildea TR, Mazzone PJ, Karnak D, Meziane M, Mehta AC. Electromagnetic navigation diagnostic bronchoscopy: a prospective study. Am J Respir Crit Care Med. 2006;174:982–9.
18. Eberhardt R, Anantham D, Herth F, Feller-Kopman D, Ernst A. Electromagnetic navigation diagnostic bronchoscopy in peripheral lung lesions. Chest. 2007;131:1800–5.
19. Anayama T, Qiu J, Chan H, Nakajima T, Weersink R, Daly M, et al. Localization of pulmonary nodules using navigation bronchoscope and a near-infrared fluorescence thoracoscope. Ann Thorac Surg. 2015;99:224–30.
20. Marshall MV, Rasmussen JC, Tan I-C, Aldrich MB, Adams KE, Wang X, et al. Near-infrared fluorescence imaging in humans with indocyanine green: a review and update. Open Surg Oncol J. 2010;2:12–25.
21. Jonak C, Skvara H, Kunstfeld R, Trautinger F, Schmid JA. Intradermal indocyanine green for in vivo fluorescence laser scanning microscopy of human skin: a pilot study. PLoS One. 2011;6:e23972.
22. Alander JT, Kaartinen I, Laakso A, Pätilä T, Spillmann T, Tuchin VV, et al. A review of indocyanine green fluorescent imaging in surgery. Int J Biomed Imaging. 2012. https://doi.org/10.1155/940585.
23. Manhire A, Charig M, Clelland C, Gleeson F, Miller R, Moss H. Guidelines for radiologically guided lung biopsy. Thorax. 2003;58:920–36.

9

The relationship between preoperative psychological evaluation and compensatory sweating

Huai-Yu Wang[1*†] (iD), Yan-Jun Zhu[1†], Jie Liu[1†], Li-Wei Li[2] and Ying-Hui Liu[1]

Abstract

Background: This study analyzes the relationship between preoperative psychological states of primary palmar hyperhidrosis patients and postoperative compensatory sweating.

Methods: We evaluated the psychological states of patients with primary palmar hyperhidrosis who received sympathectomy in our hospital from 2016 to 2017. The relationship between preoperative psychological states and postoperative compensatory sweating were assessed using Spearman's rank-order correlation.

Results: Fifty-five patients who received R4 + R3 bypass transection accepted the preoperative questionnaire survey; 35 were males and 20 were females. The average age was 24.0 ± 6.3 years (range, 14–44 years). Depression symptoms were present in 21.9% (12/55) of the patients; the incidence of anxiety was almost similar, at 23.7% (13/55). Compensatory sweating occurred in 67.3% (37/55) of the patients; of these, 56.4% (31/55) was mild and 10.9% (6/55) was moderate. None of the patients had severe compensatory sweating. There was no significant relationship between the scores of SDS, SAS, and the incidence of postoperative compensatory sweating (P>0.05). However, the psychoticism scale displayed a strong impact on the degree of compensatory sweating (P<0.05). The higher the degree of psychoticism scale, the more serious the degree of compensatory sweating.

Conclusions: The results of this study showed that patients with primary palmar hyperhidrosis are more likely to have mild or moderate mental disorders, and that postoperative compensatory sweating may impact the satisfaction of surgery. In addition, the personality characteristics of patients are related to compensatory sweating.

Keywords: Hyperhidrosis, Sympathectomy, Compensatory sweating, EPQ, Personality characteristic

Background

Primary palmar hyperhidrosis (PPH) refers to a chronic disease in which hands sweat more than normal due to emotional stress. The symptoms of this kind of sweating mainly appear in childhood and adolescence [1], characterized as mild, moderate, or severe. At present, the specific pathogenesis of this disease is still unclear; however, it is mostly believed to be associated with sympathetic nervous system dysfunction caused by certain genetic factors [2]. PPH often causes embarrassment among afflicted patients; some develop serious social

psychological problems, which may affect the quality of life and even lead to lifelong mental disorders [3–5].

One of the most popular treatment of PPH in recent years is endoscopic thoracic sympathectomy [6, 7]. It is used worldwide and has been proven to be safe and effective. However, compensatory sweating (CS) sometimes affects the quality of life postoperatively [8]. Current views are that the incidence of CS varies from 3 to 98%, and seems to be dependent on the height of the sympathetic chain resection. However, clinical evidence has shown that the incidence of CS varies even among patients with the same level of resection [9]. So far, no study has focused on the relationship between preoperative psychological state of the patient and CS.

In this study, we evaluated the degree of depression, anxiety, and personality characteristics of patients with

---

* Correspondence: 444584398@qq.com
†Huai-Yu Wang and Yan-Jun Zhu contributed equally to this work.
¹Thoracic Surgery Department of General Hospital of Air-Force PLA, No.30 Fucheng Road, Haidian District, Beijing PC: 100142, China
Full list of author information is available at the end of the article

severe PPH, and assessed whether these psychological factors have an impact on morbidity and postoperative satisfaction.

Methods

This was a cross-sectional study, which included pediatric and adult patients with severe PPH who received treatment in our hospital from 2016 to 2017. Patients who were unable to complete the questionnaire independently were excluded.

All patients were assessed by the same preoperative psychologist in the same office. Each patient had to complete three copies of questionnaires independently: the Self-Rating Depression Scale (SDS), invented by Zung in 1965 [10]; Self-Rating Anxiety Scale (SAS), invented by Zung in 1971 [11]; and Eysenck Personality Questionnaire (EPQ), invented by Eysenck in 1981 [12]. The EPQ comprises 50 items to be answered in a binary manner ('yes'/'no'). The responses define three independent personality dimensions: (i) E dimension refers to extraversion, characterized by enjoyment of social interactions and in novel activities and a tendency towards impulsive behavior; (ii) N dimension refers to neuroticism, defined by feelings of anxiety, depressed mood, and guilt; and (iii) P dimension refers to psychoticism, defined as cold, impersonal, lacking in sympathy, emotionality, empathy, and insight combined with a tendency of paranoid ideas against oneself. These personality dimensions are complemented by a social desirability scale evaluating the tendency to respond in a manner that is assumed to be viewed favorably by others. Following completion of the questionnaires in an independent and comfortable environment, doctors would receive the feedback which was then sealed; only the researchers can utilize these personal data henceforth.

Thoracoscopic sympathectomy was performed on all patients by the same surgical team with the patient in the Semi-Fowler's position with both arms elevated and supported to 90° under general anesthesia using a single lumen endotracheal tube. The costal pleura on the surface of the sympathetic chain were transected at the level of the fourth rib bed (R4 sympathectomy) with diathermy. In order to amputate the potential bypass nerve fibers, we extended the transection range by approximately 2 cm laterally along the surface of the corresponding rib. Then, the bypass of R3 was also transected with diathermy; however, the sympathetic chain of R3 was preserved. A temporary 10-Fr chest tube was inserted into the pleural cavity through the surgical incision and connected to a water seal system. After re-inflating the lungs, the chest tube was quickly removed and the incision was closed. We routinely conducted the operation on the right side first, in view of the imbalanced innervation of the heart by bilateral

sympathetic nerves. The same procedure was performed on the contralateral site. A postoperative routine chest X-ray was obtained for all patients the following day. Most of the patients were discharged on the same day. Patients underwent follow-up 6 months after operation. The follow-up questionnaire included assessment of improvement after treatment, CS, and quality of life.

The clinical presentation of CS can be classified as mild, moderate, or severe [13]. Mild CS is sweating that occurs in small amounts, and is triggered by ambient heat, psychological stress, or physical exercise. The sweat that forms does not flow, is tolerable, and does not cause embarrassment or the need to change clothes. Moderate CS is sweating that occurs in moderate amounts, with similar triggering factors as mild CS. The sweat coalesces into droplets that flow, although not necessitating a change of clothes. Therefore, the sweating, although uncomfortable, does not embarrass the patient. Severe or intense CS is when sweating occurs in large amounts, with similar triggering factors and mild and moderate CS. The sweat droplets that form flow profusely, requiring a change of clothes one or more times a day.

All descriptive statistics are expressed as the mean ± standard deviation (SD) for continuous variables. Correlations between variables were analyzed using Spearman's rank-order correlation. A p value of < 0.05 was considered to be statistically significant at the 0.05 level. Statistical analyses were performed using the SPSS statistical software version 19.0 (SPSS, Inc., Chicago, IL, USA).

Results

A total of 55 patients accepted the preoperative questionnaire survey; 35 were males and 20 were females. The average age was 24.0 ± 6.3 years (range, 14 – 44 years). The patients' age distribution were as follows: 56.4% (31/55) between the ages of 20 and 29 years, 9.1% (5/55) between 30 and 39 years, 29.1% (16/55) between 10 to 19 years, and 5.4% (3/55) over the age of 40 years (Table 1).

Depression symptoms were present in 21.9% (12/55) of PPH patients; the incidence of anxiety was almost similar, at 23.7% (13/55). Almost 40% (22/55) of the patients had at least one mental disorder; 5.4% (3/55) had two. Fortunately, none exhibited severe depression or anxiety; however, the incidence of moderate and mild depression was 5.5% (3/55) and 16.4% (9/55), respectively. The prevalence of moderate and mild anxiety was 5.5% (3/55) and 18.2% (10/55), respectively (Table 2).

No patients had postoperative pneumothorax, hemothorax, Horner's syndrome, and recurrence of palmar hyperhidrosis. CS occurred in 67.3% (37/55) of the patients; of these, 56.4% (31/55) was mild and 10.9% (6/55) was moderate. None of the patients had severe CS.

Table 1 Characteristics of patients with PPH and follow-up results after surgery

Variable	n	(%)
Age groups (years)		
10-19	16	(29.1)
20-29	31	(56.4)
30-39	5	(9.1)
Over 40	3	(5.4)
Gender		
Male	35	(63.6)
Female	20	(36.4)
CS		
Severe	0	0
Moderate	6	(10.9)
Mild	31	(56.4)
CS affected area		
Back	30	(54.5)
Prothorax	20	(36.4)
Thigh	7	(12.7)
Shank	3	(5.5)
Hip	4	(7.3)
Craniofacial	2	(3.6)
Axillary	1	(1.8)

CS compensating sweating; PPH primary palmar hyperhidrosis

The regions involved in CS were the back in 54.5% (30/55), protothorax 36.4%(20/55), thigh 12.7% (7/55), shank 5.5% (3/55), hip 7.3% (4/55), head 3.6% (2/55), and axillary 1.8% (1/55). Of the 55 patients, 43.6% (24/55) had CS in more than two regions. The degree of CS was significantly dependent on the satisfaction of the patients ($P<0.05$).

There was no significant relationship between the scores of SDS, SAS, and the incidence of postoperative CS ($P>0.05$) (Tables 3 and 4). However, there was something peculiar with regards to the EPQ scales. Although the E and N scale had no impact on the degree of CS

Table 2 Prevalence for depression and anxiety levels in PPH patients

Variable	n	(%)
Depression		
Severe	0	0
Moderate	3	(5.5)
Mild	9	(16.4)
Anxiety		
Severe	0	0
Moderate	3	(5.5)
Mild	10	(18.2)

PPH primary palmar hyperhidrosis

Table 3 Relationship between CS and SDS scale

CS state	SDS			P value
	Mild	Moderate	Severe	
None	14	4	0	0.943
Mild	24	4	3	
Moderate	5	1	0	

CS compensatory sweating; SDS Self-Rating Depression Scale

($P>0.05$) (Tables 5 and 6), the P scale displayed a strong impact on the degree of CS (P<0.05), the higher the degree of P scale, the more serious the degree of CS (Table 7).

Discussion

In this study, we found that the incidence of PPH had nothing to do with gender. Patients under 20-29 years old preferred to go to a doctor; this finding was consistent with the results of the studies by Fenilli, Kauffman, and Wolosker [14–16].

Endoscopic thoracic sympathectomy is currently one of the most common treatment for PPH. In this study, the cure rate of PPH was 100%. No patient complained of relapse.

While CS is a common postoperative complication among patients with PPH, its etiology is still unclear. The location in which CS occurs is also not fixed; in this study, the site of CS occurrence was widely varied, including the back (54.5%), protothorax (36.4%), thigh (12.7%), shank (5.5%), hip (7.3%), head (3.6%), and axilla (1.8%). Of the 55 patients, 43.6% had CS in more than 2 regions.

Approximately 21.9% of the patients in this study had combined mild or moderate depression, compared to the worldwide incidence of depression, which is approximately 16% [17]. According to a study in Brazil, the incidence of depression in patients with chronic disease was 15-61% [18]. In this study, 23.7% of the patients had preoperatively combined mild and moderate anxiety. In the general population, the incidence of anxiety is approximately 16%; however, when combined with other chronic diseases, the incidence of anxiety increased to 18-35% [19, 20]. The incidence of depression and anxiety among patients with PPH was slightly higher than the general population, although with a lower degree. In

Table 4 Relationship between CS and SAS scale

CS state	SAS			P value
	Mild	Moderate	Severe	
None	13	4	1	0.567
Mild	24	5	2	
Moderate	5	1	0	

CS compensatory sweating; SAS Self-Rating Anxiety Scale

Table 5 Relationship between CS and E scale of EPQ

CS state	E scale of EPQ			P value
	Mild	Moderate	Severe	
None	0	12	6	0.263
Mild	3	21	7	
Moderate	0	5	1	

CS compensatory sweating; *EPQ* Eysenck Personality Questionnaire

Table 7 Relation between CS and P scale of EPQ

CS state	P scale of EPQ			P value
	Mild	Moderate	Severe	
None	11	6	1	< 0.05*
Mild	1	29	1	
Moderate	0	2	4	

CS compensatory sweating; *EPQ* Eysenck Personality Questionnaire

terms of CS, gender did not affect the incidence of depression and anxiety. Preoperative depression and anxiety did not affect the incidence of postoperative CS.

The EPQ score for PPH patients, especially the P dimension, had a certain relation with postoperative CS. While the E, and N scale scores had no obvious relation with the postoperative CS, the P scale score showed an obvious relation; the higher the P scale score, the more severe the postoperative CS. The P scale refers to psychoticism, defined as cold, impersonal, lacking in sympathy, emotionality, empathy, and insight combined with a tendency of paranoid ideas against oneself.

To some extent, there are many subjective factors in the evaluation of sweating. At present, we have not identified the etiology of CS; therefore, we could not exclude the fact that patients may have exaggerated their CS during evaluation. Compared with the SDS and SAS scales, the EPQ scale evaluates the personality characteristics of patients; these indicators can reflect the personality of patients in a more stable way. The state of depression and anxiety may be caused by the symptoms of the disease. Operations are usually associated with a quick and obvious effect, while the state of depression and anxiety may improve compared with the preoperative state. However, we should be aware that neither SDS nor SAS can represent the patients' persistent mental state. However, personality traits are gradually formed as a person ages, and thus cannot be altered by an operation. Therefore, the EPQ scale is able to reflect personality traits' effect on sweating more accurately. Personality traits are gradually formed as a person ages, and thus cannot be altered by an operation. Therefore, the EPQ scale is able to reflect personality traits' effect on sweating more accurately. So we suggest that all patients with PPH should take psychological states evaluation preoperatively. And predominant high level P scale may

be considered as a relative contraindication for endoscopic thoracic sympathectomy. For these patients, we should recommend medication therapy, such as oxybutynin as first line of treatment [16].

Conclusions

The results of this study showed that patients with PPH are more likely to have mild or moderate mental disorder, and that postoperative CS may impact the satisfaction of surgery. In addition, the personality characteristics of patients are related to CS. All patients with PPH should take psychological states evaluation preoperatively. And certain psychic characteristics may be considered as a relative contraindication for surgery.

Abbreviations
CS: Compensatory sweating; EPQ: Eysenck Personality Questionnaire; PPH: Primary palmar hyperhidrosis; SAS: Self-Rating Anxiety Scale; SDS: Self-Rating Depression Scale

Acknowledgements
We would like to thank Editage [www.editage.cn] for English language editing.

Authors' contributions
WHY, LJ and ZYJ conceived of the study and contributed to revision and final approval of the manuscript. WHY and ZYJ also performed all surgical procedure. LJ and LYH contributed to data collection. WHY, ZYJ and LLW participated in background literature review and drafting. All authors contributed to proofreading of the manuscript. All authors read and approved the final manuscript.

Competing interests
The authors declare that they have no competing interests.

Table 6 Relationship between CS and N scale of EPQ

CS state	N scale of EPQ			P value
	Mild	Moderate	Severe	
None	1	14	3	0.659
Mild	2	21	8	
Moderate	0	5	1	

CS compensatory sweating; *EPQ* Eysenck Personality Questionnaire

Author details
[1]Thoracic Surgery Department of General Hospital of Air-Force PLA, No.30 Fucheng Road, Haidian District, Beijing PC: 100142, China. [2]Nuclear Medicine Department of General Hospital of Air-Force PLA, No.30 Fucheng Road,Haidian District, Beijing 100142, China.

References

1. Benson RA, et al. Diagnosis and management of hyperhidrosis. BMJ. 2013; 347:f6800.

2. Shih CJ, Wu JJ, Lin MT. Autonomic dysfunction in palmar hyperhidrosis. J Auton Nerv Syst. 1983;8(1):33–43.

3. Strutton DR, et al. US prevalence of hyperhidrosis and impact on individuals with axillary hyperhidrosis: results from a national survey. J Am Acad Dermatol. 2004;51(2):241–8.

4. Eisenach JH, Atkinson JL, Fealey RD. Hyperhidrosis: evolving therapies for a well-established phenomenon. Mayo Clin Proc. 2005;80(5):657–66.

5. Lee HH, et al. Efficacy of glycopyrrolate in primary hyperhidrosis patients. Korean J Pain. 2012;25(1):28–32.

6. Chen YB, et al. Uniportal versus biportal video-assisted thoracoscopic sympathectomy for palmar hyperhidrosis. Chin Med J. 2009;122(13):1525–8.

7. Georghiou GP, et al. Minimally invasive thoracoscopic sympathectomy for palmar hyperhidrosis via a transaxillary single-port approach. Interact Cardiovasc Thorac Surg. 2004;3(3):437–41.

8. Cerfolio RJ, et al. The Society of Thoracic Surgeons expert consensus for the surgical treatment of hyperhidrosis. Ann Thorac Surg. 2011;91(5):1642–8.

9. Li X, et al. Epidemiological survey of primary palmar hyperhidrosis in adolescents. Chin Med J. 2007;120(24):2215–7.

10. Zung WW. A self-rating depression scale. Arch Gen Psychiatry. 1965;12:63–70.

11. Zung WW. A rating instrument for anxiety disorders. Psychosomatics. 1971; 12(6):371–9.

12. Eysenck HJ. Personality and psychosomatic diseases. Act Nerv Super (Praha). 1981;23(2):112–29.

13. Liu Y, Yang J, Liu J, et al. Surgical treatment of primary palmar hyperhidrosis: a prospective randomized study comparing T3 and T4 sympathicotomy. Eur J Cardiothorac Surg. 2009;35:398–402.

14. Felini R, et al. Prevalence of hyperhidrosis in the adult population of Blumenau-SC, Brazil. An Bras Dermatol. 2009;84(4):361–6.

15. Kauffman P, Campos JR. Video-assisted thoracic sympathectomy for the treatment of axillary hyperhidrosis. J Bras Pneumol. 2011;37(1):4–5.

16. Wolosker N, et al. The use of oxybutynin for treating axillary hyperhidrosis. Ann Vasc Surg. 2011;25(8):1057–62.

17. Kessler RC, et al. Age differences in the prevalence and co-morbidity of DSM-IV major depressive episodes: results from the WHO world mental health survey initiative. Depress Anxiety. 2010;27(4):351–64.

18. Kessler RC, et al. The epidemiology of major depressive disorder: results from the National Comorbidity Survey Replication (NCS-R). JAMA. 2003; 289(23):3095–105.

19. Telles-Correia D, Barbosa A. Anxiety and depression in medicine: models and measurement. Acta Medica Port. 2009;22(1):89–98.

20. Somers JM, et al. Prevalence and incidence studies of anxiety disorders: a systematic review of the literature. Can J Psychiatr. 2006;51(2):100–13.

10

Total arterial revascularization in patients with acute myocardial infarction–feasibility and outcomes

Philippe Grieshaber[1]*⬤, Lukas Oster[2], Tobias Schneider[1], Victoria Johnson[3], Coskun Orhan[1], Peter Roth[1], Bernd Niemann[1] and Andreas Böning[1]

Abstract

Background: In acute situations such as acute myocardial infarction (AMI) with indication for coronary artery bypass grafting (CABG), total arterial revascularization (TAR) is often rejected in favour of saphenous vein (SV) grafting, which is assumed to allow for quicker vessel harvesting, a simpler anastomosis technique, and thus quicker revascularization and fewer bleeding complications. The aim of this study was to evaluate whether reluctance to apply TAR in AMI is still justified from a technical point of view in the current era and whether superiority of TAR results is also evident in emergency patients with AMI undergoing CABG.

Methods: In this retrospective analysis of 434 consecutive patients undergoing CABG for AMI with either TAR or with a combination of one internal mammary artery and SV grafts between 2008 and 2014, procedural data, short-term and mid-term outcome were compared. Propensity score matching of the groups was performed.

Results: After propensity score matching, 250 patients were included in the analysis (TAR group: $n = 98$; SV group $n = 152$). The procedural time (TAR group: 211 min vs. SV group: 200 min, $p = 0.46$) did not differ between the groups. Erythrocyte transfusion rates were higher in the SV group (76% vs. 57%; $p < 0.001$). Rates of re-exploration for bleeding did not differ. Thirty-day mortality rates were comparable (TAR group: 3.4% vs. SV group: 4.5%, $p = 0.68$). Kaplan-Meier analysis until 7 years postoperatively revealed a tendency for improved survival after TAR (75% vs. 62%; log-rank $p = 0.12$).

Conclusion: TAR neither impairs rapid revascularization nor reduces its safety in patients with AMI. It may result in improved long-term outcome and should be preferred in the clinical setting of AMI.

Keywords: Acute myocardial infarction, Coronary artery disease, Coronary artery bypass grafting surgery, Revascularization, Total arterial revascularization

Background

The use of arterial grafts for coronary artery bypass grafting surgery (CABG), particularly bilateral internal mammary arteries (BIMA), is recommended due to the superior patency of these grafts compared with saphenous vein grafts (SV grafts) [1]. In real-world practice, however, the utilization of total arterial revascularization (TAR) lags behind these recommendations [2–5]. Reasons for reluctance to conduct total arterial CABG even in stable patients include the increased technical demand, the increased operation time, and fear of bleeding complications and impaired wound healing [6–8]. In patients undergoing CABG for acute myocardial infarction (AMI), large-scale data on TAR rates is limited, and rates ranging from 2 to 58% have been described [9, 10]. In the unstable situation of AMI, the above-mentioned arguments against total arterial CABG might play an even more important role for decision-making, as patients with AMI undergoing urgent or emergent surgery would be expected to benefit from short operation times and rapid revascularization afforded by use of venous grafting. Furthermore, AMI patients are frequently administered dual antiplatelet therapy (DAPT) preoperatively, resulting in increased risk of bleeding complications [11–13].

* Correspondence: Philippe.grieshaber@chiru.med.uni-giessen.de
[1]Department of Adult and Pediatric Cardiovascular Surgery, University Hospital Giessen, Rudolf-Buchheim-Str. 7, DE-35392 Giessen, Germany
Full list of author information is available at the end of the article

It is currently unclear whether these concerns about the use of TAR in patients with AMI are valid in the current era of surgical myocardial revascularization. Furthermore, the possible effect of total arterial CABG on long-term outcome in AMI patients has never been explicitly investigated.

Methods

Study population

We conducted a retrospective, single-centre study comparing patients undergoing total arterial CABG (total arterial revascularization group [TAR group]) or CABG with a combination of one internal mammary artery (IMA) and saphenous vein grafts (saphenous vein graft group [SV group]). Adult patients with a diagnosis of AMI (non-ST-segment elevation myocardial infarction [NSTEMI] or ST-segment-elevation myocardial infarction [STEMI]) within a period of 5 days or less before CABG without concomitant procedures (e.g. valve surgery) between 01/2008 and 12/2014 were included in the analysis. Patients with low cardiac output syndrome (LCOS) or cardiogenic shock at the time of surgery were excluded. The local ethics committee approved the study.

Data collection, follow-up, definitions

Patients were identified according to the inclusion criteria from institutional patient records, and their baseline characteristics and perioperative data from the patient records and from data transferred to the nationwide quality assurance system (BQS Institute for Quality and Patient Safety, Hamburg, Germany) were analysed. Long-term follow-up was conducted via telephone interviews with the patients or their family physicians.

AMI was defined according to the Third Universal Definition of AMI [14]. The time of AMI was defined as the time of symptom onset. 'Complete revascularization' was defined using the concept of anatomical complete numeric revascularization' (bypassing of all vessels ≥1 mm with hemodynamically relevant stenosis, as assessed by coronary angiography) [15]. We quantified the surgeon's experience according to the years in practice since board certification as cardiac surgeon.

Endpoints

We compared intraoperative parameters (duration of surgery, completeness of revascularization), perioperative need for invasive ventilation, perioperative transfusion requirements and bleeding complications, acute kidney injury as defined by KDIGO (Kidney disease: improving global outcomes) [16], sternal wound impairment requiring surgical therapy, postoperative duration of intensive care unit stay and hospitalization, as well as short- and mid-term survival between the groups.

Management strategy

Patients who underwent cardiac catheterization for AMI are referred to our unit immediately after completion of the angiographic diagnosis and the heart team-based decision for CABG. The timing of surgery is determined by the surgeon on duty. CABG with the goal of complete revascularization is routinely performed on-pump with cardioplegic arrest using cold-blood cardioplegia (Buckberg) [17]. Acetylsalicylic acid is started 6 h postoperatively and continued lifelong at 100 mg/day. $P2Y_{12}$ inhibitors are started on the first postoperative day and are continued for 12 months.

Statistics

An inferential statistical analysis was performed using SPSS Version 24 (IBM, Armonk, NY, USA), GraphPad Prism version 6 software (GraphPad Software, Inc., La Jolla, CA, USA), and R version 3.1.2. Patient characteristics and outcomes were compared using Fisher's exact test, Student's t-test, or Wilcoxon-Mann-Whitney test, as appropriate. Continuous variables are presented as mean ± standard deviation (SD) unless stated otherwise.

In order to correct for potential confounding baseline parameters between the TAR group and the SV group, we carried out propensity score matching of the groups. Covariates included in the matching were age, gender, body-mass index, extent of coronary artery disease, preoperative left ventricular ejection fraction, diabetes mellitus (absence thereof, presence without insulin treatment, presence with insulin treatment), and EuroSCORE II. Nearest-neighbour matching in a 1:2 (TAR group vs. SV group) fashion was then performed. The maximum caliper between matched participants was set at 0.2. Long-term survival functions were determined using Kaplan-Meier estimation and compared using the log-rank test.

Results

Baseline data

A total of 434 patients were identified according to the inclusion criteria. Of these, 293 underwent CABG using a combination of one internal mammary artery and saphenous vein grafts, 3 underwent CABG with only vein grafts, and 138 underwent CABG using TAR. Baseline characteristics between the TAR group and the SV group differed significantly, with the TAR group having a lower proportion of female patients (17% vs. 29%; $p = 0.011$), a lower mean age (59 years vs. 71 years; $p < 0.01$), a lower rate of chronic kidney disease and a lower rate of patients with severely reduced left-ventricular ejection fraction (Table 1). Consecutively, the operative risk estimation using EuroSCORE II was lower in the TAR group than in the SV group (3.4% vs. 7.2%; $p < 0.01$) (Table 1). After propensity score matching, 250 patients (TAR group: $n = 98$, SV

Table 1 Baseline characteristics of the unmatched (left) and matched (right) groups

Parameter	Unmatched study population			Matched study population		
	SV group * n = 296	TAR group * n = 138	p-value	SV group * n = 152	TAR group * n = 98	p-value
Female gender	85 (29)	24 (17)	0.011	33 (22)	21 (21)	0.96
Body mass index (kg/m²)	28 ± 4.7	28 ± 4.8	0.31	28 ± 5.0	28 ± 4.9	0.99
Age, years	71 ± 9.2	59 ± 10	< 0.01	66 ± 9.6	63 ± 9.8	0.08
NSTEMI	202 (68)	95 (69)	0.90	105 (69)	70 (71)	0.69
STEMI	94 (32)	43 (31)		47 (31)	28 (29)	
Coronary artery disease						
1 vessel	11 (3.7)	1 (0.7)	< 0.01	9 (5.9)	1 (1.0)	0.12
2 vessel	42 (14)	25 (18)		21 (14)	18 (18)	
3 vessel	243 (82)	112 (82)		122 (80)	79 (81)	
Diabetes mellitus						
Without insulin	81 (27)	26 (19)	0.054	42 (27)	20 (20)	0.19
With insulin	50 (17)	15 (11)		29 (19)	11 (11)	
Chronic kidney disease						
Stage I (GFR > 89 ml/min)	3 (1.0) 120 (41)	0 31 (22.5)	0.034	2 (1.3) 57 (38)	0 29 (30)	0.13
Stage II (GFR 60-89 ml/min)	75 (25)	10 (7.2)		21 (14)	9 (9.2)	
Stage III (GFR 30-59 ml/min)	8 (2.7) 11 (3.7)	1 (0.7) 1 (0.7)		2 (1.3)	1 (1.0) 1 (1.0)	
Stage IV (GFR 15-29 ml/min)	11 (3.7)	0		6 (3.9)	0	
Stage V (GFR < 15 ml/min)			0.046			0.092
Chronic dialysis						
Arterial hypertension	281 (95)	129 (95)	0.35	145 (95)	90 (92)	0.25
Hypercholesterinemia	195 (66)	92 (67)	0.87	101 (66)	67 (68)	0.75
Cerebral arterial occlusive disease	42 (14)	10 (14)	0.24	21 (14)	11 (11)	0.55
Peripheral arterial occlusive disease						
Fontaine I	6 (2.0)	1 (0.7)	0.078	5 (3.2)	1 (1.0)	0.46
Fontaine II	31 (10)	11 (8.0)		17 (11)	10 (10)	
Fontaine III	5 (1.7)	1 (0.7)		1 (0.7)	1 (1.0)	
Fontaine IV	7 (2.4)	1 (0.7)		2 (1.3)	1 (1.0)	
Chronic obstructive pulmonary disease	32 (11)	11 (8.0)	0.36	16 (11)	8 (8.2)	0.54
PCI before CABG	32 (11)	20 (14)	0.72	12 (7.9)	12 (12)	0.36
Preoperative LVEF						
<20%	21 (7.4)	5 (3.7)	0.047	10 (6.9)	4 (4.2)	0.18
20–30%	27 (9.5)	4 (3.0)		8 (5.6)	3 (3.2)	
31–50%	99 (35)	45 (33)		57 (40)	29 (31)	
>50%	137 (48)	81 (60)		69 (48)	59 (62)	
EuroSCORE II	7.2 ± 8.1	3.4 ± 4.6	**< 0.01**	5.3 ± 6.1	4.8 ± 5.3	0.14

Abbreviations: *CABG* coronary artery bypass grafting, *GFR* glomerular filtration rate, *LVEF* left-ventricular ejection fraction, *NSTEMI* non-ST-segment elevation myocardial infarction, *PCI* percutaneous coronary intervention, *SV* saphenous vein grafts, *STEMI* ST-segment-elevation myocardial infarction, *TAR* total arterial revascularization
ªContinuous variables: mean ± SD; categorical variables: n (%)

group: n = 152) remained in the analysis. The differences in baseline characteristics were eliminated (Table 1). All results described in the following refer to the matched groups. All patients received antiplatelet therapy before surgery, and 33% in the TAR group and 34% in the SV group (p = 0.71) were on DAPT at the time of surgery. Otherwise, tirofiban was used for bridging until 4 h before surgery (TAR group: 65% vs. SV group: 60%; p = 0.41).

Intraoperative data

The procedures were conducted at a median of 72 h after symptom onset by eight surgeons with a mean experience of 6.5 ± 4.8 years since board certification. Surgeon experience differed significantly between the groups (TAR group: 7.2 ± 4.8 years vs. SV group: 6.0 ± 4.6 years; $p = 0.042$). In 86% of TAR procedures, BIMA grafting was applied, and 14% of patients received a combination of IMA and radial artery grafts. The total procedural times (TAR group: 211 ± 54 min vs. SV group: 200 ± 52 min; $p = 0.46$) did not differ significantly between the groups. The time on cardiopulmonary bypass (CPB) was significantly shorter in the TAR group (84 ± 36 min vs. 96 ± 43 min; $p = 0.048$) and the duration of cardioplegic arrest was similar in the two groups (TAR group: 57 ± 20 min vs. SV group: 58 ± 21 min; $p = 0.79$); however, the distribution of these phases was different, with a longer time to CPB in the TAR group (89 ± 20 min. vs. 45 ± 31 min.; $p = 0.04$) (Fig. 1). This discrepancy can be explained by procedural differences, as the harvesting of both IMA is performed sequentially, whereas the preparation of one IMA and vein grafts is usually carried out simultaneously. Interestingly, the time from the end of CPB to skin closure was significantly reduced in the TAR group (36 ± 10 min vs. 59 ± 15 min, $p = 0.042$). The number of coronary anastomoses did not differ between the groups, and complete revascularization was achieved in 99% (SV group) and 97% (TAR group; $p = 0.69$), respectively (Table 2).

The surgeon's experience had a significant inverse correlation with the total duration of the procedure (2.9 min per year of experience), cardiopulmonary bypass time (2.3 min per year of experience), and cardioplegic arrest time (1.5 min per year of experience). There were no significant differences in this relationship between TAR and SV groups (Fig. 2).

Perioperative outcomes

Fifty-seven percent of TAR group patients received erythrocyte transfusion compared with 76% of SV group patients ($p = 0.001$). Platelet transfusion occurred in 36% (TAR group) and 37% (SV group; $p = 0.86$), respectively. Fresh frozen plasma was transfused in 22% of TAR group patients and 30% of SV group patients ($p = 0.21$). In those patients who received transfusions, the median amount of transfused erythrocyte units was higher in the SV group compared with the TAR group (2 vs. 1 unit; $p = 0.041$). The amounts of platelet and fresh frozen plasma transfusions were comparable in both groups (Table 3). The rate of re-explorations due to bleeding was slightly lower in the TAR group than in the SV group (3.1% vs. 5.9%; $p = 0.30$) but this was not statistically significant. Interestingly, surgical revisions for sternal wound healing impairment were not significantly increased in the TAR group (4.0%) compared with in the SV group (2.6%; $p = 0.52$). Serum levels of troponin I and creatine kinase-isoform MB (CK-MB) increased postoperatively, which was followed by a decline until postoperative day 4. The biomarker levels of the TAR group were slightly lower than those of the SV group, but this difference was not statistically significant (Fig. 3). Postoperative intermittent atrial fibrillation occurred less frequently in the TAR group than on the SV group (10% vs. 19%, $p = 0.059$). Acute kidney injury occurred similarly in both groups. Duration of invasive ventilation and rates of tracheostomies for long-term ventilation were comparable in both groups. Consecutively, the median durations of postoperative intensive care unit

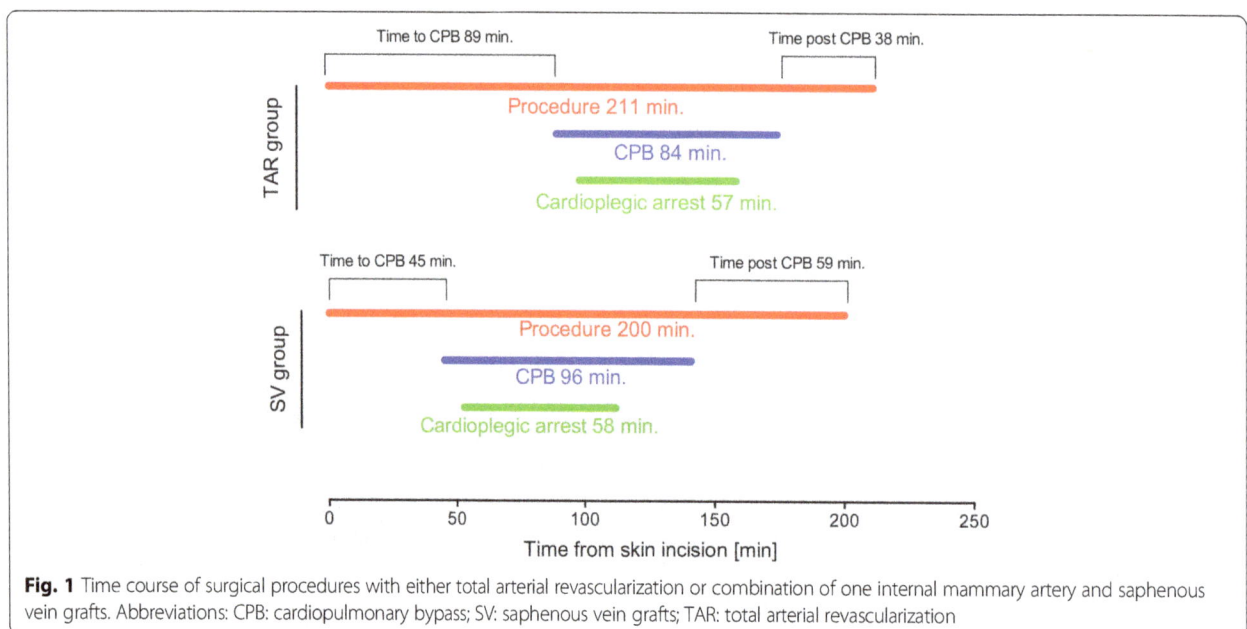

Fig. 1 Time course of surgical procedures with either total arterial revascularization or combination of one internal mammary artery and saphenous vein grafts. Abbreviations: CPB: cardiopulmonary bypass; SV: saphenous vein grafts; TAR: total arterial revascularization

Table 2 Preoperative and intraoperative data

Parameter	SV group * n = 152	TAR group * n = 98	p-value
Antiplatelet therapy			
ASA	137 (93)	86 (91)	0.44
Ticagrelor	9 (6.1)	10 (11)	0.20
Prasugrel	3 (2.0)	3 (3.2)	0.57
Clopidogrel	44 (30)	20 (22)	0.16
DAPT	51 (34)	32 (33)	0.71
Tirofiban	90 (60)	61 (65)	0.41
Vitamin K antagonists	6 (4.1)	1 (1.0)	0.082
Time interval symptom onset to operation (h)**	72 ± 5.1	72 ± 5.3	0.85
Grafts			
LIMA	147 (97)	98 (100)	**< 0.001**
RIMA	2 (1.3)	84 (86)	
Radial artery	0	18 (18)	
Saphenous vein	152 (100)	0	
Coronary anastomoses			
Total	3.8 ± 1.1	3.6 ± 1.0	0.11
Arterial grafts	1.5 ± 0.6	3.6 ± 1.0	**< 0.001**
Venous grafts	2.3 ± 1.0	0	**< 0.001**
Target vessels			
LAD	151 (99)	98 (100)	0.42
RCX	132 (89)	87 (89)	0.59
RCA	116 (76)	80 (82)	0.32
Complete revascularization [n; %]	149 (99)	95 (97)	0.69

Abbreviations: *CABG* coronary artery bypass grafting, *DAPT* dual antiplatelet therapy, *LAD* left anterior descending artery, *LVEF* left ventricular ejection fraction, *NSTEMI* non-ST-segment elevation myocardial infarction, *PCI* percutaneous coronary intervention, *RCA* right coronary artery, *RCX* Ramus circumflexus, *SV* saphenous vein grafts, *STEMI* ST-segment-elevation myocardial infarction, *TAR* total arterial revascularization
[a]Continuous variables: mean ± SD; categorical variables: n (%)
[b]Median ± SD

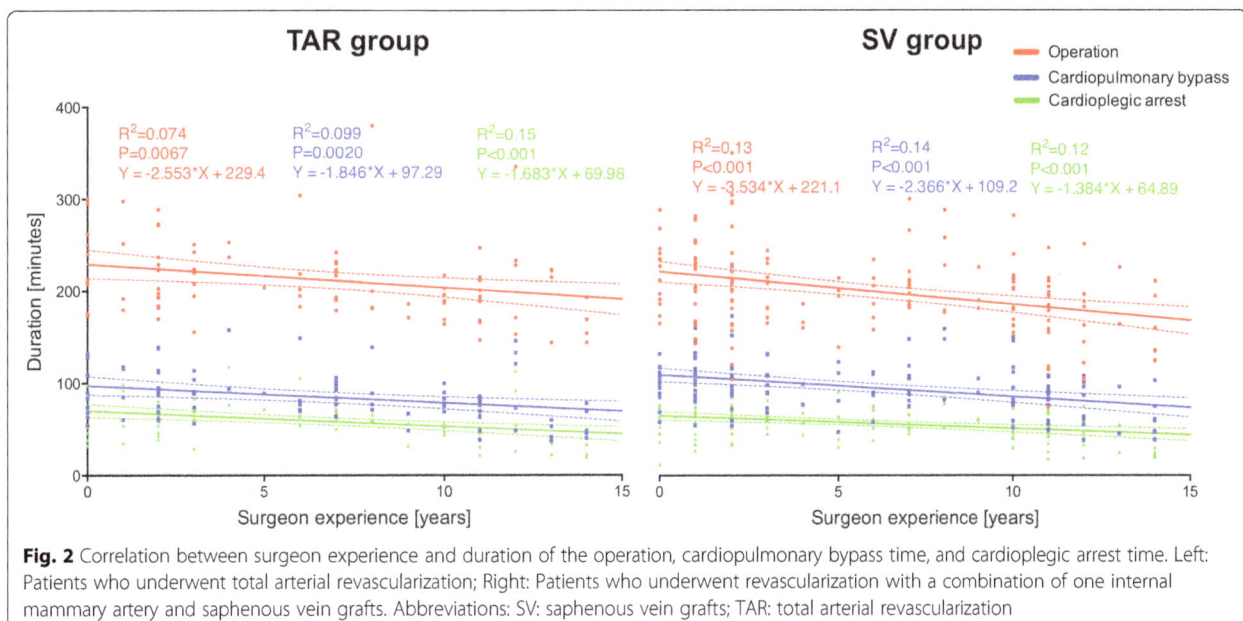

Fig. 2 Correlation between surgeon experience and duration of the operation, cardiopulmonary bypass time, and cardioplegic arrest time. Left: Patients who underwent total arterial revascularization; Right: Patients who underwent revascularization with a combination of one internal mammary artery and saphenous vein grafts. Abbreviations: SV: saphenous vein grafts; TAR: total arterial revascularization

Table 3 Perioperative outcomes

Parameter	SV group * n = 152	TAR group * n = 98	p-value
Transfusions			
Erythrocytes			
Rate	116 (76)	56 (57)	< 0.001
Amount (units)**	2 ± 2.6	1 ± 2.7	0.041
Platelets			
Rate	56 (37)	35 (36)	0.86
Amount (units)**	0 ± 1.0	0 ± 0.90	0.33
Fresh frozen plasma			
Rate	45 (30)	22 (22)	0.21
Amount (units)**	0 ± 2.0	0 ± 2.0	0.46
Re-thoracotomy for bleeding	9 (5.9)	3 (3.1)	0.30
Sternal wound healing impairment requiring surgical revision	4 (2.6)	4 (4.0)	0.52
Superficial	2 (1.3)	3 (3.0)	
Deep	2 (1.3)	1 (1.0)	
Duration of invasive ventilation (hours)**	14 ± 58	10 ± 73	0.61
Postoperative tracheostomy	11 (7.2)	5 (5.1)	0.30
New onset atrial fibrillation	29 (19)	10 (10)	0.059
Stroke (>Rankin1)	3 (2.0)	0	0.1
Acute kidney injury			
KDIGO I	59 (40)	32 (33)	0.17
KDIGO II	11 (7.5)	4 (4.1)	
KDIGO III	6 (3.9)	5 (5.1)	
Postoperative dialysis	6 (3.9)	5 (5.1)	0.69
Postoperative length of ICU stay (hours)**	73 ± 81	46 ± 93	0.28
Postoperative length of hospital stay (days) **	10 ± 4.5	10 ± 3.4	0.58
30-day all-cause mortality	6 (4.5)	3 (3.4)	0.68

Abbreviations: *ECLS* extracorporeal life support, *KDIGO* Kidney disease: improving global outcomes, *SV* saphenous vein grafts, *TAR* total arterial revascularization
[a]Continuous variables: mean ± SD; categorical variables: n (%)
[b]Median ± SD

stay and postoperative hospitalization were similar in both groups. Other postoperative data were comparable between the groups (Table 3).

Mortality and long-term follow up

Mortality at 30 days postoperatively was 4.5% in the SV group and 3.4% in the TAR group ($p = 0.68$).. Further follow-up was complete for 92% of patients with a median follow-up time of 3.7 ± 2.5 years. Kaplan-Meier estimation of survival showed a tendency for improved survival in the TAR group (log-rank $p = 0.12$) with survival curves beginning to diverge from 4 years postoperatively onwards. The overall survival probability at 7 years postoperatively was 75% in the TAR group and 62% in the SV group, respectively (Fig. 4). Symptom-driven repeat coronary angiography was reported by 17% of patients in the TAR group compared with 21% of patients in the SVG group ($p = 0.45$).

Redo-CABG was performed in 2 patients (1.3%) in the SV group and 1 patient (1.0%) in the TAR group ($p = 0.64$).

Discussion

The main finding of this analysis is that CABG using TAR is feasible in patients with AMI as it provides revascularization quality and patient safety like that of CABG using a combination of IMA and SV without increasing the time required for revascularization. Perioperative outcomes did not differ significantly between the groups. Bleeding complications and transfusion requirements were not higher after TAR than after revascularization using IMA/SV; in contrast, the proportion of patients who did not receive any red blood cell transfusion was higher in the TAR group. Postoperative atrial fibrillation was less frequent in the TAR group, possibly due to reduced red blood cell transfusion as demonstrated by previous studies [18, 19].

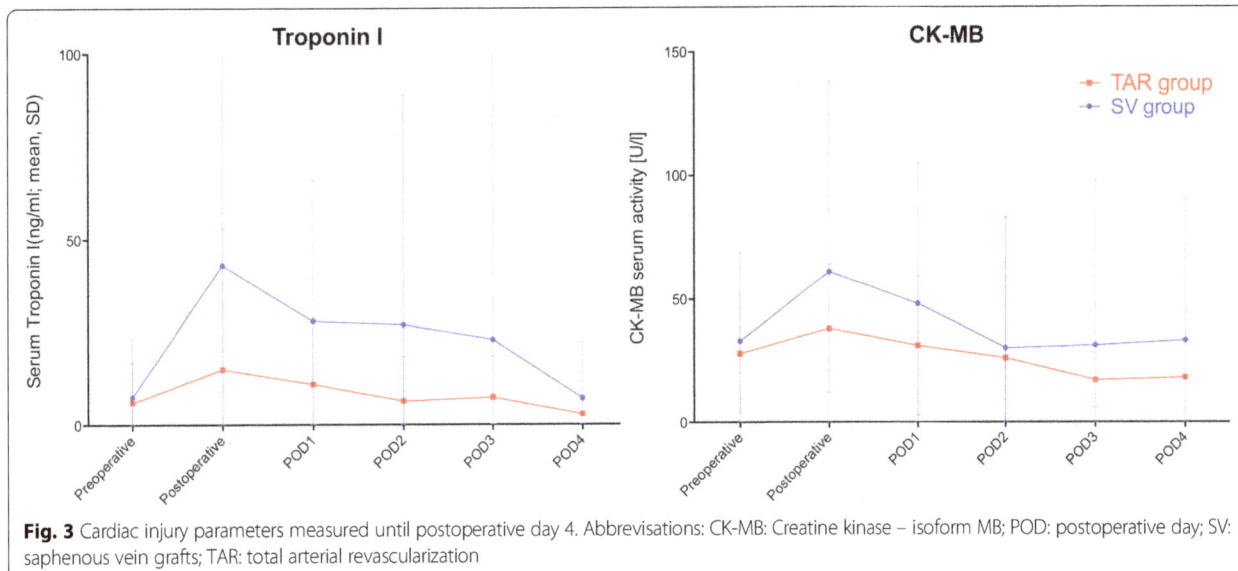

Fig. 3 Cardiac injury parameters measured until postoperative day 4. Abbrevisations: CK-MB: Creatine kinase – isoform MB; POD: postoperative day; SV: saphenous vein grafts; TAR: total arterial revascularization

Nevertheless, if transfusions were necessary, the amount of transfused erythrocyte units was rather high. This might be explained by the high rate of patients with DAPT at the time of surgery [11].

The mean time of surgeon experience was slightly higher in the TAR group, probably reflecting that more experienced surgeons tend to perform this more challenging technique in urgent or emergent clinical settings. Moreover, the increased surgeon experience in the TAR group might result in better surgical results, although recent data did not confirm this assumption for CABG procedures

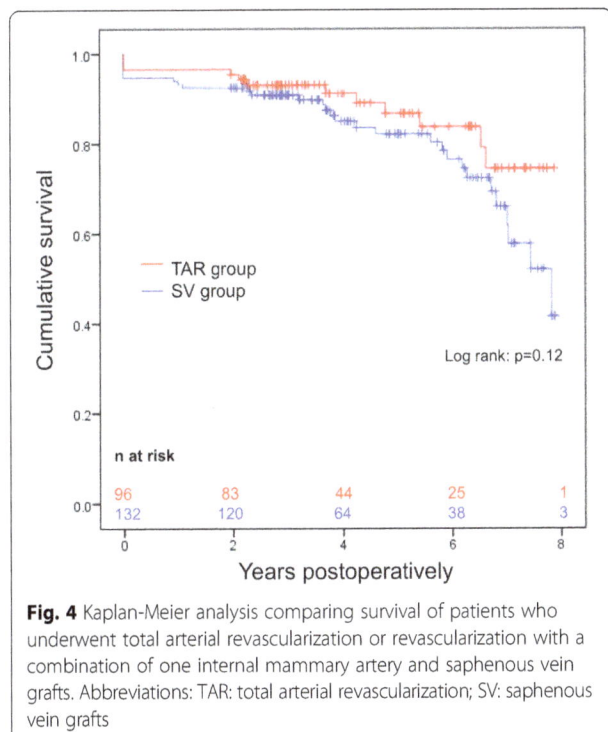

Fig. 4 Kaplan-Meier analysis comparing survival of patients who underwent total arterial revascularization or revascularization with a combination of one internal mammary artery and saphenous vein grafts. Abbreviations: TAR: total arterial revascularization; SV: saphenous vein grafts

[20–22]. Surprisingly, analysis of procedural duration revealed that the total duration of the surgical procedures involving total arterial CABG and CABG using vein grafts were similar. Our data show that the surgeon's experience has a significant influence on the duration of the procedure but that the amount is of questionable relevance. The longer phase of graft preparation in the TAR group was balanced by a shorter post-CPB phase in the TAR group. The reduction in reperfusion time and post-CPB time might be partly explained by the greater experience of the surgeons involved, leading to more efficient management at the end of the operation; however, the shorter time could additionally be explained by more rapid bypass graft function of arterial grafts compared with vein grafts, possibly resulting in quicker hemodynamic stabilization. Data on flow properties of arterial bypass grafts compared those of with vein grafts in the immediate intraoperative phase are limited: Spence et al. showed in a canine model that mammary artery graft flow is not impaired by competitive flow from the native vessel [23]. As competitive flow from either the native vessel or collaterals is frequently observed in the early and late postoperative phase, resilience of the grafts may influence their immediate and long-term function [24]. Concerning the immediate function, Weber et al. described improved intraoperative pulsatility indices and a tendency for reduced perioperative myocardial infarctions when using IMA grafts compared with vein grafts [25]. We cannot substantiate our assumption of improved immediate bypass graft function, as flow measurements were not routinely carried out at our institution. Furthermore, although the postoperative increase in serum levels of cardiac biomarkers was somewhat less in the TAR group than in the SV group (possibly reflecting reduced cardiac injury resulting from improved bypass function), this difference was not statistically significant.

We were also surprised to observe that the most technically challenging phase of the procedure, the completion of the coronary anastomoses during cardioplegic arrest, required the same amount of time in the two groups, which is not in keeping with the reluctance to perform TAR due to more difficult and prolonged completion of coronary anastomoses. In fact, the present data should encourage surgeons to commit themselves early to TAR concepts, as these are feasible without loss of time in experienced hands.

Data from the postoperative follow-up period of up to 7 years did not show significant differences in survival between the groups; however, there was a tendency for improved survival in the TAR group from 4 years onwards. The rate of reported symptom-driven repeat coronary catheterizations were non-significantly lower in the TAR group. Unfortunately, there is no information available about the results of these coronary catheterizations and interventions performed. Redo-CABG occurred similarly in both groups. Previous studies have demonstrated that differences in graft patency between SV and IMA grafts become evident only after 4–8 years [26, 27, 28]. A survival benefit after TAR in the mid- or long-term has been shown in pooled analyses [29, 30]. Our observation is in accordance with the recently published work by Taggart et al. showing no significant survival benefit after bilateral IMA versus single IMA grafting after 5 years [31]. A longer-term follow-up of the patients will be required to confirm these observations.

Several limitations of this study should be mentioned. First, patients with LCOS prior to surgery were excluded from this analysis, as CABG in these patients frequently does not follow the standardized sequence of operative steps. These patients are often placed on CPB prior to graft harvesting, and BIMA preparation is all but ruled out in these emergency situations, and hence we did not consider these exceptional, very individual situations to be suitable for a generalizable analysis. Therefore, the results of this study cannot be applied to patients who present with LCOS before CABG. Second, CPB with cardioplegic arrest was used in all procedures. Alternative approaches include off-pump CABG or on-pump CABG with beating heart [32–34], which might reduce injury and inflammation associated with CPB and cardioplegic arrest. CPB with cardioplegic arrest, however, provides hemodynamic stability during the procedure with optimized exposure for accurate anastomosing. To date there are no data available showing superiority of one strategy over the other.

Although the logistical and technical aspects (procedural times, completeness of revascularization) of our study are not likely to be biased by the study design, outcome data of this retrospective, propensity-matched analysis should be considered with caution. Unknown confounders might reduce comparability of the groups and bias outcome data.

Conclusion

TAR should be considered the standard of care in hemodynamically stable patients with AMI undergoing CABG, as it is equally safe and rapid compared with the use of combinations of IMA and vein grafts. Reluctance to apply TAR in these patients due to fear of protracted revascularization and bleeding complications is no longer justified. Long-term outcome may be improved after TAR, but these observations remain to be confirmed in a longer-term study.

Abbreviations
AMI: Acute myocardial infarction; BIMA: Bilateral internal mammary artery; CABG: Coronary artery bypass grafting surgery; CK-MB: Creatine kinase, isoform MB; CPB: Cardiopulmonary bypass; LCOS: Low cardiac output syndrome; NSTEMI: Non-ST-segment elevation myocardial infarction; OR: Odds ratio; SD: Standard deviation; STEMI: ST-segment-elevation myocardial infarction; SV: Saphenous vein grafts; TAR: Total arterial revascularization

Acknowledgements
T The authors thank Irina Oswald for excellent assistance during patient follow-up and Dr. Elizabeth Martinson for language editing of the manuscript.

Funding
This is an investigator-initiated project without external funding.
The authors of this manuscript received external funding for other research projects from the following sources:
PG: The German Heart Foundation, the University Hospital Giessen and Marburg Research Fund, the Von-Behring-Röntgen-Foundation.
LO: none
TS: none
VJ: none
CO: none
PR: none
BN: The German Heart Foundation, the University Hospital Giessen and Marburg Research Fund, the Von-Behring-Röntgen-Foundation.
AB: The German Heart Foundation, the University Hospital Giessen and Marburg Research Fund, the Von-Behring-Röntgen-Foundation.

Authors' contributions
PG initiated and led the study, coordinated data collection and analysis as well as drafting of the manuscript. LO and TS carried out data collection and data anlysis and contributed in drafting the manuscript. PG, LO, TS, VJ, CO, PR, BN and AB drafted parts of the manuscript and all authors revised the manuscript critically and approved the manuscript finally.

Competing interests
The authors of this manuscript have research support from The German Heart Foundation, the University Hospital Giessen and Marburg Research Fund, the Von-Behring-Röntgen-Foundation (PG, BN and AB). The authors declare that there are no conflicting financial or non-financial interests. All authors confirm that they had full control of the design and the methods of the study, the data analysis and the production of the written report.

Author details
[1]Department of Adult and Pediatric Cardiovascular Surgery, University Hospital Giessen, Rudolf-Buchheim-Str. 7, DE-35392 Giessen, Germany. [2]Department of Anaesthesiology, Sana Hospital Berlin-Lichtenberg, Berlin, Germany. [3]Department of Cardiology and Angiology, University Hospital Giessen, Giessen, Germany.

References
1. Kolh P, Windecker S, Alfonso F, Collet J-P, Cremer J, Falk V, Filippatos G, Hamm C, Head SJ, Jüni P, Kappetein AP, Kastrati A, Knuuti J, Landmesser U, Laufer G, Neumann F-J, Richter DJ, Schauerte P, Sousa Uva M, Stefanini GG, Taggart DP, Torracca L, Valgimigli M, Wijns W, Witkowski A, ESC Committee for Practice Guidelines, Zamorano JL, Achenbach S, Baumgartner H, Bax JJ, Bueno H, Dean V, Deaton C, Erol Ç, Fagard R, Ferrari R, Hasdai D, Hoes AW, Kirchhof P, Knuuti J, Kolh P, Lancellotti P, Linhart A, Nihoyannopoulos P, Piepoli MF, Ponikowski P, Sirnes PA, Tamargo JL, Tendera M, Torbicki A, Wijns W, Windecker S, Committee EACTSCG, Sousa Uva M, Achenbach S, Pepper J, Anyanwu A, Badimon L, Bauersachs J, Baumbach A, Beygui F, Bonaros N, De Carlo M, Deaton C, Dobrev D, Dunning J, Eeckhout E, Gielen S, Hasdai D, Kirchhof P, Luckraz H, Mahrholdt H, Montalescot G, Paparella D, Rastan AJ, Sanmartin M, Sergeant P, Silber S, Tamargo J, ten Berg J, Thiele H, van Geuns R-J, Wagner H-O, Wassmann S, Wendler O, Zamorano JL. 2014 ESC/EACTS guidelines on myocardial revascularization: the task force on myocardial revascularization of the European Society of Cardiology (ESC) and the European Association for Cardio-Thoracic Surgery (EACTS). Developed with the special contribution of the European Association of Percutaneous Cardiovascular Interventions (EAPCI). Eur J Cardio-Thorac Surg Off J Eur Assoc Cardio-Thorac Surg. 2014;46:517–92. https://doi.org/10.1093/ejcts/ezu366.
2. Mohr FW, Rastan AJ, Serruys PW, Kappetein AP, Holmes DR, Pomar JL, Westaby S, Leadley K, Dawkins KD, Mack MJ. Complex coronary anatomy in coronary artery bypass graft surgery: impact of complex coronary anatomy in modern bypass surgery? Lessons learned from the SYNTAX trial after two years. J Thorac Cardiovasc Surg. 2011;141:130–40. https://doi.org/10.1016/j.jtcvs.2010.07.094.
3. ElBardissi AW, Aranki SF, Sheng S, O'Brien SM, Greenberg CC, Gammie JS. Trends in isolated coronary artery bypass grafting: an analysis of the Society of Thoracic Surgeons adult cardiac surgery database. J Thorac Cardiovasc Surg. 2012;143:273–81. https://doi.org/10.1016/j.jtcvs.2011.10.029.
4. Itagaki S, Cavallaro P, Adams DH, Chikwe J. Bilateral internal mammary artery grafts, mortality and morbidity: an analysis of 1 526 360 coronary bypass operations. Heart. 2013;99:849–53. https://doi.org/10.1136/heartjnl-2013-303672.
5. Tabata M, Grab JD, Khalpey Z, Edwards FH, O'Brien SM, Cohn LH, Bolman RM. Prevalence and variability of internal mammary artery graft use in contemporary multivessel coronary artery bypass graft surgery. Circulation. 2009;120:935–40. https://doi.org/10.1161/CIRCULATIONAHA.108.832444.
6. Deutsch O, Gansera L, Wunderlich M, Eichinger W, Gansera B. Does bilateral ITA grafting increase Perioperative complications? Outcome of 6,476 patients with bilateral versus 5,020 patients with single ITA bypass. Thorac Cardiovasc Surg. 2015;64:188–94. https://doi.org/10.1055/s-0035-1558992.
7. Benedetto U, Altman DG, Gerry S, Gray A, Lees B, Pawlaczyk R, Flather M, Taggart DP. Pedicled and skeletonized single and bilateral internal thoracic artery grafts and the incidence of sternal wound complications: insights from the arterial revascularization trial. J Thorac Cardiovasc Surg. 2016;152:270–6. https://doi.org/10.1016/j.jtcvs.2016.03.056.
8. Tavolacci M-P, Merle V, Josset V, Bouchart F, Litzler P-Y, Tabley A, Bessou J-P,

Czernichow P. Mediastinitis after coronary artery bypass graft surgery: influence of the mammary grafting for diabetic patients. J Hosp Infect. 2003; 55:21–5. https://doi.org/10.1016/S0195-6701(03)00116-6.
9. Nichols EL, McCullough JN, Ross CS, Kramer RS, Westbrook BM, Klemperer JD, Leavitt BJ, Brown JR, Olmstead E, Hernandez F, Sardella GL, Frumiento C, Malenka D, DiScipio A. Optimal timing from myocardial infarction to coronary artery bypass grafting on hospital mortality. Ann Thorac Surg. 2017;103:162–71. https://doi.org/10.1016/j.athoracsur.2016.05.116.
10. Locker C, Mohr R, Paz Y, Kramer A, Lev-Ran O, Pevni D, Shapira I. Myocardial revascularization for acute myocardial infarction: benefits and drawbacks of avoiding cardiopulmonary bypass. Ann Thorac Surg. 2003;76:771–6. https://doi.org/10.1016/S0003-4975(03)00732-X.
11. Nagashima Z, Tsukahara K, Uchida K, Hibi K, Karube N, Ebina T, Imoto K, Kimura K, Umemura S. Impact of preoperative dual antiplatelet therapy on bleeding complications in patients with acute coronary syndromes who undergo urgent coronary artery bypass grafting. J Cardiol. 2017;69:156–61. https://doi.org/10.1016/j.jjcc.2016.02.013.
12. Mahla E, Prueller F, Farzi S, Pregartner G, Raggam RB, Beran E, Toller W, Berghold A, Tantry US, Gurbel PA. Does platelet reactivity predict bleeding in patients needing urgent coronary artery bypass grafting during dual Antiplatelet therapy? Ann Thorac Surg. 2016;102:2010–7. https://doi.org/10.1016/j.athoracsur.2016.05.003.
13. Siller-Matula JM, Petre A, Delle-Karth G, Huber K, Ay C, Lordkipanidzé M, Caterina RD, Kolh P, Mahla E, Gersh BJ. Impact of preoperative use of P2Y12 receptor inhibitors on clinical outcomes in cardiac and non-cardiac surgery: a systematic review and meta-analysis. Eur Heart J Acute Cardiovasc Care. 2015:2048872615585516. https://doi.org/10.1177/2048872615585516.
14. Thygesen K, Alpert JS, Jaffe AS, Simoons ML, Chaitman BR, White HD. Third universal definition of myocardial infarction. Circulation. 2012;126:2020–35. https://doi.org/10.1161/CIR.0b013e31826e1058.
15. Ong ATL, Serruys PW. Complete Revascularization. Circulation. 2006;114:249–55. https://doi.org/10.1161/CIRCULATIONAHA.106.614420.
16. Khwaja A. KDIGO clinical practice guidelines for acute kidney injury. Nephron Clin Pract. 2012;120:c179–84. https://doi.org/10.1159/000339789.
17. Böning A, Rohrbach S, Kohlhepp L, Heep M, Hagmüller S, Niemann B, Mühlfeld C. Differences in ischemic damage between young and old hearts–effects of blood cardioplegia. Exp Gerontol. 2015;67:3–8. https://doi.org/10.1016/j.exger.2015.04.012.
18. Alameddine AK, Visintainer P, Alimov VK, Rousou JA. Blood transfusion and the risk of atrial fibrillation after cardiac surgery. J Card Surg. 2014;29:593–9. https://doi.org/10.1111/jocs.12383.
19. Koch CG, Li L, Van Wagoner DR, Duncan AI, Gillinov AM, Blackstone EH. Red cell transfusion is associated with an increased risk for postoperative Atrial fibrillation. Ann Thorac Surg. 2006;82:1747–56. https://doi.org/10.1016/j.athoracsur.2006.05.045.
20. Yount KW, Yarboro LT, Narahari AK, Ghanta RK, Tribble CG, Kron IL, Kern JA, Ailawadi G. Outcomes of trainees performing coronary artery bypass grafting: does resident experience matter? Ann Thorac Surg. 2017;103:975–81. https://doi.org/10.1016/j.athoracsur.2016.10.016.
21. Ch'ng SL, Cochrane AD, Wolfe R, Reid C, Smith CI, Smith JA. Procedure-specific cardiac surgeon volume associated with patient outcome following valve surgery, but not isolated CABG surgery. Heart Lung Circ. 2015;24:583–9. https://doi.org/10.1016/j.hlc.2014.11.014.
22. Burt BM, ElBardissi AW, Huckman RS, Cohn LH, Cevasco MW, Rawn JD, Aranki SF, Byrne JG. Influence of experience and the surgical learning curve on long-term patient outcomes in cardiac surgery. J Thorac Cardiovasc Surg. 2015;150:1061–1068.e3. https://doi.org/10.1016/j.jtcvs.2015.07.068.
23. Spence PA, Lust RM, Zeri RS, Jolly SR, Mehta PM, Otaki M, Sun YS, Chitwood WR. Competitive flow from a fully patent coronary artery does not limit acute mammary graft flow. Ann Thorac Surg. 1992;54:21–5.
24. Glineur D, Hanet C. Competitive flow in coronary bypass surgery: is it a problem? Curr Opin Cardiol. 2012;27:620–8. https://doi.org/10.1097/HCO.0b013e3283583000.
25. Weber A, Tavakoli R, Genoni M. Superior flow pattern of internal thoracic artery over Saphenous vein grafts during OPCAB procedures. J Card Surg. 2009;24:2–5. https://doi.org/10.1111/j.1540-8191.2008.00730.x.
26. Fitzgibbon GM, Kafka HP, Leach AJ, Keon WJ, Hooper GD, Burton JR. Coronary bypass graft fate and patient outcome: angiographic follow-up of 5,065 grafts related to survival and reoperation in 1,388 patients during 25 years. J Am Coll Cardiol. 1996;28:616–26. https://doi.org/10.1016/0735-1097(96)00206-9.

27. Goldman S, Zadina K, Moritz T, Ovitt T, Sethi G, Copeland JG, Thottapurathu L, Krasnicka B, Ellis N, Anderson RJ, Henderson W. Long-term patency of saphenous vein and left internal mammary artery grafts after coronary artery bypass surgery: results from a Department of Veterans Affairs Cooperative Study. J Am Coll Cardiol. 2004;44:2149–56. https://doi.org/10.1016/j.jacc.2004.08.064.

28. Gansera B, Schmidtler F, Angelis I, Kiask T, Kemkes BM, Botzenhardt F. Patency of internal thoracic artery compared to vein grafts - postoperative angiographic findings in 1189 symptomatic patients in 12 years. Thorac Cardiovasc Surg. 2007;55:412–7. https://doi.org/10.1055/s-2007-965372.

29. Weiss AJ, Zhao S, Tian DH, Taggart DP, Yan TD. A meta-analysis comparing bilateral internal mammary artery with left internal mammary artery for coronary artery bypass grafting. Ann Cardiothorac Surg. 2013;2:390–400. https://doi.org/10.3978/2399.

30. Taggart DP, D'Amico R, Altman DG. Effect of arterial revascularisation on survival: a systematic review of studies comparing bilateral and single internal mammary arteries. Lancet. 2001;358:870–5. https://doi.org/10.1016/S0140-6736(01)06069-X.

31. Taggart DP, Altman DG, Gray AM, Lees B, Gerry S, Benedetto U, Flather M. Randomized trial of bilateral versus single internal-thoracic-artery grafts. N Engl J Med. 2016;375:2540–9. https://doi.org/10.1056/NEJMoa1610021.

32. Miyahara K, Matsuura A, Takemura H, Saito S, Sawaki S, Yoshioka T, Ito H. On-pump beating-heart coronary artery bypass grafting after acute myocardial infarction has lower mortality and morbidity. J Thorac Cardiovasc Surg. 2008;135:521–6. https://doi.org/10.1016/j.jtcvs.2007.10.006.

33. Gp V, Cs D, No T, Vh T, As E. Acute myocardial infarction: OPCAB is an alternative approach for treatment. Heart Surg Forum. 2001;4:147–50.

34. Nishi H, Sakaguchi T, Miyagawa S, Yoshikawa Y, Fukushima S, Yoshioka D, Saito T, Toda K, Sawa Y. Optimal coronary artery bypass grafting strategy for acute coronary syndrome. Gen Thorac Cardiovasc Surg. 2014;62:357–63. https://doi.org/10.1007/s11748-013-0358-6.

11

Anxiety after Sympathectomy in patients with primary palmar hyperhidrosis may prolong the duration of compensatory hyperhidrosis

Kai Qian, Yong-Geng Feng, Jing-Hai Zhou, Ru-Wen Wang, Qun-You Tan* and Bo Deng*

Abstract

Background: Compensatory hyperhidrosis (CH) is a frequent side effect after sympathectomy for the treatment of primary palmar hyperhidrosis. We determined the effects of demographic and clinical factors which may increase the duration of CH (DCH).

Methods: One hundred twenty-two patients who had undergone sympathectomies from 2014 to 2016 were retrospectively reviewed. Anxiety was evaluated using the State and Trait Anxiety Inventory score. Follow-up evaluations continued until CH remitted. A Cox proportional hazards model was used to determine the association between DCH and variables.

Results: DCH ranged from 5 to 27 weeks (median, 11.47 weeks). Severe CH (HR = 0.318, 95% CI, 0.136–0.741) and exacerbated anxiety 1 month post-operatively (HR = 0.816, 95% CI, 0.746–0.893) may prolong CH. A positive correlation between post-operative anxiety and DCH was common in patients with moderate or severe CH, and in cases with forearm CH.

Conclusions: Pre- and post-operative anxiety should be evaluated, and anti-anxiety treatment is offered to patients with moderate-to-severe CH to shorten the DCH.

Keywords: Anxiety, Palmar hyperhidrosis, Compensatory hyperhidrosis

Background

Primary palmar hyperhidrosis (PH) is a condition marked by excessive perspiration, which can be exacerbated by stress and anxiety [1]. Sympathectomy by video-assisted thoracic surgery (VATS) has been used in PH treatment with acceptable results [2]; however, post-operative compensatory hyperhidrosis (CH) is a frequent side effect (morbidity, 44–86% [3]) that significantly lowers the quality of life [4]. CH can result from aberrant function of the sympathetic nervous system after surgery [5], which destroys the nerve flex arch between the sympathetic nervous system and hypothalamus [6]. A systemic review suggested that, as compared with other levels, a T3 or T3–4

sympathectomy can offer better efficacy and satisfaction rate and result in less post-operative CH [7]. Fortunately, post-operative CH will be gradually and finally obliterated [8]; however, the clinical or demographic factors may prolong the duration of CH (DCH) remain unclear.

CH may lead to severe anxiety [9]. Conversely, we speculate that anxiety may affect DCH following sympathectomy. Therefore, we sought to analyze these clinical and demographic factors, including anxiety, which may prolong the DCH.

Methods

Patients

The study protocol was reviewed and approved by the Research Ethics Board in Daping Hospital (Chongqing City, P.R. China) [reference no. 20160809], and informed consent was written and obtained from all patients.

* Correspondence: tanqy001@163.com; superdb@163.com
Department of Thoracic Surgery, Institute of Surgery Research, Daping Hospital, Army Medical University, Chongqing 400042, People's Republic of China

From September 2014 to September 2016, there were 122 patients with severe PH, as defined by United States Skin Association [10, 11], who underwent bilateral multiple-level VATS sympathectomy (Table 1). The exclusion criteria were as follows: (i) patients accepted botulinum toxin treatment and Chinese herb treatment prior to operation; (ii) patients with uncorrected bleeding diatheses (international normalized ratio>1.7 and platelet count < 50,000/dL); (iii) pre-operative acute inflammation (serum C-reactive protein concentration > 10 mg/L; white blood cell count > 10×10^9/L); (iv) patients were diagnosed with secondary hyperhidrosis or other neuromuscular diseases; and (v) patients were pregnant or lactating.

The follow-up strategy is shown in Fig. 1. Post-operatively, patients were confirmed to have or not have CH, which was defined as new onset post-operative or worsening sweating in the lower extremities, trunk, axillae, face, and groin [2]. All patients were queried via questionnaire (Hyperhidrosis Disease Severity Scale) [12], as shown in Additional file 1: Table S1. Follow-up was discontinued in patients when CH remitted.

Bilateral sympathectomy by VATS

General anesthesia and a double-lumen endotracheal tube placement was performed. During the operation, patients were placed in the supine position with exposure of both axillary regions. A 1-cm incision was made at the third intercostal space on the anterior axillary line, and a 5-mm diameter thoracoscope (0° telescope; Karl Storz, Germany) was placed via a 12-mm trocar. To identify anatomic landmarks, pneumothoraces were induced in all patients via temporary apnea [13]. An electrocautery hook was inserted to isolate and cut the sympathetic chains at T2–3, T2–4, or T3–4 (Table 1). After sympathectomy, the lung was confirmed to be re-expanded after air was evacuated from the pleural cavity via a 16-Fr catheter [14]. Chest drainage tubes were not placed in all of the patients.

Anxiety evaluation

Anxiety was evaluated using State-Trait Anxiety Inventory (STAI) [15], differentiating temporary "state-anxiety"(SAI) from long-term quality of "trait-anxiety"(TAI). The STAI can be used in clinical settings to diagnose anxiety and to distinguish anxiety from depressive syndromes. The STAI can be obtained from the publisher (Mind Garden, 855 Oak Grove Avenue, Suite 215, Menlo Park, CA 94025; USA, URL, http://www.mindgarden.com/index.htm). SAI is the temporary and changeable feeling induced by the arousal of the autonomic nervous system (e.g., how a person is feeling at the time of a perceived threat) [16]. TAI is viewed as a predisposition to anxiety, which is a relatively stable personality characteristic [17]. SAI and TAI were measured using a 4-point rating scale for 20 items (1, 'not at all'; 2, 'mild'; 3, 'moderate'; and 4, 'very') [18]. Total scores of SAI and TAI varied between 20 and 80.

Statistical analysis

Kolmogorov–Smirnov test was used for determination of the distribution. The Fisher exact test was used for categorical variables. The t-test or Mann–Whitney U test was used for continuous variables. Univariate and multivariate analyses were performed using a Cox proportional hazards model to determine associations between DCH and potential impact factors. Parameters demonstrating a statistically significant effect on DCH in the univariate Cox model were included for analysis in the multivariate model with forward and stepwise selection. Hazard ratios (HRs) were estimated as relative risk with corresponding 95% confident intervals (CIs). Statistical analyses were performed with SPSS (version 23.0, IBM Corp.: Armonk, NY), with a two-sided $P < 0.05$ considered statistically significant for all reports. The XLSTAT® (Addinsoft company, Pairs, France) was used to assess statistical power.

Results

Clinical and demographic characteristics of patients with CH

Among the 122 patients, 57 (46.72%) developed CH after sympathectomies (Table 1). Post-operative follow-up was discontinued until CH remitted, ranging from 5 to 27 weeks (median duration, 11.47 weeks). We chose 1 month post-operatively as the time point to evaluate the psychologic status for the following reasons: (i) anxiety resulting from surgery has resolved; and (ii) CH in some cases resolved within 5 weeks.

The body mass index (BMI) of the CH group were significantly lower, as compared with the non-CH group, even though the BMIs in either group were within the normal range (Table 1). Table 1 shows significant severe pre-operative anxiety status (SAI-p) of the patients with CH as compared with patients without CH ($p < 0.05$).

Clinical factors prolonged CH

The univariate Cox model indicated that four factors significantly may increase DCH, i.e., CH degree (HR = 0.098; 95% CI, 0.045–0.216), SAI-p (HR = 0.908; 95% CI, 0.854–0.966), SAI-1 m (HR = 0.773; 95% CI, 0.716–0.843), sympathectomy level (HR = 1.698; 95% CI, 1.256–2.295), TAI-p (HR = 0.900; 95% CI, 0.845–0.958), and TAI-1 m (HR = 0.893; 95% CI, 0.838–0.953; Table 2).

The multivariable Cox model also showed that severe CH and a high SAI-1 m score was significantly associated with prolonged CH (HR = 0.318; 95% CI, 0.136–0.741 and HR = 0.816; 95% CI, 0.746–0.893), as shown in Table 2.

Table 1 Clinical and demographic characteristics of patients with and without CH[a]

	Patients without CH	Patients with CH	P value
	(n = 65)	(n = 57)	
Gender			0.323*
Male	40(61.54)	30(52.6)	
Female	25(38.46)	27(47.4)	
Age[years]			0.440*
Mean	21.65	21.33	
SD	5.001	5.601	
BMI[kg/m²]			0.006
Mean	22.86	20.04	
SD	1.47	1.784	
Location of CH[b]			–
Head, face, and neck	–	24(42.1)	
Forearm	–	24(42.1)	
Trunk and perineum	–	5(8.8)	
Calves, feet, and thighs	–	4(7.0)	
Degree of CH[c]			–
None	65(100)	0	
Mild	–	30(52.6)	
Moderate	–	16(28.1)	
Severe	–	11(19.3)	
Hresult-1 m			0.830*
Completely dry	40(61.5)	44(77.2)	
Significant improvement	25(38.5)	13(22.8)	
Improvement	0	0	
No change	0	0	
SAI-P			0.014*
Mean	37.22	39.86	
SD	3.319	5.749	
SAI-1 m			0.481*
Mean	37.51	40.19	
SD	3.355	8.037	
TAI-P			0.633*
Mean	39.80	40.54	
SD	1.725	5.558	
TAI-1 m			0.697*
Mean	39.75	40.61	
SD	1.714	5.552	

Table 1 Clinical and demographic characteristics of patients with and without CH[a] *(Continued)*

	Patients without CH	Patients with CH	P value
	(n = 65)	(n = 57)	
The method of sympathectomy			0.896*
T2-3	32(49.2)	28(49.1)	
T2–4	14(21.5)	11(19.3)	
T3–4	19(29.2)	18(31.6)	

Note: [a]Kolmogorov–Smirnov test for determination of distribution
*Mann–Whitney U test
[b]According to the rule of nines, i.e., guide for resuscitation of burn patients, the location of CH divides into 4 groups [27]
[c]Mild: CH is not noticeable, unless under detailed questioning; Moderate: CH is tolerable, but sometimes interferes with daily activities; Severe: CH is intolerable and always interferes with daily activities
Abbreviations: BMI: body mass index; CH: compensatory hyperhidrosis; Hresult-1 m: hand effects in post-operative 1 month; SAI-1 m: State Anxiety Inventory score 1 month post-operatively; SAI-P: Pre-operative State Anxiety Inventory score; TAI-1 m: Trait Anxiety Inventory score 1 month post-operatively; TAI-P: Pre-operative Trait Anxiety Inventory score

Correlation between SAI-1 m and DCH

Severe anxiety 1 month post-operatively was significantly associated with prolonged CH in the patients with moderate or severe CH ($r = 0.906$, $P = 0.000$; and $r = 0.880$, $P = 0.000$); however, there was no correlation in patients with mild CH (Fig. 2).

Severe anxiety 1 month post-operatively was significantly associated with prolonged CH in the patients with forearm CH ($r = 0.805$; $P = 0.001$) (Fig. 3a). Indeed, forearm CH appeared to be more severe compared with other anatomic areas ($P = 0.004$), as compared to Fig. 3b.

Discussion

Severe CH is one of the refractory complications after sympathectomy for PH treatment, causing patient dissatisfaction and depression [4]. The incidence of CH ranges from 33 to 85%, and CH may persist 6–12 months [19]. In the current study, CH occurred in 57 patients (46.72%) and the medium DCH was 11.47 weeks. To obtain detailed CH information, our follow-up period lasted 52 weeks, indicating a gradual decrease in the intensity of CH.

Sweating is influenced by two factors (emotional stimulation [central control] and environmental temperature [peripheral control]) [12]; however, PH was more likely triggered by emotional stimulation (anxiety and depression), but less related to environmental temperature [20]. Based on the Hospital Anxiety and Depression Scale, Braganca et al. [21] reported that anxiety, rather than depression, is main cause of primary PH. Kumagai et al. [22] showed that less anxiety was accompanied with a lower degree of CH after sympathectomy. Our study revealed more severe pre-operative anxiety in patients with CH compared to patients without CH, and severe post-

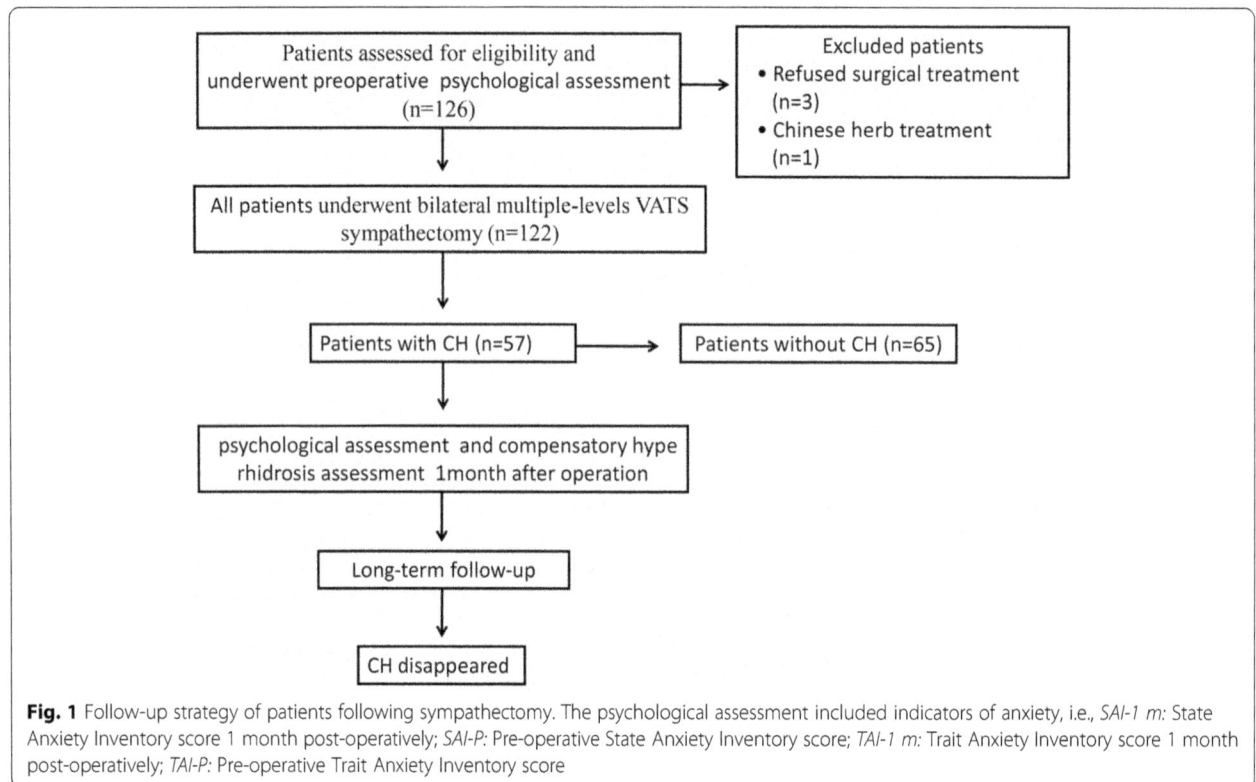

Fig. 1 Follow-up strategy of patients following sympathectomy. The psychological assessment included indicators of anxiety, i.e., *SAI-1 m:* State Anxiety Inventory score 1 month post-operatively; *SAI-P:* Pre-operative State Anxiety Inventory score; *TAI-1 m:* Trait Anxiety Inventory score 1 month post-operatively; *TAI-P:* Pre-operative Trait Anxiety Inventory score

operative anxiety may be critical to prolong DCH, especially in patients with moderate-to-severe CH.

The incidence of anxiety was reported to be higher in patients with axillary or craniofacial PH compared with other anatomic areas. Nevertheless, we found forearm CH to be more severe compared with other anatomic areas, and exacerbated anxiety resulting from CH may predispose to prolonged CH in these patients.

Before the introduction of sympathectomy, there were a variety of anti-anxiety treatments for PH, such as

hypnosis, psychotherapy [23], biofeedback [24], and tranquilizing drugs [24]. Anti-anxiety treatment may reduce negative physiologic manifestations, risk of infection, and the induction of anesthesia, but increase wound healing and promote post-operative recovery [25]. Patients who underwent psychosocial intervention following coronary artery bypass grafting were at reduced risk of adverse post-operative events [26].

In our cohort, there was one patient with insomnia caused by anxiety who was treated with eszopiclone

Table 2 Risk factors and prolonged duration of CH ($n = 57$)

Variables	Univariate analysis		Multivariate analysis	
	HR(95% CI)	P value	HR(95% CI)	P value
SAI-1 m	0.773(0.716–0.843)	0.000[a]	0.816(0.746–0.893)	0.000[b]
TAI-1 m	0.893(0.838–0.953))	0.001[c]	N.A.	0.874
SAI-P	0.908(0.854–0.966)	0.002[d]	N.A.	0.248
TAI-P	0.900(0.845–0.958)	0.001[e]	N.A.	0.453
Degree	0.098(0.045–0.216)	0.000[f]	0.318(0.136–0.741)	0.002[g]
Location	0.898(0.709–1.138)	0.374	N.A.	N.A.
Sympathectomy level	1.698(1.256–2.295)	0.001[h]	N.A.	0.751

Note: Statistical powers of the Cox model were calculated using XLSTAT (Addinsoft, Inc., New York, NY, USA) and presented as follows: [a]= 0.965; [b]= 0.978; [c]= 0.966; [d]= 0.939; [e]= 0.984; [f]= 0.104; [g]= 0.624; and [h]= 0.932. N.A. = not available

A systemic review [7] indicated a variety of CH incidences among different sympathectomy levels as follows: T2–3, 57%; T2–4, 38%; and T3–4, 6%. Therefore, we categorized the sympathectomy levels as follows: T2–3 = 1; T2–4 = 2; and T3–4 = 3

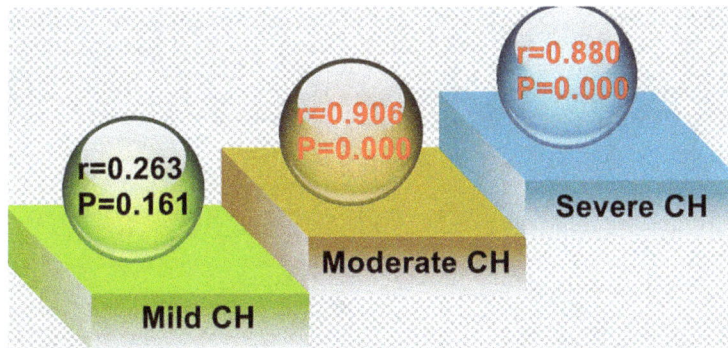

Fig. 2 Correlation between SAI-1 m and DCH. SAI-1 m may prolong DCH in the cases with moderate-to-severe CH ($r = 0.906$, $P = 0.000$; and $r = 0.880$, $P = 0.000$). *Mild:* CH is not noticeable, unless under detailed questioning; *Moderate:* CH is tolerable, but sometimes interferes with my daily activities; *Severe:* CH is intolerable and always interferes with my daily activities

(3 mg/qd) for the 10-day perioperative period. Interestingly, although the patient had severe PH preoperatively, he did not exhibit CH after sympathectomy. As a result, a randomized clinical trial is warranted to study the impact of pre-operative anti-anxiety treatment on CH and DCH.

In summary, our study has shown that pre- and post-operative anxiety should be evaluated, and anti-anxiety treatment should be administered to patients with moderate-to-severe CH in an effort to shorten the DCH.

Conclusions
Pre- and post-operative anxiety should be evaluated, and anti-anxiety treatment should be administered to patients with moderate-to-severe CH to shorten the DCH.

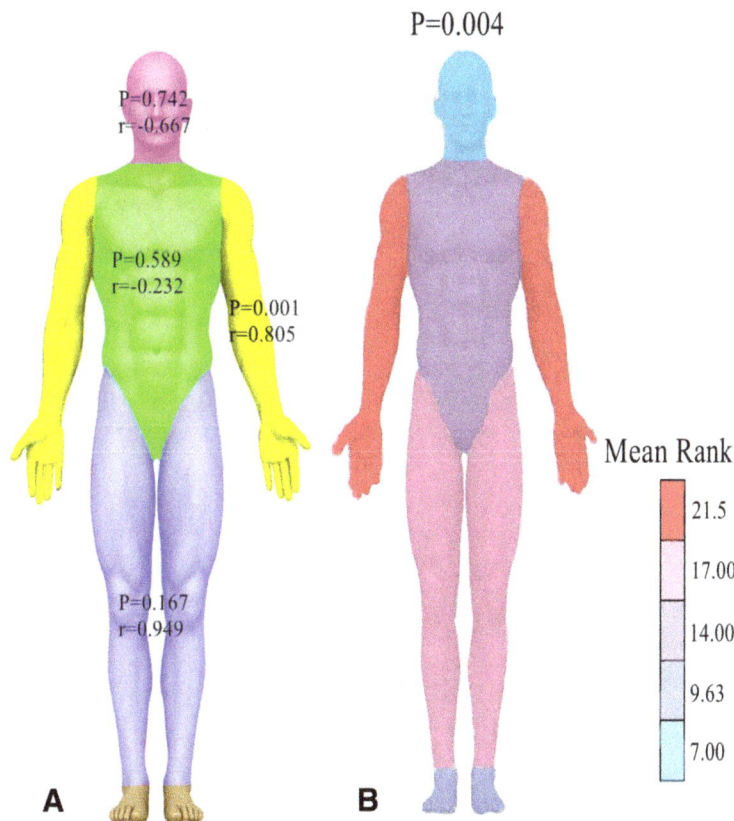

Fig. 3 a The significant positive correlation ($r = 0.805$; $P = 0.001$) between SAI-1 m and DCH was found in the patients with forearm CH, rather than other anatomic locations; (**b**): Forearm CH was more severe as compared with other anatomic areas ($P = 0.004$)

Abbreviations

BMI: Body mass index; CH: Compensatory hyperhidrosis; CI: Confidence interval; HR: Hazard radio; SAI-1 m: State Anxiety Inventory score 1 month post-operatively; SAI-P: Preoperative State Anxiety Inventory score; TAI-1 m: Trait Anxiety Inventory score 1 month post-operatively; TAI-P: Preoperative Trait Anxiety Inventory score

Acknowledgements

The author thanks Dr. Yi Deng for a critical review of the manuscript.

Authors' contributions

KQ was a major contributor in writing the manuscript. DB analyzed and interpreted the patient data regarding compensatory hyperhidrosis and anxiety. QYT gave final approval of the version of the manuscript to be published. JHZ, RWW, and YGF were involved in drafting the manuscript or revising the manuscript critically for important intellectual content. All authors read and approved the final manuscript, and made substantial contributions to conception and design.

Competing interests

The authors declare that they have no competing interests.

References

1. Zhang W, Yu D, Jiang H, et al. Video-assisted Thoracoscopic Sympathectomy for palmar hyperhidrosis: a meta-analysis of randomized controlled trials. PLoS One. 2016;11(5):e0155184.
2. Ong W, Lee A, Tan WB, et al. Long-term results of a randomized controlled trial of T2 versus T2-T3 ablation in endoscopic thoracic sympathectomy for palmar hyperhidrosis. Surg Endosc. 2016;30(3):1219–25.
3. Schick CH, Horbach T. Sequelae of endoscopic sympathetic block. Clin Auton Res. 2003;13(Suppl 1):I36–9.
4. Jeong JY, Park SS, Sim SB, et al. Prediction of compensatory hyperhidrosis with botulinum toxin a and local anesthetic. Clin Auton Res. 2015;25(4):201–5.
5. Gong TK, Kim DW. Effectiveness of oral glycopyrrolate use in compensatory hyperhidrosis patients. Korean J pain. 2013;26(1):89–93.
6. Lin CC, Telaranta T. Lin-Telaranta classification: the importance of different procedures for different indications in sympathetic surgery. Ann Chir Gynaecol. 2001;90(3):161–6.
7. Deng B, Tan QY, Jiang YG, et al. Optimization of sympathectomy to treat palmar hyperhidrosis: the systematic review and meta-analysis of studies published during the past decade. Surg Endosc. 2011;25(6):1893–901.
8. Bryant AS, Cerfolio RJ. Satisfaction and compensatory hyperhidrosis rates 5 years and longer after video-assisted thoracoscopic sympathotomy for hyperhidrosis. J Thorac Cardiovasc Surg. 2014;147(4):1160–3. e1
9. Cramer MN, Jay O. Compensatory hyperhidrosis following thoracic sympathectomy: a biophysical rationale. Am J Physiol Regul Integr Comp Physiol. 2012;302(3):R352–6.
10. Shayesteh A, Boman J, Janlert U, et al. Primary hyperhidrosis: implications on symptoms, daily life, health and alcohol consumption when treated with botulinum toxin. J Dermatol. 2016;43(8):928–33.
11. Lai YT, Yang LH, Chio CC, et al. Complications in patients with palmar hyperhidrosis treated with transthoracic endoscopic sympathectomy. Neurosurgery. 1997;41(1):110–3. discussion 13–5
12. Solish N, Bertucci V, Dansereau A, et al. A comprehensive approach to the recognition, diagnosis, and severity-based treatment of focal hyperhidrosis: recommendations of the Canadian hyperhidrosis advisory committee. Dermatol Surg. 2007;33(8):908–23.
13. Sung SW, Kim YT, Kim JH. Ultra-thin needle thoracoscopic surgery for hyperhidrosis with excellent cosmetic effects. Eur J Cardiothorac Surg. 2000; 17(6):691–6.
14. Yuncu G, Turk F, Ozturk G, et al. Comparison of only T3 and T3-T4 sympathectomy for axillary hyperhidrosis regarding treatment effect and compensatory sweating. Interact Cardiovasc Thorac Surg. 2013;17(2):263–7.
15. Babinska D, Barczynski M, Oseka T, et al. Comparison of perioperative stress in patients undergoing thyroid surgery with and without neuromonitoring-a pilot study. Langenbecks Arch Surg. 2016;
16. Gros DF, Antony MM, Simms LJ, et al. Psychometric properties of the state-trait inventory for cognitive and somatic anxiety (STICSA): comparison to the state-trait anxiety inventory (STAI). Psychol Assess. 2007;19(4):369–81.
17. Fontein-Kuipers Y, Ausems M, Bude L, et al. Factors influencing maternal distress among Dutch women with a healthy pregnancy. Women Birth. 2015;28(3):e36–43.
18. Biggs JT, Wylie LT, Ziegler VE. Validity of the Zung self-rating depression scale. British J psychiatry : the journal of mental science. 1978;132:381–5.
19. Tulay CM. Sympathectomy for palmar hyperhidrosis. Indian J surgery. 2015; 77(Suppl 2):327–9.
20. Adar R, Kurchin A, Zweig A, et al. Palmar hyperhidrosis and its surgical treatment: a report of 100 cases. Ann Surg. 1977;186(1):34–41.
21. Braganca GM, Lima SO, Pinto Neto AF, et al. Evaluation of anxiety and depression prevalence in patients with primary severe hyperhidrosis. An Bras Dermatol. 2014;89(2):230–5.
22. Kumagai K, Kawase H, Kawanishi M. Health-related quality of life after thoracoscopic sympathectomy for palmar hyperhidrosis. Ann Thorac Surg. 2005;80(2):461–6.
23. Tabet JC, Bay JW, Magdinec M. Essential hyperhidrosis. Current therapy. Cleveland Clinic quarterly. 1986;53(1):83–8.
24. Duller P, Gentry WD. Use of biofeedback in treating chronic hyperhidrosis: a preliminary report. Br J Dermatol. 1980;103(2):143–6.
25. Bradt J, Dileo C, Shim M. Music interventions for preoperative anxiety. The Cochrane database of systematic reviews. 2013;6:CD006908.
26. Heilmann C, Stotz U, Burbaum C, et al. Short-term intervention to reduce anxiety before coronary artery bypass surgery–a randomised controlled trial. J Clin Nurs. 2016;25(3–4):351–61.
27. Freshwater MF, Su CT. The second rule of nines: a guide for resuscitation of burn patients. Ann Plast Surg. 1979;2(4):298.

12

Graft protective effect and induction of CD4$^+$Foxp3$^+$ cell by Thrombomodulin on allograft arteriosclerosis in mice

Enzhi Yin[1,2†], Shigefumi Matsuyama[3,4†], Masateru Uchiyama[1,5*], Kento Kawai[5] and Masanori Niimi[1]

Abstract

Background: Thrombomodulin (TM) is a promising therapeutic natural anti-coagulant, which exerts the effects to control disseminated intravascular coagulation. However, little is known whether TM on micro-vessels could play an important role in the regulation of intimal hyperplasia. We investigated the vessel-protective effect of TM in the survival of fully major histocompatibility complex (MHC)-mismatched murine cardiac allograft transplantation.

Methods: CBA recipients transplanted with a C57BL/6 heart received intraperitoneal administration of normal saline or 0.2, 2.0, and 20.0 μg/day of TM for 7 days ($n = 5, 7, 11$, and 11, respectively). Immunohistochemical and fluorescent staining studies were performed to determine whether CD4$^+$Foxp3$^+$ regulatory T cell were generated at 2 and 4 weeks after grafting. Morphometric analysis for neointimal formation in the coronary arteries of the transplanted allograft was conducted at 2 and 4 weeks after grafting.

Results: Untreated CBA recipients rejected C57BL/6 cardiac grafts acutely (median survival time [MST], 7 days). CBA recipients exposed with the above doses had significantly prolonged allograft survival (MSTs, 17, 24 and 50 days, respectively). Morphometric assessment showed that intimal hyperplasia was clearly suppressed in the left and right coronary arteries or allografts from TM-exposed recipients 2 and 4 weeks. Immunohistochemical studies at 2 weeks showed more CD4$^+$Foxp3$^+$ cells and lower myocardial damage in the allografts from TM-exposed recipients. Notably, fluorescent staining studies demonstrated that TM-exposed recipients 4 weeks post-engraftment had strong aggregation of CD4$^+$Foxp3$^+$ cells in the intima of the coronary arteries of the cardiac allografts.

Conclusions: TM may prolong the survival of fully MHC-mismatched cardiac allografts through suppressing intimal hyperplasia and inducing the accumulation of regulatory CD4$^+$Foxp3$^+$ cells within coronary arteries.

Keywords: Thrombomodulin (CD141), graft protection, CD4$^+$Foxp3$^+$ cell, heart transplantation

Background

The coagulation cascade is a multi-step process that can cause efficient clotting even with minimal coagulatory activation. Hemostatic factors such as platelets and coagulation factors are produced in surplus of as much as ten times more than required for effective clotting; thus, even if the number of platelets were to decrease to one tenth, bleeding rarely occurs. Conversely, anti-coagulation mechanisms are much less dynamic due to the lack of a similar enhancement system and minimal circulating anti-coagulants in comparison. In comparison, even diminishing the anticoagulants to half its normal amount will render it ineffective in preventing the formation of clots. Therefore, exogenous anti-coagulants (i.e. heparin sulfate, tissue plasminogen activator, prostacyclin, nitric oxide, and thrombomodulin) are frequently administered to prevent excessive coagulation. In particular, thrombomodulin (TM) has recently been used as a promising therapeutic natural anti-coagulant drug within clinical trials.

Discovered by Esmon et al. in 1982, TM (CD141) is expressed on the endothelial cell surface of all vessels

* Correspondence: mautiya@yahoo.co.jp
†Enzhi Yin and Shigefumi Matsuyama contributed equally to this work.
[1]Department of Surgery, Teikyo University, 2-11-1 Kaga, Itabashi-ku, Tokyo 173-8605, Japan
[5]Transplantation Research Immunology Group, Nuffield Department of Surgical Sciences, University of Oxford, John Radcliffe Hospital, Oxford, UK
Full list of author information is available at the end of the article

[1]. The anti-coagulatory effects of TM can alleviate disseminated intravascular coagulation (DIC) induced by hematologic malignancy and severe infections such as sepsis [2]. It was demonstrated that TM forms a complex with thrombin that activates protein C (PC), which then inactivates Va and VIIIa factor to regulate subsequent thrombin formation [1]. After the anti-coagulatory mechanism of TM was gradually elucidated, use of recombinant human soluble TM (rTM) for the treatment of DIC and severe infections was approved in Japan in 2008, leading to many mega-studies on TM. For instance in Japan in 2007, a randomized, double-blind clinical, and phase III trial on the effects of rTM and low-dose heparin on DIC associated with hematologic malignancy or infection demonstrated that rTM could improve DIC resolution rate and clinical course of bleeding symptoms [2]. In Belgium in 2013, another randomized, double-blind, phase IIa trial on the effects of rTM on DIC associated with sepsis showed that D-dimer and pro-thrombin fragments, which are markers of the fibrinolytic system, were lower in the rTM group than in the placebo group [3]. Motivated by favorable outcomes in clinical trials and the promising effectiveness of TM on the control of coagulation and inflammation under severe conditions, we hypothesized that TM-based therapy may be effective in mediating acute rejection of heart transplantation by regulating or suppressing conditions such as myocardial destruction and micro-vasculopathy.

Generally, TM is thought to be expressed on the endothelial cell surface of all vessels. However, little is known whether TM expression on micro-vessels could play a role in the regulation of microcirculation disturbance or allograft vessel protection. In a study on pediatric heart transplant recipients, serum levels of post-transplant TM were elevated after transplantation, except in patients with severe chronic allograft vasculopathy who displayed significantly lower levels [4]. Moreover, some reports indicated the effects of TM to transplantation-associated microangiopathy after hematopoietic stem cell transplantation [5]. Taken together, these insights may indicate that the manipulation of TM concentration can mediate progression of angiopathy and that fluctuation of natural TM can be used as a clinical biomarker after transplant. Therefore, in this study we investigated whether coagulopathy and microvasculopathy play a role in the pathogenesis of allograft rejection and also whether TM-based treatment had vessel-protective effects in a model of fully MHC-mismatched murine cardiac allograft transplantation.

Methods
Animals
Male CBA (H2^k) and C57BL/6 (H2^b, B6) mice that were 8 to 12 weeks of age were purchased from Sankyo Ltd.

(Tokyo, Japan), housed in conventional facilities at the Biomedical Services Unit of Teikyo University, and used in accordance with the guidelines for animal experimentation approved by Medicine Animal Ethics Committee of Teikyo University (13-023, 7/11/2013) and the "Principles of laboratory animal care" (NIH publication, vol. 25, no. 28, revised 1996).

Heart transplantation
Heart transplantation was conducted as described previously [6]. Briefly, all heart transplantation in mice were performed by one operator who can achieve a 98% successful rate. In this experiment (donor: male B6; recipient: male CBA), fully allogeneic cardiac transplant model with transplanted heart beating over 3 days was considered as a successful and recordable model. The operation began with preparation of the recipient animal. Under an operation microscope at 15× magnification the inferior vena cava and abdominal aorta below the renal vessels were dissected free, as ligating lumbar veins and arteries between sufficient recipient vessels for anastomosis. Two Scoville-lewis clamps (Downs Surgical Ltd., London, UK) were placed around both aorta and vena cava in preparation for later occlusion of the vessels. In preparation of the donor animal, inferior vena cava, azygos vein, and the superior vena cava were ligated with 7-0 silk sutures in order. The aorta and pulmonary artery were separated and divided as far distally as possible. The pulmonary veins were ligated as a group with a single 7-0 silk sutures. The donor aorta was sutured end-to-side to the recipient abdominal aorta using 10-0 surgical suture (Kyowa Precision Instruments Crop., Tokyo, Japan) (Fig. 1). Subsequently the pulmonary artery was anastomosed to the recipient inferior vena cava. Upon release of the clamps the heart begun to fibrillate and usually within a few minutes it reverted to a sinus rhythm. Postoperatively, cardiac graft function was assessed daily by palpating the heart for evidence of

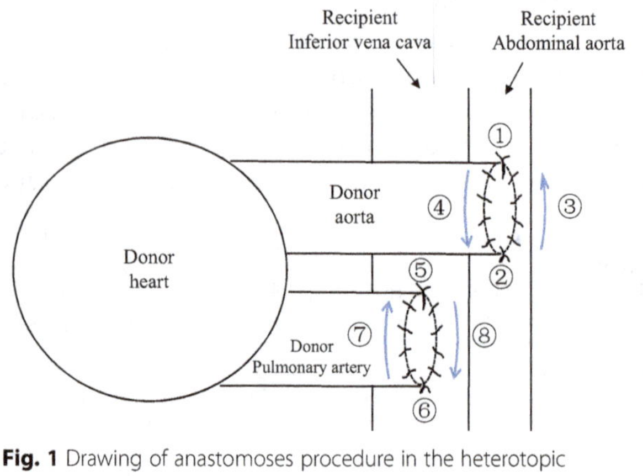

Fig. 1 Drawing of anastomoses procedure in the heterotopic cardiac grafts

contraction. Rejection was defined as complete cessation of the heartbeat and confirmed by direct visualization and histologic examination of the graft.

Measurement of TM

Transplanted CBA recipients with beating B6 heart (untreated recipients) and naïve CBA mice were prepared to evaluate the concentration of serum TM in time series. The serums from untreated recipients on day 3, 5, 7, and 10 after grafting and naïve mice were obtained. Measurement of TM was assessed by using an ELISA for TM (R&D, #MTHBD0, Mouse Thrombomodulin/BDCA-3 Quantikine ELISA Kit, MN, USA) according to the manufacturer's instructions.

Exposure to TM

Transplanted CBA recipients were intraperitoneally exposed with one dose of 0.2, 2.0, and 20.0 µg/day of TM (Asahi Kasei Pharma Corporation, Tokyo, Japan) for the replenishment of TM from the day of cardiac transplantation to 7 days afterward (n = 7, 11, and 11, respectively). Each dose of TM was diluted with normal saline (1 ml). Transplant recipients in the control group were given intraperitoneal injections of normal saline (n = 5).

Morphometric analysis of neointimal formation in allografts

The morphometric analysis was conducted as described previously [7]. Coronary artery cross-sections of donor B6 hearts from TM-exposed and untreated recipients 2 and 4 weeks after grafting were visualized by type IV collagen staining and analyzed by computer-assisted morphometry. The coronary arteries such as the left coronary artery (LCA) and the right coronary artery (RCA) were analyzed in the anatomical regions labeled clearly as the right ventricle and left ventricle as described in the previous paper [7]. All morphometric comparts including the lumen and intima were assessed by the image software (NanoZoomer Digital Pathology Virtual Slide Viewer, Hamamatsu Photonics, Hamamatsu, Shizuoka, Japan). The quantitative methodology was developed to assess the neointimal formation through the stenosis index (SI). SI was calculated as a percentage by dividing intimal area by the sum of lumen and intimal area.

Histological, immunohistochemical (IHC) and fluorescent staining studies of harvest grafts

Cardiac allografts transplanted into untreated and TM-treated CBA recipients were removed 2 weeks after grafting and studied histologically and immunohistochemically. Frozen sections (4-µm thick) were cut, mounted on silane-coated slides, and stained with hematoxylin-eosin (HE). HE staining was assessed by

grading with a semi-quantitative scale for the amount of mononuclear cell infiltration (0, no infiltration; 1, faint and limited infiltration; 2, moderate infiltration; 3, severe infiltration) [8, 9]. All graft heart slides were assessed blindly by unrelated three researchers.

IHC and fluorescent staining studies were performed to determine whether the myocardial function in the transplanted cardiac allografts was preserved and CD4$^+$Foxp3$^+$ regulatory T cells were generated. Results of double immunostaining of cardiac allografts were obtained 2 and 4 weeks after transplantation from mice exposed to 20.0 µg/day of TM. Additionally, the expression of TM (CD141) in cardiac allografts from TM-treated recipients was examined on 4 weeks after grafting. Fresh 4-µm-thick graft cryosections were fixed in ice-cold acetone and preincubated in Block Ace (Dainippon Pharmaceutical Co., Ltd., Tokyo, Japan). Samples were incubated with anti-CD4 monoclonal antibody (mAb) (RM4-5; BD Biosciences, San Jose, CA) and anti-CD141 (AF3894; R&D System) polyclonal antibody, or anti-Foxp3 mAb (FJK-16 s, eBioscience); incubated with alkaline phosphatase (ALP)-conjugated anti-rat Ig (712-055-153; Jackson ImmunoResearch Laboratories, West Grove, PA) for anti-CD4, with ALP-conjugated anti-goat Ig (705-055-003; Jackson ImmunoResearch Laboratories) for anti-CD141 and with ALP-conjugated anti-rabbit Ig (712-055-152; Jackson ImmunoResearch Laboratories) for anti-Foxp3; and developed blue with Vector Blue (Vector Laboratories, Burlingame, CA). Cryosections were then incubated with rabbit anti-mouse type IV collagen polyclonal antibody (LB1403; Cosmo Bio, Tokyo) and peroxidase-conjugated anti-rabbit Ig (55,693; Mitsubishi Chemical, Tokyo) and then developed brown with diaminobenzidine (Vector Laboratories). In IHC study, the number of infiltrating CD4$^+$ and Foxp3$^+$ cell in TM-

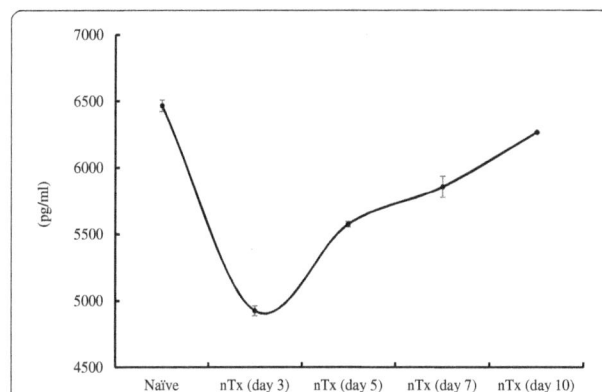

Fig. 2 Measurement of Thrombomodulin (TM) in naïve CBA mice and untreated CBA recipients. The serums from untreated recipients on day 3, 5, 7, and 10 after grafting and naïve mice were obtained. nTx, untreated

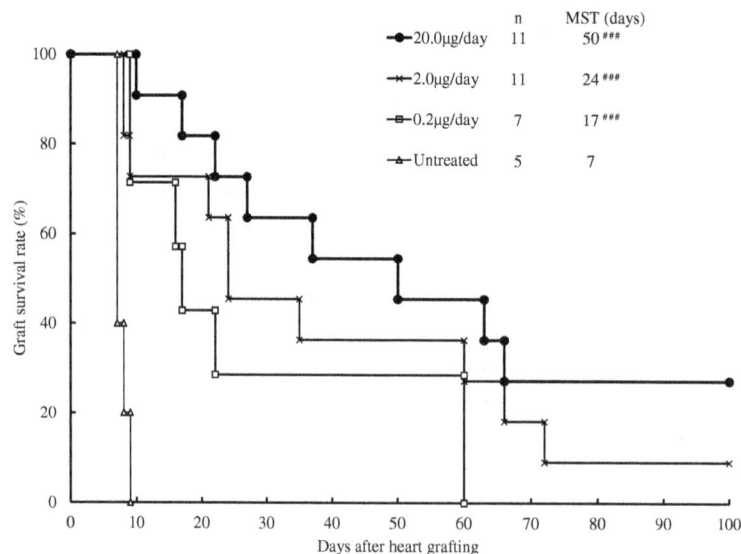

Fig. 3 Cardiac graft survivals in CBA recipients of a C57BL/6 heart that were exposed to 0.2, 2.0, and 20.0 μg/day of Thrombomodulin (TM) from the day of transplantation to 7 days afterward. MST, median survival time. ###$p < 0.001$ compared with untreated group

treated recipient or untreated recipient was counted in the area of 400 μm × 400 μm. All graft heart slides were assessed blindly by unrelated researchers.

Triple fluorescent staining studies of cardiac allograft obtained 4 weeks after grafting from mice exposed to 20.0 μg/day of TM. Fresh 4-μm-thick graft cryosections were incubated with anti-Foxp3 mAb (FJK-16 s, eBioscience); then incubated with Alexa Fluor® 594-conjugated anti-rat Ig (A-11007, Thermo Fisher Scientific, Waltham, MA,

USA) for anti-Foxp3 (shown as red in Fig. 7b). After blocking with normal rat Ig, cryosections were incubated with Alexa Fluor® 647-conjugated anti-CD4 mAb (RM4-5, BioLegend, San Diego, CA) (shown as green in Fig. 7b). Subsequently, cryosections were incubated with rabbit anti–mouse type IV collagen polyclonal antibody (LB1403; Cosmo Bio); then incubated with AMCA-conjugated anti-rabbit Ig (711-155-152, Jackson ImmunoResearch Laboratories) (shown as blue in Fig. 7b).

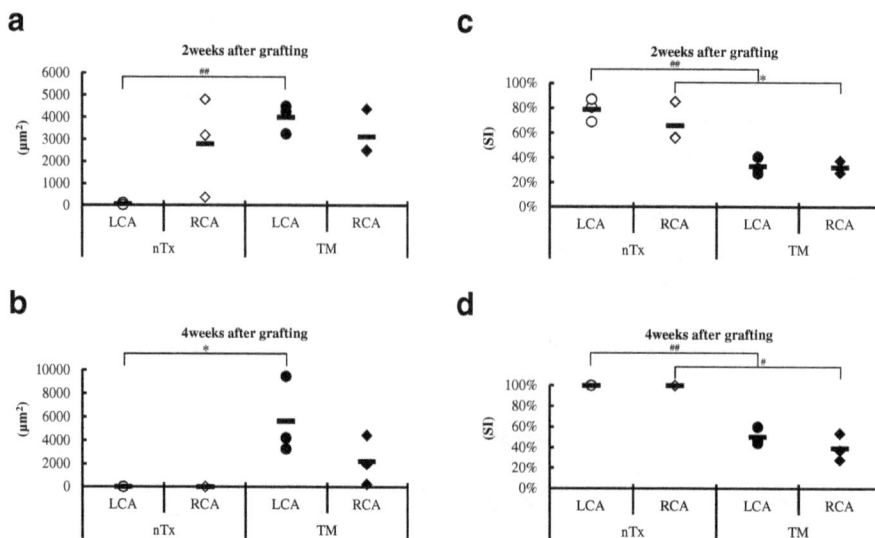

Fig. 4 Morphometric analysis of neointimal formation in transplanted cardiac graft exposed with Thrombomodulin (TM) and normal saline. **a**, **b** Results of lumen area (μm²) in the left coronary arteries (LCA) and the right coronary arteries (RCA) of each group 2 and 4 weeks after grafting. **c**, **d** Results of SI (stenosis index) in LCA and RCA of each group 2 and 4 weeks after grafting. LCA, left coronary artery; nTx, untreated; RCA, right coronary artery; SI, stenosis index. *$p < 0.05$, #$p < 0.01$, and ##$p < 0.005$ for difference between two groups

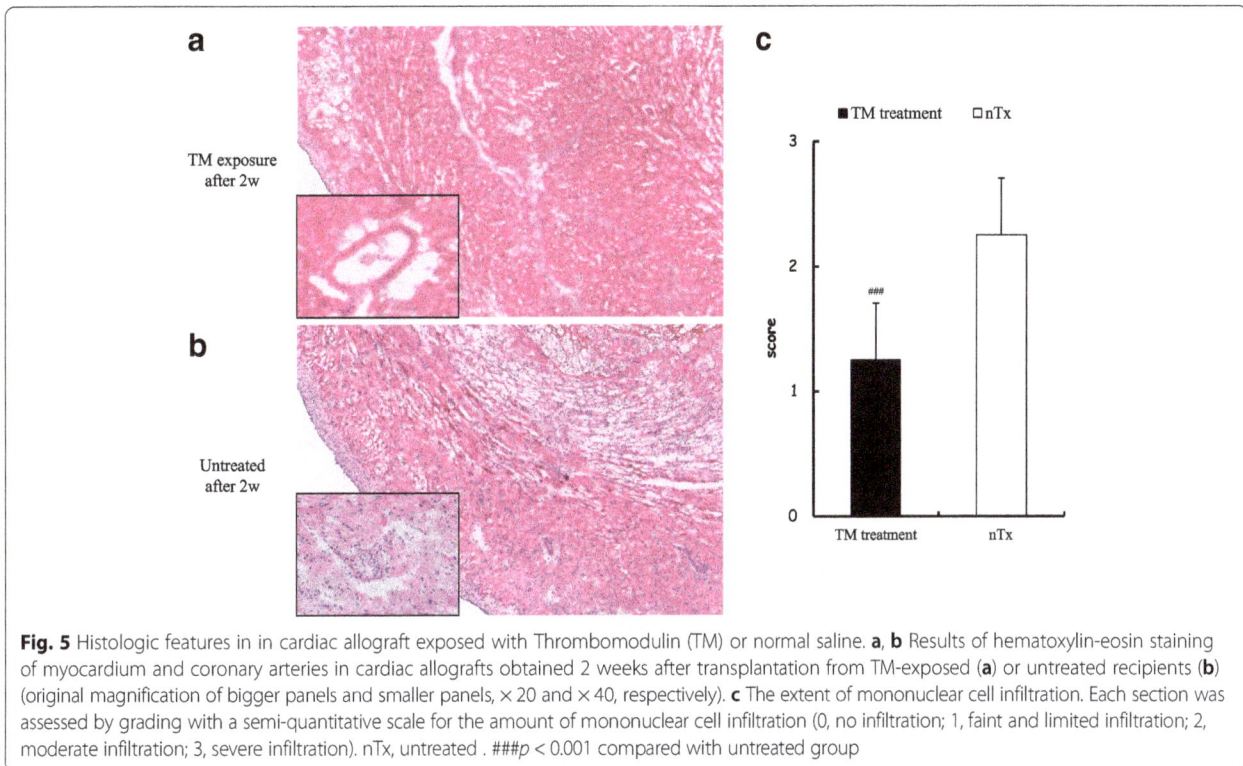

Fig. 5 Histologic features in in cardiac allograft exposed with Thrombomodulin (TM) or normal saline. **a**, **b** Results of hematoxylin-eosin staining of myocardium and coronary arteries in cardiac allografts obtained 2 weeks after transplantation from TM-exposed (**a**) or untreated recipients (**b**) (original magnification of bigger panels and smaller panels, ×20 and ×40, respectively). **c** The extent of mononuclear cell infiltration. Each section was assessed by grading with a semi-quantitative scale for the amount of mononuclear cell infiltration (0, no infiltration; 1, faint and limited infiltration; 2, moderate infiltration; 3, severe infiltration). nTx, untreated . ###$p < 0.001$ compared with untreated group

Statistical analysis

Cardiac allograft survival in two experimental groups was compared by using log-rank test. In the immunohistochemical study, the difference between two groups was assessed by an unpaired Student's t test.

A P value of less than 0.05 was regarded as significant.

Results

Fluctuation of TM

TM concentration in the serum from untreated recipients on day 3, 5, 7, 10 and naïve mice was measured ($n = 3$). TM concentration decreased the most on day 3 after transplantation and gradually recovered afterward (Fig. 2). The level of TM concentration on day 10 was similar to that in naïve mice.

Significant prolonged survival of cardiac allografts in mice exposed with TM

Untreated CBA recipients rejected B6 cardiac grafts acutely ($n = 5$) (median survival time (MST), 7 days). CBA recipients exposed with 0.2 ($n = 7$), 2.0 ($n = 11$) and 20.0 μg/day ($n = 11$) of TM had significantly prolonged allograft survival in a dose-dependent manner (MSTs, 17, 24 and 50 days, respectively, $P < 0.001$ compared with untreated group; Fig. 3).

Suppression of intimal hyperplasia in coronary arteries of donor B6 heart from TM-exposed CBA recipients

Morphometric assessment showed the degree of neointimal formation and coronary stenosis in donor B6 hearts within CBA recipients exposed with TM and normal saline ($n = 3$). LCAs of transplanted B6 heart within TM-treated recipients 2 weeks after grafting remained more patent with minimal obstruction, compared to those of untreated recipients 2 weeks after grafting (Fig. 4a and c). The transplanted B6 heart 4 weeks after grafting showed signs of fibrosis, and all the coronary arteries were stenotic. In the TM treatment group after 4 weeks, similar to the group after 2 weeks, the lumen area was preserved, and SI remained below 50% (Fig. 4b and d).

Histologic features of cardiac allografts in mice exposed with TM

Histologic examinations of cardiac allografts obtained 2 weeks after grafting showed preserved myocardial and vessel structure in TM-exposed recipients, whereas the fracture image of myocardial tissue of allografts from untreated recipients showed the progression of acute rejection (Fig. 5a and b). Moreover, there was a significant difference in the graft score grade on a semi-quantitative scale between the untreated and TM-treated allografts (Fig. 5c).

IHC examinations of cardiac allografts obtained 2 weeks after grafting showed considerable induction

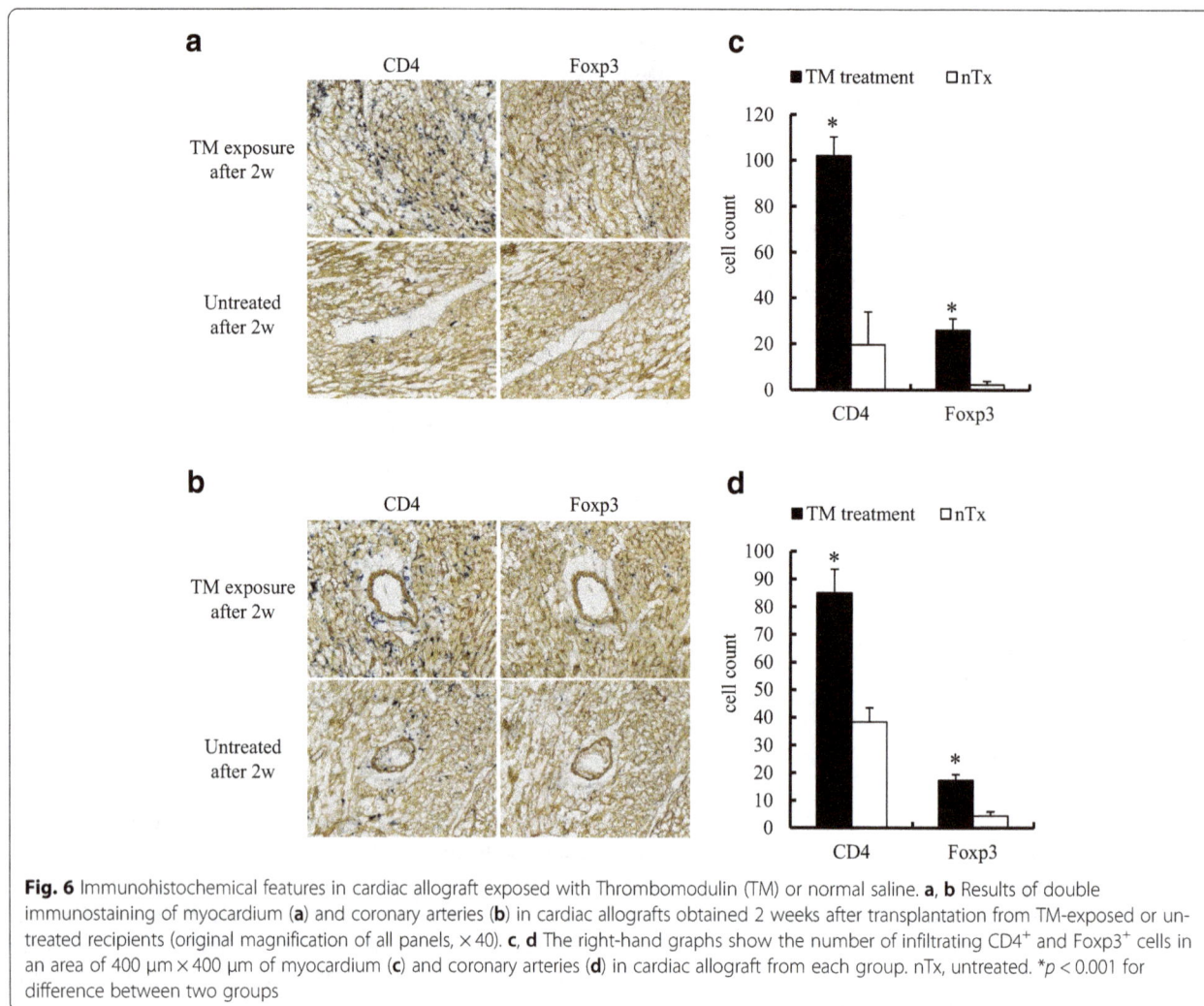

Fig. 6 Immunohistochemical features in cardiac allograft exposed with Thrombomodulin (TM) or normal saline. **a, b** Results of double immunostaining of myocardium (**a**) and coronary arteries (**b**) in cardiac allografts obtained 2 weeks after transplantation from TM-exposed or untreated recipients (original magnification of all panels, ×40). **c, d** The right-hand graphs show the number of infiltrating CD4$^+$ and Foxp3$^+$ cells in an area of 400 μm × 400 μm of myocardium (**c**) and coronary arteries (**d**) in cardiac allograft from each group. nTx, untreated. *$p < 0.001$ for difference between two groups

and infiltration of regulatory T cell-like CD4$^+$Foxp3$^+$ cells in allografts of TM-exposed recipients, whereas allografts from untreated recipients showed more aggressive inflammation, minimal infiltration of CD4$^+$Foxp3$^+$ cells, and signs indicating progression of acute rejection (Fig. 6a and c). Although TM-treated CBA recipients 2 weeks after grafting showed some progression of intimal thickening of coronary arteries in their allografts, the count of infiltration of CD4$^+$Foxp3$^+$ cells around coronary arteries was significantly more than that of untreated mice. Conversely, some vessels in allografts from untreated recipients were stenosed by 50 to 80% or completely obstructed, had less CD4$^+$Foxp3$^+$ cells, and strong filtration of CD4$^+$Foxp3$^-$ cells (Fig. 6b and d). Histologic features after 4 weeks demonstrated clear CD4$^+$Foxp3$^+$ and CD141$^+$ expression on the inner surface of coronary arteries within allografts from TM-exposed recipients relative to those of untreated recipients (Fig. 7a).

Prominent accumulation of CD4$^+$Foxp3$^+$ cells in cardiac allografts from TM-exposed mice

Fluorescent staining studies done 4 weeks after grafting clearly demonstrated that cardiac allografts from TM-exposed CBA recipients had aggregation of CD4$^+$Foxp3$^+$ cell in the myocardium of allograft (Fig. 7a). Notable, infiltration of CD4$^+$Foxp3$^+$ cells to the intima of the coronary arteries in transplanted B6 hearts was observed (Fig. 7b).

Discussion

The present study, demonstrated for the first time that TM administration during cardiac allograft transplantation can have graft-protective effects and induce CD4$^+$Foxp3$^+$ T cells within the allograft to prevent acute rejection in a murine fully MHC-mismatched model. There are several possible mechanisms by which TM administration could induce prolongation of murine cardiac allografts. Firstly, one mechanism may be through the suppression of intimal hyperplasia and

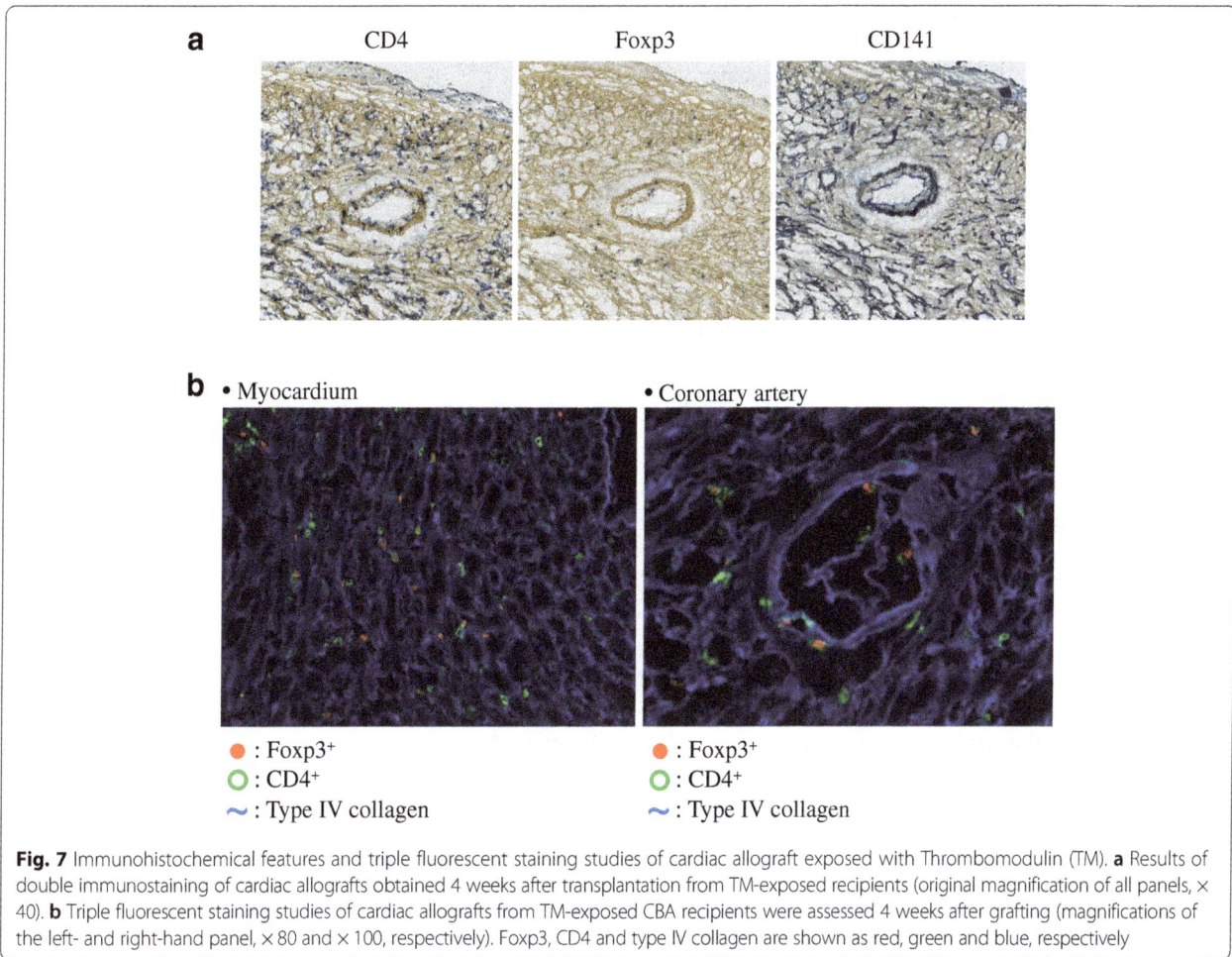

Fig. 7 Immunohistochemical features and triple fluorescent staining studies of cardiac allograft exposed with Thrombomodulin (TM). **a** Results of double immunostaining of cardiac allografts obtained 4 weeks after transplantation from TM-exposed recipients (original magnification of all panels, × 40). **b** Triple fluorescent staining studies of cardiac allografts from TM-exposed CBA recipients were assessed 4 weeks after grafting (magnifications of the left- and right-hand panel, × 80 and × 100, respectively). Foxp3, CD4 and type IV collagen are shown as red, green and blue, respectively

arteriosclerosis within the coronary arteries of the allograft. This is supported by previous studies that have elucidated its activity within transplantation-associated micro-angiopathy [5] and engraftment syndrome after hematopoietic stem cell transplantation [10]. Moreover, another report has demonstrated that TM overexpression limits neointimal formation in common femoral arteries of the rabbit model [11]. In our IHC study, the TM-treated group demonstrated preserved myocardial structure at 2 weeks post-transplantation and showed a significant statistical difference compared to the control group that had all rejected their grafts by 2 weeks (Fig. 5). Additionally, the vascular structure within the coronary artery in the TM treatment group was maintained and infiltration of inflammatory cells such as monocytes into the coronary arteries was suppressed (Fig. 5). In concordance with our IHC results, both the LCA and RCA in the control group 2 weeks after grafting were narrowed by an average of 60 to 80%, whereas the stenosis rate of the TM treatment group was limited to about 30% (Fig. 4). This disparity was even more distinct after 4 weeks. The allografts of the untreated group 4 weeks after grafting

showed progression of fibrosis and almost all the coronary arteries were occluded, whereas TM treatment held the coronary stenosis rate at 40 to 50%, suggesting that the graft protective effect could continue up to 3 weeks after administration of TM. However, there were no findings to suggest that the effect of TM remained beyond 3 weeks from the end of TM administration, so it was conceivable that there would be other mechanisms in play to explain the vascular protective effects after 4 weeks post-engraftment.

Our previous studies have demonstrated that substantial accumulation of inducible CD4+Foxp3+ regulatory T cells was observed around the coronary arteries of prolonged grafts [12–14]. Thus, based on the previous findings, it was reasoned that a second mechanism by which TM can protect the graft is through the generation of regulatory CD4+Foxp3+ T cell. From the IHC staining, it was observed that CD4+Foxp3+ cells accumulated in the myocardium and around the coronary arteries of allografts in the TM-treated recipients at 2 weeks after grafting (Fig. 6). After 4 weeks, while assessment of pathological staining became difficult in the untreated group due to severe fibrosis, CD4$^+$Foxp3$^+$ cells and CD141 expression in the myocardium and around the coronary arteries of allografts within TM-treated recipients were maintained while it was not in the untreated group. TM's effect on CD4$^+$Foxp3$^+$ cells has also been documented in previous reports. rTM administration to murine acute respiratory distress syndrome (ARDS) model has been shown to induce prolongation of survival time and ameliorate development of ARDS through increasing regulatory T cell in the lung [15]. Moreover, in another study, it was shown to alleviate GVHD via increasing splenic regulatory T cell [16]. Based on our previous data, it can be reasoned that inducible CD4$^+$Foxp3$^+$ Treg do not disappear in a short period of time [17, 18]. From the findings in this study that demonstrate that the general structure of the allograft was maintained even three weeks after termination of TM administration, it can be concluded that TM may generate CD4$^+$Foxp3$^+$ regulatory T cells that infiltrate transplanted cardiac allografts and that greater aggregation of these cells around coronary arteries may lead to the prolongation of allograft survival.

There are some limitations to this study. First, 50% of TM-treated recipients did not show the prolongation of allograft for more than 100 days after grafting. We determined the term of 7 days of TM administration according to previous studies on TM treatment for DIC that have only administered TM up to 7 days from the onset of DIC and the fact that 90% of our transplanted recipients rejected allografts acutely within 8 days. Future work which extends the administration period or optimizes TM dosage may yield enlightening results. Second, the correlation between blood concentration of TM administrated and graft survival after TM administration is unknown. Considering the minute difference of MST, it might be necessary to evaluate the TM concentration after administration in time series. Finally, the present study was conducted using a small number of mice with a limited follow-up period. If the efficiency of TM pointed out by this study is observed in the long-term, a longer observation period and detailed analysis of these recipients is required.

Conclusion

In summary, TM prolonged survival of fully MHC-mismatched cardiac allograft through the suppression of intimal hyperplasia and inducing the accumulation of regulatory CD4$^+$Foxp3$^+$ cell within the coronary arteries. Further research which optimizes the TM regimen after allograft transplantation may lead to even greater outcomes.

Abbreviations

ALP: Alkaline phosphatase; C57BL/6: B6; DIC: Disseminated intravascular coagulation; HE: Hematoxylin-eosin; IHC: Immunohistochemical; LCA: Left coronary artery; mAb: Monoclonal antibody; MHC: Major histocompatibility complex; MST: Median survival time; PC: Protein C; RCA: Right coronary artery; rTM: Recombinant human soluble thrombomodulin; SI: Stenosis index; TM: Thrombomodulin

Acknowledgements

The authors thank Prof. Kenjiro Matsuno and Mr. Hisashi Ueta, Department of Anatomy (Macro), Dokkyo University, Tochigi, Japan for technical assistance with the immunohistochemistry studies, and Prof. Toshio Nakaki and Dr. Nobuko Matsumura, Department of Pharmacology, Teikyo University School of Medicine, Tokyo, Japan for technical assistance with histological studies.

Funding

This work was supported by JSPS KAKENHI Grant Number 15 K19927.

Authors' contributions

MU and MN designed the research, analyzed the data, and was the major contributor in writing the manuscript. EY and SM carried out the research. Collected the data and analyzed the data. KK provided the editorial effort. All authors read and approved the final manuscript.

Competing interests

All authors declare that they have no competing interests.

Author details

[1]Department of Surgery, Teikyo University, 2-11-1 Kaga, Itabashi-ku, Tokyo 173-8605, Japan. [2]Department of Cardiovascular Surgery, The 2nd Affiliated Hospital of Harbin Medical University, Harbin, China. [3]Department of Cardiovascular Surgery, New Tokyo Hospital, Chiba, Japan. [4]Department of Cardiovascular Surgery, Teikyo University, Tokyo, Japan. [5]Transplantation Research Immunology Group, Nuffield Department of Surgical Sciences, University of Oxford, John Radcliffe Hospital, Oxford, UK.

References

1. Esmon NL, Owen WG, Esmon CT. Isolation of a membrane-bound cofactor for thrombin-catalyzed activation of protein C. J Biol Chem. 1982;257:859–64.
2. Saito H, Maruyama I, Shimazaki S, Yamamoto Y, Aikawa N, Ohno R, et al. Efficacy and safety of recombinant human soluble thrombomodulin (ART-123) in disseminated intravascular coagulation: results of a phase III, randomized, double-blind clinical trial. J Thromb Haemost. 2007;5:31–41.
3. Vincent JL, Ramesh MK, Ernest D, LaRosa SP, Pachl J, Aikawa N, et al. A randomized, double-blind, placebo-controlled, phase 2b study to evaluate the safety and efficacy of recombinant human soluble thrombomodulin, ART-123, in patients with sepsis and suspected disseminated intravascular coagulation. Crit Care Med. 2013;41:2069–79.
4. Fenton M, Simmonds J, Shah V, Brogan P, Klein N, Deanfield J, et al. Inflammatory cytokines, endothelial function, and chronic allograft vasculopathy in children: an investigation of the donor and recipient vasculature after heart transplantation. Am J Transplant. 2016;16:1559–68.
5. Sakai M, Ikezoe T, Bandobashi K, Togitani K, Yokoyama A. Successful treatment of transplantation-associated thrombotic microangiopathy with recombinant human soluble thrombomodulin. Bone Marrow Transplant. 2010;45:803–5.
6. Niimi M. The technique for heterotopic cardiac transplantation in mice: experience of 3000 operations by one surgeon. J Heart Lung Transplant. 2001;20:1123–8.
7. Armstrong AT, Strauch AR, Starling RC, Sedmak DD, Orosz CG. Morphometric analysis of neointimal formation in murine cardiac allografts: II. Rate and location of lesion development. Transplantation. 1997;64:322–8.
8. Stewart S, Winters GL, Fishbein MC, Tazelaar HD, Kobashigawa J, Abrams J, et al. Revision of the 1990 working formulation for the standardization of nomenclature in the diagnosis of heart rejection. J Heart Lung Transplant. 2005;24:1710–20.

9. Billingham ME, Cary NR, Hammond ME, Kemnitz J, Marboe C, McCallister HA, et al. A working formulation for the standardization of nomenclature in the diagnosis of heart and lung rejection: heart rejection study group. The international society for heart transplantation. J Heart Transplant. 1990;9:587–93.

10. Ikezoe T, Takeuchi A, Taniguchi A, Togitani K, Yokoyama A. Recombinant human soluble thrombomodulin counteracts capillary leakage associated with engraftment syndrome. Bone Marrow Transplant. 2011;46:616–8.

11. Waugh JM, Li-Hawkins J, Yuksel E, Kuo MD, Cifra PN, Hilfiker PR, et al. Thrombomodulin overexpression to limit neointima formation. Circulation. 2000;102:332–7.

12. Uchiyama M, Jin X, Yin E, Shimokawa T, Niimi M. Treadmill exercise induces murine cardiac allograft survival and generates regulatory T cell. Transpl Int. 2015;28:352–62.

13. Uchiyama M, Yin E, Yanagisawa T, Jin X, Hara M, Matsuyama S, et al. Yogurt feeding induced the prolongation of fully major histocompatibility complex-mismatched murine cardiac graft survival by induction of CD4 +Foxp3+ cells. Transplant Proc. 2017;49:1477–82.

14. Uchiyama M, Jin X, Zhang Q, Hirai T, Bashuda H, Watanabe T, et al. Danazol induces prolonged survival of fully allogeneic cardiac grafts and maintains the generation of regulatory CD4[+] cells in mice. Transpl Int. 2012;25:357–65.

15. Kudo D, Toyama M, Aoyagi T, Akahori Y, Yamamoto H, Ishii K, et al. Involvement of high mobility group box 1 and the therapeutic effect of recombinant thrombomodulin in a mouse model of severe acute respiratory distress syndrome. Clin Exp Immunol. 2013;173:276–87.

16. Ikezoe T, Yang J, Nishioka C, Yokoyama A. Thrombomodulin alleviates murine GVHD in association with an increase in the proportion of regulatory T cells in the spleen. Bone Marrow Transplant. 2015;50:113–20.

17. Uchiyama M, Jin X, Matsuda H, Bashuda H, Imazuru T, Shimokawa T, et al. An agonistic anti-BTLA mAb (3C10) induced generation of IL-10-dependent regulatory CD4[+] T cells and prolongation of murine cardiac allograft. Transplantation. 2014;97:301–9.

18. Uchiyama M, Jin X, Zhang Q, Hirai T, Amano A, Bashuda H, et al. Auditory stimulation of opera music induced prolongation of murine cardiac allograft survival and maintained generation of regulatory CD4[+]CD25[+] cells. J Cardiothorac Surg. 2012;7:26.

13

Risk factors and treatment of pneumothorax secondary to granulomatosis with polyangiitis: a clinical analysis of 25 cases

Xuhua Shi, Yongfeng Zhang and Yuewu Lu[*] ⓘD

Abstract

Objectives: To investigate the risk factors and treatment strategies for pneumothorax secondary to granulomatosis with polyangiitis (GPA).

Method: Retrospective analysis of cases with pneumothorax secondary to GPA from our own practice and published on literature.

Results: A total of 25 patients, 18 males and 7 females, mean age 44 ± 15.7 years, were analyzed. Diagnosis included pneumothorax (11 cases), hydropneumothorax ($n = 5$), empyema ($n = 8$) and hemopneumothorax ($n = 1$). 88% (22/25) patients showed single/multiple pulmonary/ subpleural nodules with/without cavitation on chest imaging. Erythrocyte sedimentation rate and C-reactive protein were both elevated. Corticosteroids and immunosuppressive agents were used in 16 cases. Five cases received steroid pulse therapy, of which 4 patients survived. Pleural drainage was effective in some patients. Seven patients underwent surgical operations. In the 10 fatal cases, infection and respiratory failure were the most common cause. Lung biopsy/ autopsy showed lung/pleural necrotizing granulomatous vasculitis, breaking into the chest cavity, pleural fibrosis, bronchial pleural fistula, etc. The mean age in the death group was greater than the survival group (53 ± 12.9 years vs 40.1 ± 14.7 years, $p = 0.05$), the ineffective pleural drainage was also higher in the death group (5/5 vs 0/7, $p = 0.01$).

Conclusions: Pneumothorax was seen in the active GPA, due to a variety of reasons, and gave rise to high fatality rate. Aggressive treatment of GPA can improve the prognosis. Older and lack of response for pleural drainage indicates poor prognosis.

Keywords: Granulomatosis with Polyangiitis, Wegener's granulomatosis, Pneumothorax

Background

Granulomatosis with polyangiitis (GPA), also known as Wegener's granulomatosis, is a necrotizing granulomatous vasculitis, most commonly involving lung (Fig. 1), upper respiratory tract, and kidney [1]. When the respiratory system is involved, lung imaging study usually shows nodules, infiltrates, alveolar hemorrhage [2]. When pleural is involved, the patient can present with pleurisy, pleural effusion and thickening. Pneumothorax is a rare but serious complication, when occurred, can be categorized into pneumothorax, hydropneumothorax, empyema, hemopneumothorax, etc [3, 4]. So far there were only 20 cases of pneumothorax reported and the clinical presentation varied. Also, the cause and risk factors of GPA associated pneumothorax are unclear, and there is no consensus on important aspects of treatment strategy, such as, when the pneumothorax or infection is developed, how should treatment for the primary disease be adjusted? How to appropriately apply the pleural drainage and other surgical interventions? We encountered one case of GPA associated hydropneumothorax in our clinic who recovered after undergone active treatment of the primary disease

* Correspondence: sxhherosci@sina.com; llyyww615@sina.com
Department of Rheumatology and Immunology, Beijing Chao-Yang Hospital, Capital Medical University, 8 Gongren Tiyuchang Nanlu, Chaoyang District, Beijing 100020, China

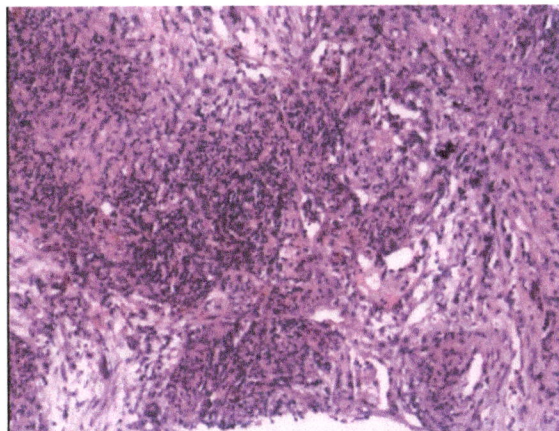

Fig. 1 The microscopic features of pulmonary nodule obtained by percutaneous lung biopsy in a patient with granulomatous vasculitis (GPA). There are more infiltrating lymphocytes, neutrophils and eosinophils in fibrous tissues. Granulomas composed of tissue cells and inflammatory cells are also visible. There are prominent inflammatory cell infiltration and granuloma in the wall of small vessels. HE staining, 100×

and pleural drainage. The incidence of GPA associated pneumothorax is low. However, if not treated properly the fatality rate can be quite high. Currently there is still no cohort-based research. Therefore, we conducted a retrospective analysis of our case and all cases reported in the literature [4–24], aiming to identify the risk factors of GPA associated pneumothorax and explore the important principles of its clinical management once occurred, to guide the optimal treatment of the patients.

Materials and methods

Because it is a retrospective research, the period of observation spans from 1978 (the first case) to 2015 (the last case). The patients came from two sources. The first was the case diagnosed and treated in our clinic. The second source included cases reported in the literature identified from the search of major databases, including: Chinese Biomedical Literature Database (CBM), Pubmed, EMBASE, and BIOSIS Preview. The searching key words were "pneumothorax", "multi-vessel granulomatous inflammation" and "Wegener's granulomatosis." Full text articles were retrieved for review. All procedures performed in studies involving human participants were in accordance with the ethical standards of the institutional and/or national research committee and with the 1964 Helsinki declaration and its later amendments or comparable ethical standards.

Given the small number of reported cases and wide time span covered by the search, we went over the papers carefully, excluded the cases of pneumothorax unrelated to GPA (for example, pneumothorax caused by lung biopsy during the disease diagnosis). One lung imaging study included 31 cases of Wegener's

granulomatosis confirmed by clinical and pathology examination, but only had 1 case complicated by pneumothorax. We carefully reviewed and collected information on each patient's clinical diagnoses, gender, age, time from disease onset to the development of pneumothorax, diagnosis of pneumothorax, the type of pneumothorax (pneumothorax, hydropneumothorax, empyema, hemopneumothorax), clinical presentations, laboratory test results (including anti-neutrophil cytoplasmic antibodies, anti-PR3 antibody, erythrocyte sedimentation rate, C-reactive protein), lung imaging findings (X ray / CT), corticosteroids and immunosuppressants treatment, pleural drainage, surgery, infection (infection site, pathogens, etc.), biopsy / autopsy pathology results. Four cases were reported from non-English literature, for which the information was gathered from the abstract written in English.

Case analysis included general patient characteristics (gender, age, duration of disease, type of pneumothorax, lung imaging findings, extrapulmonary manifestations, laboratory results, treatment and prognosis), infection (infection site, pathogens, etc.), biopsy / autopsy pathology results (lungs and other organs), as well as comparison between death and survived patients. This analysis included patients who met the 1990 American College of Rheumatology (ACR) classification criteria for Wegener's granulomatosis [1, 25] defined as follows: 1) Nasal or oral inflammation: development of painful or painless oral ulcers or purulent or bloody nasal discharge; 2) Abnormal chest radiograph: chest radiograph showing the presence of nodules, fixed infiltrates, or cavities; 3) Urinary sediment: microhematuria (>5 red blood cells per high power field) or red cell casts in urine sediment; 4) Granulomatous inflammation on biopsy: histologic changes showing granulomatous inflammation within the wall of an artery or in the perivascular or extravascular area (artery or arteriole). Patients need to meet at least 2 criteria to be diagnosed as Wegener's granulomatosis. The cases diagnosed before 1990 were confirmed with biopsy showing necrotizing granulomatous vasculitis.

Statistical analysis

The general characteristics of the patients were summarized with descriptive statistics. Age, duration, anti-PR3, erythrocyte sedimentation rate (ESR) and C-reactive protein (CRP) were expressed as mean ± standard deviation, and were compared between death group and survival group using independent t-test. Categorical variables, including sex, types of pneumothorax, chest imaging (nodules, cavity, pulmonary hemorrhage), extrapulmonary manifestations (fever, skin lesions, nasal and sinus involvement, oral ulcers, renal involvement, nervous system involvement, arthralgia / arthritis, parotid swelling), positived ANCA, pleural drainage, surgery, spontaneous absorption, death, infection site, pathogens, biopsy site and pathology, therapy and interruption of treatment, risk factors for pneumothorax secondary to GPA, were summarized as percentage, and were analyzed between death group and survival group using chi-square test.

Results

The first case in the series was from our clinic. The patient had sinusitis for 20 years, purulent nasal discharge, hemoptysis for 3 years, repeated skin ulcers for 2 years, difficulty in breathing for 2 months before being hospitalized. At admission, lung CT showed bilateral multiple nodules with/without cavity (biopsy indicated granulomatous inflammation). Right cavity ruptured and resulted in hydropneumothorax. C-ANCA was positive, the level of anti-PR3 was 150.5RU/ml. The condition improved after pleural drainage and treatment with corticosteroids and cyclophosphamide, cyclosporine A. The rest of the series included 1 case from the Chinese Biomedical Literature Database, and 23 cases from PubMed, EMBASE, BIOSIS Preview databases. The total was 25 cases.

The average age of the case series was 44 years, with a male to female ratio of 2.6: 1. The disease duration ranged from 1 month to 18 years. In 8 patients GPA was diagnosed after the occurrence of pneumothorax. The type of pneumothorax included pneumothorax, hydropneumothorax, empyema, hemopneumothorax. Respiratory symptoms presented were cough (5 cases), chest tightness and shortness of breath (9 cases), dyspnea (10 cases), and hemoptysis (2 cases). The majority of patients (88%) showed single or multiple nodules with/without cavitation on lung imaging. All patients had extrapulmonary manifestations, including fever, ear and nose involvement, neurologic symptoms, glomerulonephritis, and skin lesion. Most patients were treated with glucocorticoid (steroid pulse therapy for some patients) and immunosuppressive agents. In certain patients the medications were interrupted after the diagnosis of pneumothorax / infection and resulted in two deaths. None of the patients in the survivors group stopped the medication. Also, in the survivor group, about one-third patients received corticosteroid pulse therapy, while this was only 10% in the death group. Some patients did not undergo pleural drainage and successfully recovered from spontaneous absorption. The effects of pleural drainage were also mixed. Seven patients underwent surgeries, including pulmonary cavity resection, pulmonary lobectomy, and partial pleurectomy, etc. Four patients underwent surgery because the lung failed to re-expand or there were large persistent air volume leaks after pleural drainage and the details were not recorded properly. The fatality rate was high due to infection, respiratory failure, sepsis, respiratory arrest (Table 1). Infection involved the lungs, thoracic cavity, blood circulation, etc. Pseudomonas aeruginosa

Table 1 General characteristics of patients with pneumothorax secondary to GPA

Clinical features	Results
Male/Female (case)	18(72%)/7(28%)
Age(year)	44 ± 15.7(16~70)
Duration (weeks)	26 ± 51.0(0.83~216)
Pneumothorax type (case)	
Pneumothorax	11(44%)
hydropneumothorax	5 (20)
empyema[a]	8 (32%)
Hemopneumothorax	1 (4%)
Chest Imaging(n)	
Nodules (Multi/Single)	22(88%)
Cavity	21(84%)
Pulmonary hemorrhage	1 (4%)
Extrapulmonary manifestations (n)	
Fever	11(44%)
Skin lesions (purpura, gangrene, ulcers, etc.)	7 (28%)
Nasal and sinus involvement	15(60%)
Oral ulcers	5 (20%)
Glomerulonephritis and other	13(52%)
Nervous system (facial paralysis, mononeuropathy, etc.)	6 (24%)
Arthralgia/arthritis	11(44%)
Parotid swelling	2 (8%)
Laboratory tests	
ANCA-positive(n)	13/20(65%)
Anti-PR3(RU/ml)	176 ± 145.3(26~411)
ESR (mm/h)	92 ± 31.6(24~145)
CRP (mg/dl)	20 ± 27.4(2.35~90)
Pleural drainage(n)	16
Surgery(n)	7 (28%)
Spontaneous absorption(n)	4 (16%)
Death	10(40%)

Note: ANCA, anti-neutrophil cytoplasmic antibodies; anti-PR3, anti-proteinase 3 antibody; ESR, erythrocyte sedimentation rate; CRP, C-reactive protein
[a]These cases with empyema showed a clear pneumothorax at chest X-ray or CT scan

were frequently detected (Table 2). Biopsy/autopsy showed lung nodules, pleural necrotizing granulomatous vasculitis, breaking into the pleural cavity, pleural fibrosis, and bronchial pleural fistula (Table 3). The average age of death group was greater than the average age of survivor group ($53 ± 12.9$ years vs $40.1 ± 14.7$ years, $p = 0.05$). In the death group, lack of response to pleural drainage which refers to the failure of the lung to re-expand or large persistent air volume leaks, was more common than that in the survivors (5/5 vs 0/7, $p = 0.01$) (Table 4).

Table 2 Infection in patients with pneumothorax secondary to GPA

The site of infection and pathogens	n = 20
The site of infection	
Lung	4 (20%)
Pleural	9 (45%)
Blood	3 (15%)
Parotid	1 (5%)
Pathogens	
Pseudomonas aeruginosa	5 (25%)
Hemolytic streptococcus	2 (10%)
Proteus	1 (5%)
Bacteroides fragilis	1 (5%)
Streptococcus faecalis	1 (5%)
Candida albicans	1 (5%)
Aspergillus niger	1 (5%)

Note: A total of 20 cases

Discussion

The incidence of pneumothorax in patients with GPA is low. So far, there were only individual case reports in the literature. Our analysis is the first systematic review of these cases. The results showed that pneumothorax secondary to GPA may be caused by many factors, is associated with high risk of fatality. Older age and non-response to pleural drainage indicate poor prognosis, and effective treatment of primary disease is very important to improve the prognosis.

There are different opinions for the cause of pneumothorax. Our analysis showed GPA associated pneumothorax is a collective effect of multiple factors (Table 5), rather than a single cause. First, 88% of patients in the analysis had pulmonary nodules, more frequent than the reported 40–70% in the general GPA patients [26]. Also,

Table 3 Biopsy/autopsy results of patients with pneumothorax secondary to GPA

Biopsy site and pathology	Cases (n, %)
Lung (12 cases)	
Pulmonary nodules necrotizing granulomatous vasculitis	6/12(50.0%)
bronchial pleural fistula	2/12(16.7%)
Pleural necrotizing granulomatous vasculitis	1/12(8.3%)
Subpleural blister and fibrosis, pulmonary fibrosis and elastic tissue hyperplasia	1/12(8.3%)
Nose (necrotizing granulomatous vasculitis)	8
Skin (leukocytoclastic vasculitis)	2
Parotid (necrotizing granulomatous vasculitis)	1
Oral (necrotizing granulomatous vasculitis)	1

Note: lung biopsy/autopsy in a total of 12 cases

21 out of 22 patients with pulmonary nodules had cavity, well above the 49% identified in general GPA patients population, [3] suggesting that breaking into the pleural cavity from cavitary nodule may be the main reason for the occurrence of pneumothorax (Fig. 2), especially cavitary nodules close to the pleura [9, 13, 17, 18]. Secondly, this analysis found that positive microbial culture of sputum and pleural drainage are common, and the same pathogen may be identified from both tests (in our patient, Aspergillus niger was detected from both sputum and pleural fluid drainage samples). This suggests that the secondary infection in the nodule cavity may contribute to the occurrence of pneumothorax, especially empyema in GPA patients [7]. The secondary infection is associated with cavity formation, and use of corticosteroids and immunosuppressants [8] not only increases the risk of infection, but also delays the wound healing after lung biopsy, thus causes pneumothorax [4]. Thirdly, the results of lung pathological examination in 2 patients showed bronchial pleural fistula is a pathological feature for pneumothorax [5, 8]. In addition, the disease progression itself involving the pleura may be a potential factor in the development of pneumothorax [3, 16]. In this analysis pleural biopsy revealed necrotizing granulomas and vasculitis. Epstein DM has reported a pneumothorax patient who did not have pulmonary manifestations at the diagnosis, but showed multiple pulmonary nodules one year later, suggesting pneumothorax may be caused by the primary disease itself that involves the pleura, and the emergence of pneumothorax indicates the likelihood of pulmonary lesion in the future [6]. Many patients in this analysis also had extrapulmonary manifestations. Inflammatory markers such as ESR, CRP were significantly increased, suggesting many of them were at the active stage of vasculitis when pneumothorax occurred. In only 1 patient who was confirmed GPA 18 years ago through nasal biopsy, wedge resection of lung and pleura partial resection were performed after the diagnosis of pneumothorax. Pathology exam showed subpleural blister with significant fibrosis, pulmonary fibroelastosis, no sign of vasculitis, and the pneumothorax may be caused by fibrous tissue traction [19]. Therefore, there are a few reasons and risk factors for pneumothorax in GPA patients. Breaking of nodule into the pleural cavity is the most common cause. Pneumothorax may occur at any time during the disease progression, while the majority of patients were in the active stage when it occurred.

This analysis also showed the prognosis of GPA patients complicated with pneumothorax is poor, and the fatality rate could be 40%, much higher than the general GPA patients [27]. The average age of patients who later died was higher than the survivors. Severe/ recurrent infections, respiratory failure were among the common causes of death. Lung infections, pleural cavity infections,

Table 4 Patients characteristics related to morality

Clinical features	Death group(n = 10)	Survival group (n = 12)	P value
Male/Female(n)	7(70.0%)/3(30.0%)	8(80.0%)/4(40.0%)	1.000
Age (years)	53 ± 12.9(33~70)	40 ± 14.7(25~70)	0.050
Duration (weeks)	19 ± 24.8(10~48)	34 ± 69.2(0.83~216)	0.547
Extrapulmonary manifestations (n)			
Fever	3 (30.0%)	7 (58.3%)	0.231
Skin lesions (purpura, gangrene, ulceration)	3 (30.0%)	3 (25.0%)	1.000
Ear (hearing loss, otitis media)	2 (20.0%)	4 (33.3%)	0.646
Nasal and sinus involvement	5 (50.0%)	7 (58.3%)	1.000
Oral ulceration	4 (40.0%)	1 (8.3%)	0.135
glomerulonephritis	6 (60.0%)	6 (50.0%)	0.691
Nervous system (facial paralysis, multiple mononeuropathy, etc.)	3 (30.0%)	1 (8.3%)	0.293
Arthralgia/arthritis	4 (40.0%)	4 (33.3%)	1.000
Parotid swelling and pain	2 (20.0%)	0 (0.0%)	0.195
ESR(mm/h)	104 ± 26.7	82 ± 33.9	0.233
Infection(n)	6 (60.0%)	3 (25.0%)	0.192
Corticosteroids and Immunosuppressants (n)			
steroid pulse therapy	1 (10.0%)	4 (33.3%)	0.323
treatment interruption	2/4(50.0%)	0/8(0.0%)	0.091
Non-response to Pleural drainage (n)	5/5 (100%)	0/7 (0.0%)	0.010
Surgery(n)	2 (20.0%)	5 (41.7%)	0.381

Note: 3 cases without prognostic information, n = 22 cases; ESR, erythrocyte sedimentation rate

blood infections are the most common forms of infection, and the most common pathogen is Pseudomonas aeruginosa. We also found, in certain patients the use of corticosteroids and immunosuppressive agents were interrupted or reduced after the development of pneumothorax/ infection with an intention to control the risk of infection [14]. However, this did not seem to improve the prognosis. We believe because most patients are in the active stage

Table 5 Risk factors for pneumothorax secondary to GPA

Risk factors	N
Active stage of Granulomatous vasculitis	19/20(95.0%)[a]
Pulmonary nodules broke into the chest cavity	15
Pleural necrotizing granulomatous vasculitis	1/12 (8.3%)[b]
Bronchial pleural fistula	2/12 (16.7%)[b]
Lesions fibrosis with pleural cohesion	1/12 (8.3%)[b]
Secondary infection in nodule cavity	3
Lesions fibrosis due to immunosuppressant	1
Delayed wound healing due to Glucocorticoid	2
Others	1

[a]Based on symptoms, laboratory tests, pathology
[b]Lung biopsy in 12 cases

of vasculitis, the treatment for primary disease should be maintained and unnecessary interruption is not recommended [9]. Treatment of primary disease may increase the risk of infection. If infection is present, it is recommended that sensitive antibiotics be given besides the treatment of primary disease to improve the prognosis [17–19]. In addition, pleural drainage can remove pleural effusion and help lung recruitment, but our analysis showed that not all patients benefit from pleural drainage, especially in the death group where the procedure showed ineffective for all patients. Therefore, we speculate that lack of response to pleural drainage may be an indicator of poor prognosis. On the other hand, in some patients who did not undergo pleural drainage, pneumothorax was absorbed spontaneously after the treatment of primary disease. So, pleural drainage should be decided based on the situation of the patients. If the patient is in general good state and has no obvious respiratory symptoms, decreased oxygenation, pleural drainage may not be necessary [16]. If the patient's condition is urgent, chest tube should be promptly placed. For patients not responding to pleural drainage, thoracotomy should be performed [21]. Also, for patients complicated with pleural infection, adequate drainage is essential [20]. Otherwise, extubation

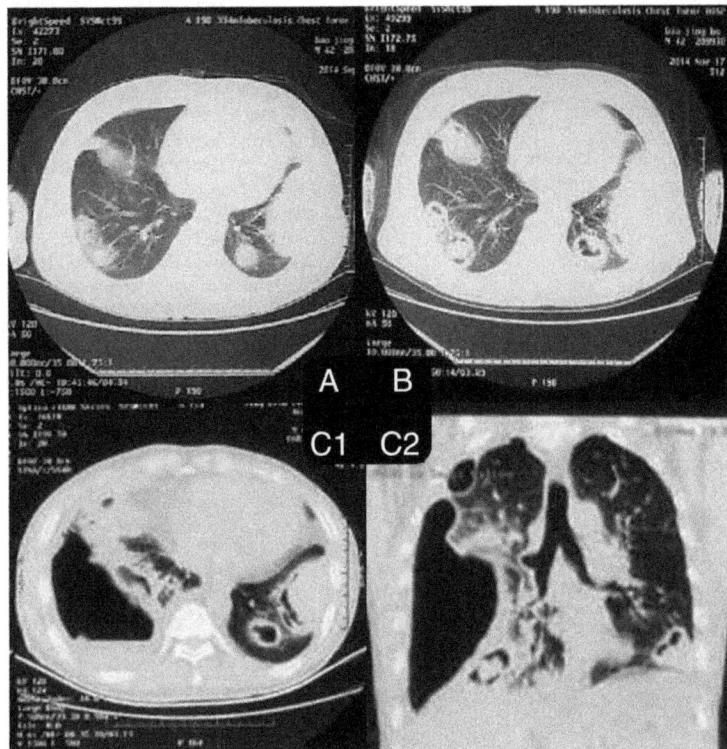

Fig. 2 The bilateral fixed nodules, cavitation, right hydropneumothorax in a patient with granulomatous vasculitis (GPA)

should be considered to reduce the risk of infection. Due to the small sample size, it is still unclear whether there are differences between different thoracic surgical methods. The common purpose of different surgical methods is to achieve lung expansion and to repair persistent air leaks. Therefore, video-assisted thoracic surgery (VATS) is recommended in order to reduce the damage to the patient. Not all nodules require operative resection except in those with cavity inside and adjacent to pleural. Similarly, pleurodesis is not always necessary and should be determined according to the patient's actual conditions. According to my own understanding and experience, lung expansion and cessation of air leaks after surgical/immunosupressive therapy and the effective control of severe complications such as infection are most important factors for a better prognosis. Different surgical methods do not have significant impact on the prognosis.

In summary, pneumothorax secondary to GPA generally occurs during active phase of the disease, and is caused by a variety of reasons. Aggressive treatment of primary disease can improve the prognosis. Pleural drainage should be considered based on the condition of patients, and ineffective pleural drainage indicates poor prognosis. The incidence of pneumothorax secondary to GPA is low but the case fatality rate is high. Here we

reported the first retrospective analysis of a large case series of GPA associated pneumothorax, provided a comprehensive review of the risk factors for pneumothorax, and analyzed the advantages and disadvantages of the main treatment approaches. We think the information can help clinicians identify high-risk patients for pneumothorax and make rational treatment decisions. Because this study was a retrospective analysis, limited to the number of cases reported in the literature, the results may not be generalizable to all GPA patients. Physicians should make decisions based on each patient's condition.

Conclusions

Pneumothorax was seen in the active GPA, due to a variety of reasons, and gave rise to high fatality rate. Aggressive treatment of GPA can improve the prognosis. Older and lack of response for pleural drainage indicates poor prognosis.

Abbreviations

ACR: American College of Rheumatology; CBM: Chinese Biomedical Literature Database; CRP: C-reactive protein; ESR: Erythrocyte sedimentation rate; GPA: Granulomatosis with polyangiitis

Acknowledgements

No.

Funding
No.

Authors' contributions
YL contributed to experimental design, coordination and interpreted the data. XS analyzed results and drafted the manuscript. YZ collected data of research. All authors read and approved the final manuscript.

Competing interests
The authors declare that they have no competing interests.

References

1. Lutalo PM, D'Cruz DP. Diagnosis and classification of granulomatosis with polyangiitis (aka Wegener's granulomatosis). J Autoimmun. 2014;48-49:94–8.

2. Abdou NI, Kullman GJ, Hoffman GS, Sharp GC, Specks U, McDonald T, Garrity J, Goeken JA, Allen NB. Wegener's granulomatosis: survey of 701 patients in North America. Changes in outcome in the 1990s. J Rheumatol. 2002;29(2):309–16.

3. Cordier JF, Valeyre D, Guillevin L, Loire R, Brechot JM. Pulmonary Wegener's granulomatosis. A clinical and imaging study of 77 cases. Chest. 1990;97(4):906–12.

4. Sezer I, Kocabas H, Melikoglu MA, Budak BS, Ozbudak IH, Butun B. Spontaneous pneumothorax in Wegener's granulomatosis: a case report. Mod Rheumatol. 2008;18(1):76–80.

5. Maguire R, Fauci AS, Doppman JL, Wolff SM. Unusual radiographic features of Wegener's granulomatosis. AJR Am J Roentgenol. 1978;130(2):233–8.

6. Epstein DM, Gefter WB, Miller WT, Gohel V, Bonavita JA. Spontaneous pneumothorax: an uncommon manifestation of Wegener granulomatosis. Radiology. 1980;135(2):327–8.

7. Jaspan T, Davison AM, Walker WC. Spontaneous pneumothorax in Wegener's granulomatosis. Thorax. 1982;37(10):774–5.

8. Wolffenbuttel BH, Weber RF, Kho GS. Pyopneumothorax: a rare complication of Wegener's granulomatosis. Eur J Respir Dis. 1985;67(3):223–7.

9. Ogawa M, Azemoto R, Makino Y, Mori Y, Ueda S, Wakashin M, Ohto M. Pneumothorax in a patient with Wegener's granulomatosis during treatment with immunosuppressive agents. J Intern Med. 1991;229(2):189–92.

10. Zhiren Li XB, Zhen J. The rare pulmonary manifestations of Wegener's granulomatosis(report of 2 cases and literature review). Chinese Journal of Practical Internal Medicine. 1992;04:216–7.

11. Courthaliac C, Aumaitre O, Andre M, Kemeny JL, Janicot H, Gilain L, Michel JL. Features of tomodensitometry in the development of pleuropulmonary lesions related to Wegener's granulomatosis. Rev Med Interne. 1999;20(7):571–8.

12. Tsushima K, Tanaka H, Urushihata K, Ogasawara H, Gono H, Takashi S, Tsukadaira A, Yamamoto H, Kaneki T, Yamaguchi S, et al. A case of limited Wegener granulomatosis with hypereosinophilia. Nihon Kokyuki Gakkai Zasshi. 2000;38(12):937–42.

13. Michel J, Courthaliac C, Andre M, Lhoste A, Aumaitre O. Quid? Pneumothorax complicating Wegener disease with rupture of pleura of cavitary nodule. J Radiol. 2001;82(1):73–5.

14. Bulbul Y, Ozlu T, Oztuna F. Wegener's granulomatosis with parotid gland involvement and pneumothorax. Med Princ Pract. 2003;12(2):133–7.

15. Imamoglu M, Bahadir O, Reis A. Parotid gland involvement as an initial presentation of Wegener's granulomatosis. Otolaryngol Head Neck Surg. 2003;129(4):451–3.

16. Shimizu T, Ohara T, Ito S, Nakano M, Tsutsui N, Sato T, Suzuki E, Gejyo F. A case of Wegener's granulomatosis complicated with seropneumothorax. Mod Rheumatol. 2003;13(2):181–4.

17. Delevaux I, Khellaf M, Andre M, Michel JL, Piette JC, Aumaitre O. Spontaneous pneumothorax in Wegener granulomatosis. Chest. 2005;128(4):3074–5.

18. Ates A, Karaaslan Y, Yildiz G, Gunesen O, Han S. A case of Wegener's granulomatosis complicated with hydropneumothorax. J Clin Rheumatol. 2006;12(5):264–5.

19. Storelli E, Casali C, Natali P, Rossi G, Morandi U. Unusual pathogenesis of spontaneous pneumothorax secondary to Wegener's granulomatosis. Ann Thorac Surg. 2007;84(1):288–90.

20. Belhassen-Garcia M, Velasco-Tirado V, Alvela-Suarez L, Carpio-Perez A, Lledias JP, Novoa N, Iglesias-Gomez A, Cordero-Sanchez M. Spontaneous pneumothorax in Wegener's granulomatosis: case report and literature review. Semin Arthritis Rheum. 2011;41(3):455–60.

21. Kahraman H, Inci MF, Tokur M, Cetin GY. Spontaneous pneumothorax in a patient with granulomatosis with polyangiitis. BMJ Case Rep. 2012;2012

22. Kosalka J, Bazan-Socha S, Zugaj A, Ignacak M, Zuk J, Sokolowska B, Musial J. Granulomatosis with polyangiitis (Wegener's granulomatosis) with hard palate and bronchial perforations treated with rituximab - a case report. Pneumonol Alergol Pol. 2014;82(5):454–7.

23. Pinto B, Dhir V, Singh PK, Gowda KK, Sharma A. Granulomatosis with polyangiitis and severe respiratory involvement. J Emerg Med. 2014;47(3):e79–81.

24. Shi XH, Zhang YF, Lu YW. Successful treatment of granulomatosis with polyangiitis with hydropneumothorax using corticosteroids and immunosuppressant. Exp Ther Med. 2017;13(6):3586–90.

25. Leavitt RY, Fauci AS, Bloch DA, Michel BA, Hunder GG, Arend WP, Calabrese LH, Fries JF, Lie JT, Lightfoot RW Jr, et al. The American College of Rheumatology 1990 criteria for the classification of Wegener's granulomatosis. Arthritis Rheum. 1990;33(8):1101–7.

26. Ananthakrishnan L, Sharma N, Kanne JP. Wegener's granulomatosis in the chest: high-resolution CT findings. AJR Am J Roentgenol. 2009;192(3):676–82.

27. Comarmond C, Cacoub P. Granulomatosis with polyangiitis (Wegener): clinical aspects and treatment. Autoimmun Rev. 2014;13(11):1121–5.

14

The role of epithelial-mesenchymal transition in the post-lung transplantation bronchiolitis obliterans

Chong Zhang, Yuequn Niu, Li Yu, Wang Lv, Haichao Xu, Abudumailamu Abuduwufuer, Jinlin Cao and Jian Hu[*]

Abstract

Background: Many patients who receive lung transplantation (LT) operations develop varying degrees of bronchiolitis obliterans (BO) after the surgeries. Epithelial-mesenchymal transition (EMT) is considered to be related to the process of bronchiolitis obliterans. In this study we simulated the pathological process of post-lung transplantation bronchiolitis obliterans, and explored the correlation between BO and EMT of small airway epithelial cells.

Methods: We transplanted the left lungs of F344 rats to Lewis rats by the Tri-cuff anastomosis and established the allogeneic rat left lung orthotopic transplantation model. Cyclosporine and lipopolysaccharide were administrated appropriately after the surgery. The histological structure and the expression levels of the EMT markers was observed with the methods of HE staining, Masson staining and immunohistochemistry. The analysis of enumeration data was performed using Fisher's Exact test and Spearman's rank correlation was used for the correlation analysis.

Results: Inflammatory cell infiltration, fibroplasia of bronchiole walls and significant lumen stenosis were found in the pulmonary mesenchyme of the transplanted lungs. The positive expression rate of E-cadherin in the transplanted lungs was 38.50% (5/13), significantly lower than that in the normal lung tissues [87.50% (7/8)] ($P < 0.05$), while the positive expression rate of Vimentin was 76.92% (10/13) which is significantly higher than that in the normal lung tissues [25.00% (2/8)] ($P < 0.05$). And a negative correlation existed between the expression levels of E-cadherin and Vimentin ($r = -0.750, P < 0.01$).

Conclusions: In the disease model we established in this study, we found pathological changes that met BO characteristics happened in the transplanted lungs. Meanwhile, the small airway epithelial cells of transplanted lungs underwent an epithelial-mesenchymal transition, which indicated a role of EMT in the BO airway remodeling.

Keywords: Lung transplantation, Chronic rejection, Bronchiolitis obliterans, Epithelial-mesenchymal transition, E-cadherin, Vimentin

Background

Up to now, lung transplantation (LT) is the only effective method in the treatment of terminal pulmonary disease, but chronic dysfunction of transplanted lungs related to chronic graft rejection limits the long-term effect of LT [1]. The development of chronic lung allograft dysfunction (CLAD), with the Bronchiolitis obliterans (BO) being the most common manifestation, is considered to be a major player in the process of chronic graft failure and the most frequent cause of long-term morbidity and mortality after LT [2, 3]. As a process of chronic airway rejection, BO is manifested in the fibroplasia and occlusion of small airway, leading to persistent decline of lung function. Approximately 68% of lung transplant patients showed varying degrees of BO within 3 months after surgery [4]. The structural alteration of the terminal bronchioles is a main cause of the airway obstruction in the process of BO [5]. Since the principal pathological change of BO is airway remodeling, inhibition of which could be the key of future clinical management of post-lung transplantation BO.

EMT refers to a process that epithelial cells lose their original epithelial features and obtain some mesenchymal

* Correspondence: dr_hujian@zju.edu.cn
Department of Thoracic Surgery, First Affiliated Hospital of Zhejiang University, No. 79 Qingchun Road, Zhejiang, Hangzhou 310003, China

characteristics, such as losing cell adhesion, gaining the ability to migrate and extending to a spindle shape similar to fibroblasts in morphology. Then the epithelial cells stretch out pseudopodia, separate themselves from the surrounding cells, break through the basement membrane and become new mesenchymal cells [6, 7]. In terms of surface markers, EMT is characterized by lost expression of E-cadherin, decreased expression of epithelial markers, and increased expression of mesenchymal markers such as Vimentin and smooth muscle actin (SMA) in cells [8]. E-cadherin, a calcium-dependent cell surface protein, which can promote the adhesion between the epithelial cells, is the main protein to anchor the adhesion junction between epithelial cells. The expression of E-cadherin decreases in the process of embryonic development, tissue fibrosis and cancer [9]. On the contrary, Vimentin, which is only found in mesenchymal cells, is a kind of intermediate filament protein, attached to nucleus, endoplasmic reticulum, and the sides or end of mitochondrion, making great contribution to support and anchor organelles in the protoplasm and playing an important role in the cell shape maintenance. [10]. Current studies have showed that EMT is involved in the BO airway remodeling [11, 12]. Thus, further exploration of the mechanism and pathological significance of EMT may provide novel targets for treatment of post-lung transplantation bronchiolitis obliterans.

In the present study, a left lung orthotopic transplantation model was successfully established in rats. We then further explored the histological structure changes in BO and detected the expression levels of the several essential EMT markers. We found EMT took part in the process of airway remodeling in the post-lung transplantation BO, which provided a potential target for the future treatment of BO after the lung transplantation surgery.

Methods

Both male and female healthy SPF (specific pathogen free) F344 and Lewis rats, weighted 200-250 g, were included as the donors and recipients of the lung transplantation surgery. The weight of the donor and the corresponding recipient was controlled as close as possible. The rats were all fed in SPF environment. Temperature of the animal room was 20–22 °C and photoperiod was 12 h. The rats adapted themselves to the environment for a week before the experiments, drinking and eating freely. The ones with normal behavior and showed no adverse reactions were included in the surgery. The rats were divided into 2 groups. F344 rats with sham operations were grouped as normal control and Lewis rats received allogeneic left lung orthotopic transplantation [F344-to-Lewis] were grouped as the experimental group.

We established the allogeneic lung transplantation model. F344 rats (donors) with intraperitoneal injection of atropine 0.25 mg were anesthetized with intraperitoneal injection of chloral hydrate (10 vol%) 4 ml/kg, and connected to a small animal ventilator after the tracheal intubation. Then abdominal median incisions were made and the rats were injected with heparin 1000 U/kg via inferior vena cava. Next we cut open the diaphragm and the anterior chest wall to sufficiently expose the cardio-pulmonary tissues. The lung lavage was performed using 4 °C improved Euro-Collins solution and the perfusion continued until the lung tissues were pale and the perfusates were clear and translucent. Then we separated the left lung hilum, sheared off the left pulmonary artery, left pulmonary vein and left bronchus, and fixed a cannula to each broken end by ligation. The donor lungs were preserved in 4 °C improved Euro-Collins solution and set aside.

Lewis rats (recipients) received the same operations of anesthesia, intubation and ventilation surgery as the donor rats. We got into the chest via an incision in the left fourth intercostal space and separated the hilum. Then we clamped the pulmonary artery and pulmonary vein by microvascular clamp and sheared them off from the distal end. Next, the pulmonary artery and pulmonary vein of the donor lung were inserted into the corresponding vessels of the recipient and fixed by ligation. Afterwards the vein and artery were opened in sequence. Then we clamped the bronchus, sheared it off from the distal end, removed the original lung and put the donor lung into the original position in the thoracic cavity. After that we inserted the bronchus of the donor lung into the corresponding broken end and fixed it by ligation. Finally the lung was ventilated to recover. The criterions of successful anastomosis: (1) no blood or air leaking from the three anastomotic stomas; (2) the pulmonary artery and pulmonary vein were both filled; (3) the lung presented as pink, uniform and elastic. Finally we put into the thoracic drainage tube and performed sternal closure and anesthesia recovery.

We randomly chose healthy F344 rats to perform sham operation, which only included the thoracotomy and sternal closure surgery while the lung transplantation was not performed. The operation of anesthesia, intubation, ventilation, incision cutting, sternal closure and anesthesia recovery were all the same as that of the recipients described previously.

Next, we established the BO model [13]. From the first day after the surgery, the rats from experimental group were given intraperitoneal injection of cyclosporine (5 mg/kg•d) for 10 days in order to reduce the acute rejection. At the 28th day after the surgery, the rats from experimental group were given intratracheal administration with lipopolysaccharide (0.5 mg/kg) while the treatment of the control group was intratracheal administration of PBS at the 28th day after the sham operation.

The rats from both control and experimental group were killed at the 90th day after the surgery and their left lungs were taken out and fixed by 10% Formalin. The paraffin sections of the samples were made and examined by HE staining, Masson staining and immunohistochemistry.

Following dewaxing and hydration according to the normal protocols, HE staining and Masson staining were performed. After mounting, the histological structure was observed and the differences between experimental group and control group were compared.

Streptavidin-peroxidase (SP) was used to perform the examination. Paraffin embedded sections with normal dehydration were performed antigen retrieval. The primary antibodies (Vimentin and E-cadherin), secondary antibody (mouse anti-rabbit IgG) and SP complex were dropwise added in sequence. Then we examined the expression levels of Vimentin and E-cadherin after 30 min incubation in 37 °C incubator. In 5 high power fields of each section, two experienced researchers independently analyzed and evaluated the levels of positive expression rates of Vimentin and E-cadherin, which were considered as yellow or brown granules appeared in the cells. The staining results were analyzed with staining intensity and positive cell number both taken into consideration. Immunoreactive score (IRS) was calculated by SI × PP. SI stands for staining intensity: 0 for no color, 1 for light yellow, 2 for brown, and 3 for dark brown. PP stands for the percentage of positive cells: 0 for no positive cells, 1 for less than 10%, 2 for 10 to 50%, 3 for 50 to 75%, and 4 for more than 75%. We set IRS ≤ 3 for negative and IRS > 3 for positive. Finally, the qualitative results of immunohistochemistry were determined by the overall conditions of the five random fields: Vimentin (+), Vimentin (−), E-cadherin (+), E-cadherin (−).

All of the experiment data were analyzed using SPSS 20 software. The analysis of enumeration data was performed using Fisher's Exact test and the Spearman's rank correlation was for the correlation analysis. $P < 0.05$ was considered significant.

Results

There were 13 rats for the successful modeling of experimental group and 8 sham-operated F344 rats for the control group. The HE staining results of tissue sections of healthy lungs and transplanted lungs were shown in Fig. 1. In the sections of healthy lungs, the wall of bronchiole had longitudinal plicae and were covered by pseudostratified ciliated columnar epithelium; there were no significant abnormality or just mild inflammatory cell infiltration that can be seen in histomorphology. On the contrary, the sections of transplanted lungs showed obviously abnormal bronchiole epithelium, which had hypertrophic mucosa and clear plicae. Peripheral inflammatory cell infiltration, stroma deposition and hyperplasia of fibrous tissue were found in submucosa. It was also visible for lamellar inflammatory exudate or even granulation tissues in the bronchiole lumen; and the lumen also had stenosis at different levels.

The Masson staining sections of healthy and transplanted lung tissues were shown in Fig. 2. In the healthy lung tissue sections, the muscularis of bronchiole tunica media was thin and the smooth muscle was arranged in an undivided circle. However in the transplanted lung tissue sections, the muscularis of bronchiole tunica media became thick and the arrangement of smooth muscle was disordered. From there evident hyperplasia of fibrous tissue was also found.

The immunohistochemistry results of E-cadherin and Vimentin expression were shown in Figs. 3 and 4. The overall qualitative result of 21 rats' lung tissue specimens illustrated that there were 38.50% (5/13) of lung transplanted rats showed a positive expression of E-cadherin while it was 87.50% (7/8) of that in the healthy ones; and the difference between two groups was significant ($P < 0.05$). As for Vimentin, the positive expression rate of transplanted lung tissue sections was 76.92% (10/13) while in the healthy lung tissues it was 25.00% (2/8) and the significant difference existed between the two groups as well ($P < 0.05$). Spearman's rank correlation analysis of the qualitative results of E-cadherin and Vimentin expression levels in the 21 lung tissue

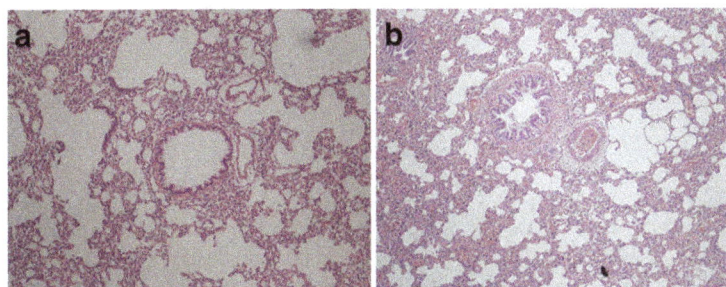

Fig. 1 HE staining results of lung tissue sections in two groups. **a** Healthy lung in 100×; **b** transplanted lung in 100×

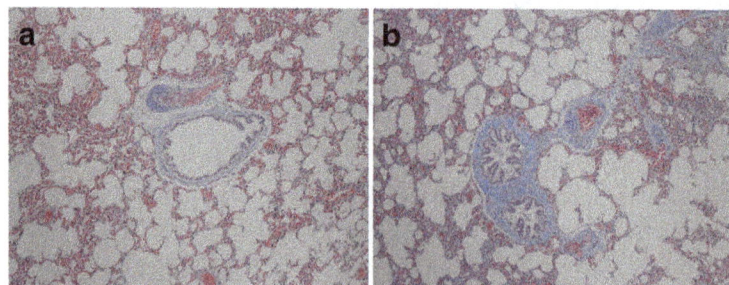

Fig. 2 Masson staining results of lung tissue sections in two groups. **a** Healthy lung in 100×; **b** transplanted lung in 100×

specimens demonstrated a negative correlation between them ($r = -0.750$, $P < 0.01$).

Discussion

Lung transplantation (LT) is the only effective method in the treatment of terminal pulmonary disease, but the chronic dysfunction of transplanted lung remains to be a problem waiting to be solved with great urgency. According to its clinical manifestation and pathological characteristics, current studies believe that the chronic dysfunction is closely related to the self-inflammatory process, including bronchiolitis obliterans, chronic vascular rejection, post-transplantation large airway inflammation, chronic bronchiolitis, chronic lung stroma fibrosis and chronic pleurisy [14]. Among all of these, our study mainly discussed about the post-transplantation bronchiolitis obliterans.

Bronchiolitis obliterans is a chronic airway disease which mainly manifests as infiltration of airway neutrophils and macrophages. Conditions like oxidative stress and the imbalance of protease and antiprotease can lead to the release of many inflammatory mediators, such as TNF-α、IL-6、IL-8、IL-1. The inflammatory mediators finally causes airway mucus hypersecretion, airway smooth muscle hypertrophy, increased collagen synthesis and hyperplasia of airway microvessels, namely the airway remodeling. Airway remodeling is the key pathological change in the process of lung function decline caused by BO. In the transplanted lungs we found evidently abnormal bronchiole epithelium, which had hypertrophic mucosa and clear plicae. Peripheral inflammatory cell infiltration, stroma deposition and hyperplasia of fibrous tissue were found in submucosa. It was also visible for lamellar inflammatory exudate or even granulation tissue in the bronchiole lumen; and the lumen also had stenosis at different levels. These are the characteristics of airway remodeling and in accordance with pathological changes of BO. Therefore, we successfully established the model of post-lung transplantation BO.

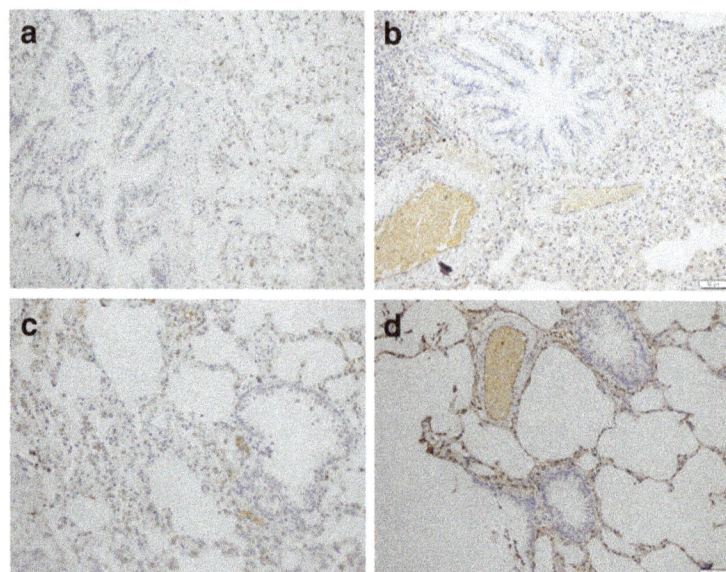

Fig. 3 The expression of E-cadherin in lung tissue sections of the two groups; **a** transplanted lung, SI = 1, PP = 2, IRS = 2, E-cadherin (−); **b** transplanted lung, SI = 1, PP = 4, IRS = 4, E-cadherin (+); **c** healthy lung, SI = 1, PP = 3, IRS = 3, E-cadherin (−); **d** healthy lung, SI = 2, PP = 3, IRS = 6, E-cadherin (+). Notes: immunohistochemistry (200×); IRS for immunoreactive score, SI for staining intensity, PP for percentage of positive cells

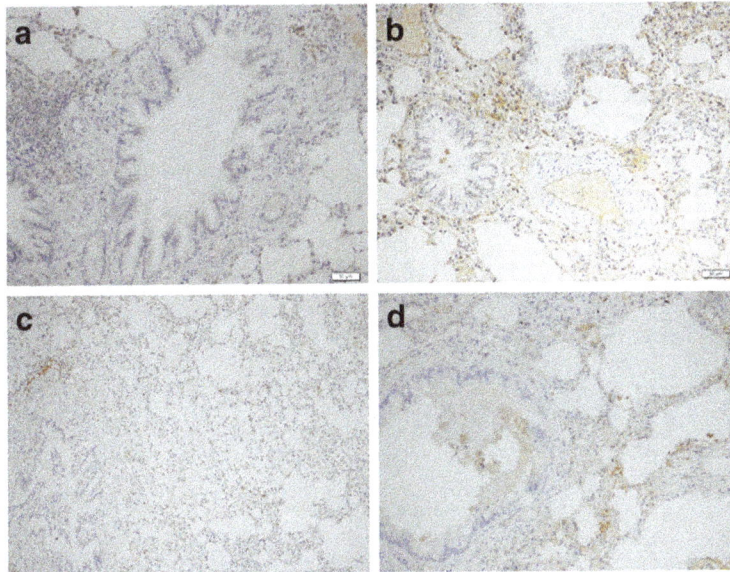

Fig. 4 The expression of Vimentin in lung tissue sections of the two groups; **a** transplanted lung, SI = 2, PP = 1, IRS = 2, Vimentin (–); **b** transplanted lung, SI = 1.5, PP = 4, IRS = 6, Vimentin (+); **c** healthy lung, SI = 1, PP = 3, IRS = 3, Vimentin (–); **d** healthy lung, SI = 1, PP = 4, IRS = 4, Vimentin (+). Notes: immunohistochemistry (200×); IRS for immunoreactive score, SI for staining intensity, PP for percentage of positive cells

In addition, we also explored the correlation between EMT and the airway remodeling. At present, many studies have demonstrated that EMT is associated with airway epithelial remodeling [15–17]. By observing a mouse asthma model, Johnson et al. [16] have found absence of E-cadherin expression, appearance of mesenchymal related indicators and thickening of smooth muscle in mouse airway epithelial cells after a 15-week exposure of dust mites. This work illustrated that EMT was involved in the process of asthma airway remodeling. The study of Sohal et al. [17] also demonstrated a close correlation between EMT and chronic obstructive pulmonary disease (COPD) airway remodeling. They found that cells in the cracks of basement membrane of COPD group expressed the mesenchymal cell markers such as S100A4, Vimentin and MMP9. Further immunohistochemistry analysis showed that there were correspondingly 13.8% and 7% of COPD sufferers' basement epithelial cells and cells in reticular basement membrane simultaneously expressing keratin and S100A4, which means that EMT existed in the airway of COPD sufferers. Our immunohistochemistry results showed decreased E-cadherin expression and significantly increased Vimentin expression in transplanted lungs compared to normal lung tissues, which means an EMT process happened. Thus, the airway remodeling after lung transplantation is also related to EMT.

In our study, we noted that the BO pathological changes happened along with EMT in transplanted lung tissues, which testified EMT was involved in the small airway remodeling of BO. Inevitably, this study has a few limitations. The most important point among these is the relatively small sample size. In consideration of the complexity of the development and progress of BO after lung transplantation, small sample of a rat model has its natural drawbacks to present full understanding of such a huge issue. Secondly, although we tried to ensure that the experimental animal characteristics and the experimental conditions are similar, some common factors in animal model, such as various pathophysiological mechanisms, different responses to drugs, variations induced by techniques, differences in genetic regulation and anatomical differences, might have potential effects on this disease model. In addition, adding a Lewis to Lewis transplantation group as another control group would increase the reliability of the conclusions. Besides, it is also a pity that we still can't identify the exact position of EMT in BO though they are existing simultaneously. We still don't know whether that EMT is one of the causes of BO or it is only an accompanying phenomenon in the process of BO genesis and development. If EMT promotes the genesis and development of BO, then suppressing EMT may inhibit the progression of BO; while if EMT is just an accompanying phenomenon in the process of BO genesis and development, then further exploration of the mechanism of EMT is needed for the potential clues of post-lung transplantation BO.

Conclusions

Although there were still some deficiencies, we believe that the established disease model in our study provided convincing evidences to prove that EMT is involved in the BO airway remodeling. However the role of EMT in BO still remains unknown and the specific relations between them is still remained to be explored. Further study of the mechanism and pathological significance of EMT in the transplanted lungs after lung transplantation may reveal novel targets for the prevention and treatment of post-lung transplantation bronchiolitis obliterans.

Abbreviations

BO: Bronchiolitis obliterans; CLAD: Chronic lung allograft dysfunction; COPD: Chronic obstructive pulmonary disease; EMT: Epithelial-mesenchymal transition; HE: Hematoxylin-eosin; IgG: Immunoglobulin G; IL: Interleukine; IRS: Immunoreactive score; LT: Lung transplantation; MMP: Matrix metalloproteinase; MUC5AC: Mucin 5 AC; PP: Percentage of positive cells; SI: Staining intensity; SMA: Smooth muscle actin; SP: Streptavidin-peroxidase; SPF: Specific pathogen free; TNF: Tumor necrosis factor

Acknowledgements
Not applicable.

Funding
This work was supported by the General Program of National Natural Science Foundation of China [grant number 81373161]; General Program of Medical and Health Research of Zhejiang Province [grant number 2012KYA081; 2013KYB095]; Research Program of Public Welfare Technology (Experimental Animals) of Zhejiang Province [grant number 2016C37124] and General Research Program of Education Department Zhejiang Province [grant number Y201017002].

Authors' contributions
CZ, WL and JH contributed to the conception of the study. WL, AA and JC gave valuable suggestions to the experiments. CZ, LY and HX performed all the experiments and statistical analyses. YN, CZ and JH drafted the manuscript. All authors read and approved the final manuscript.

Competing interests
The authors declare that they have no competing interests.

References

1. Weigt SS, DerHovanessian A, Wallace WD, Lynch JP 3rd, Belperio JA. Bronchiolitis obliterans syndrome: the Achilles' heel of lung transplantation. Semin Respir Crit Care Med. 2013;34(3):336–51.
2. Verleden GM, Vos R, Dupont L, Van Raemdonck DE, Vanaudenaerde BM, Verleden SE. Are we near to an effective drug treatment for bronchiolitis obliterans? Expert Opin Pharmacother. 2014;15(15):2117–20.
3. Fiser SM, Tribble CG, Long SM, Kaza AK, Kern JA, Jones DR, et al. Ischemia-reperfusion injury after lung transplantation increases risk of late bronchiolitis obliterans syndrome. Ann Thorac Surg. 2002;73(4):1041–7.
4. Estenne M, Maurer JR, Boehler A, Egan JJ, Frost A, Hertz M, et al. Bronchiolitis obliterans syndrome 2001: an update of the diagnostic criteria. J Heart Lung Transplant. 2002;21:297–310.
5. Thompson BR, Hodgson YM, Kotsimbos T, Liakakos P, Ellis MJ, Snell GI, Verbanck S. Bronchiolitis obliterans syndrome leads to a functional deterioration of the acinus post lung transplant. Thorax. 2014;69(5):487–8.
6. Kalluri REMT. When epithelial cells decide to become mesenchymal-like cells. J Clin Invest. 2009;119(6):1417–9.
7. Kalluri R, Weinberg RA. The basics of epithelial-mesenchymal transition. J Clin Invest. 2009;119(6):1420–8.
8. Smith BN, Bhowmick NA. Role of EMT in Metastasis and Therapy Resistance. J Clin Med. 2016;27(5):2.
9. Zeisberg M, Neilson EG. Biomarkers for epithelial-mesenchymal transitions. J Clin Invest. 2009;119:1429–37.
10. Chen K, Jiang P, Deng S, Wang N. Expression of thyroid transcription factor-1 and vimentin in neonatal mice with bronchopulmonary dysplasia. Nan Fang Yi Ke Da Xue Xue Bao. 2012;32(8):1111–5.
11. Borthwick LA, Parker SM, Brougham KA, Johnson GE, Gorowiec MR, Ward C, et al. Epithelial to mesenchymal transition (EMT) and airway remodelling after human lung transplantation. Thorax. 2009;64(9):770–7.
12. Gardner A, Fisher AJ, Richter C, Johnson GE, Moisey EJ, Brodlie M, et al. The critical role of TAK1 in accentuated epithelial to mesenchymal transition in obliterative bronchiolitis after lung transplantation. Am J Pathol. 2012;180(6):2293–308.
13. Atanasova S, Hirschburger M, Jonigk D, Obert M, Petri K, Evers A, et al. A relevant experimental model for human bronchiolitis obliterans syndrome. J Heart Lung Transplant. 2013;32:1131–9.
14. Snell GI, Westall GP. The contribution of airway ischemia and vascular remodelling to the pathophysiology of bronchiolitis obliterans syndrome and chronic lung allograft dysfunction. Curr Opin Organ Transplant. 2010;15:558–62.
15. Hackett TL, Warner SM, Stefanowicz D, Shaheen F, Pechkovsky DV, Murray LA, et al. Induction of epithelial-mesenchymal transition in primary airway epithelial cells from patients with asthma by transforming growth factor-beta1. Am J Respir Crit Care Med. 2009;180:122–33.
16. Johnson JR, Roos A, Berg T, Nord M, Fuxe J. Chronic respiratory aeroallergen exposure in mice induces epithelial-mesenchymal transition in the large airways. PLoS One. 2011;6:e16175.
17. Sohal SS, Ward C, Danial W, Wood-Baker R, Walters EH. Recent advances in understanding inflammation and remodeling in the airways in chronic obstructive pulmonary disease. Expert Rev Respir Med. 2013;7:275–88.

15

The fortune cookie flap for aesthetic reconstruction after chest keloid resection

Tae Hwan Park*⬥, Jang Won Lee and Chan Woo Kim

Abstract

Background: Generally, the recurrence rate of keloids is unacceptably high after surgical excision alone. Nevertheless, surgical reduction of keloids is inevitable in many cases. The reconstruction of extensive soft tissue defects following complete keloid resection is challenging to surgeons. In this study, we present our clinical experience using a novel fortune cookie flap for treating chest keloids. This flap provides an excellent surgical option that maintains natural appearance with minimal donor-site morbidity.

Methods: We retrospectively reviewed the data from 3 consecutive cases of reconstruction using the fortune cookie flap following resection of chest keloids between March and December, 2017.

Results: Successful reconstructions were performed without any major complications. The mean dimensions of the reconstructed defect were 5.0 × 4.2 cm, while the mean dimensions of the flap were 7.7 × 5.7 cm.

Conclusions: Owing to its simplicity, reliability, versatility, minimal morbidity and excellent aesthetics, the fortune cookie flap is as an excellent option for reconstruction following complete keloid resection on the chest.

Keywords: Keloid, Fortune cookie, Keystone, Perforator, Flap

Background

Generally, the recurrence rate of keloids is unacceptably high after surgical excision alone. Nevertheless, surgical reduction of keloids is inevitable in many cases. The reconstruction of extensive soft tissue defects following complete keloid resection is challenging to surgeons. Specifically in a chest keloid, the tissue mobility is relatively limited; therefore, it is generally accepted that reconstruction after resection of chest keloids is a great burden to surgeons [1]. For this reason, some physicians prefer intralesional excision to preclude any surgical defect that cannot be closed primarily and therefore requires a second surgical procedure, such as flap surgery or skin grafting [2]. On the other hand, skin grafting in patients with keloid is a great concern to both the patient and physician because there is a significant risk of the original keloid recurring and of new keloid formation at the distant donor site.

The keystone flap is a gaining popularity because of its versatility in covering various defects, while offering stable vascularity of the perforator flaps and a relatively easy harvest. Very recently, the authors have presented a series of aesthetic reconstruction after resection of retro-auricular keloids with the traditional keystone flap [3]. However, the traditional keystone flap cannot be successfully used in every anatomical region, even in sizeable defects following complete keloid excision. In this study, we present our clinical experiences using a novel fortune cookie flap for patients with resected chest keloid.

Methods

Data collection

We reviewed all patients who underwent the fortune cookie flap for surgical defect following complete keloid resection in 2017. This study was approved by the Institutional Review Board of the CHA University and

* Correspondence: hard-piano@hanmail.net
Department of Plastic and Reconstructive Surgery, CHA Bundang Medical Center, CHA University, 59 Yatap-ro, Bundang-gu, Seongnam, Gyeonggi 13496, Republic of Korea

conducted in accordance with the Declaration of Helsinki. A comprehensive review of the basic demographic data, medical histories, wound sites and sizes, wound culture results and complications was performed. Appropriate statistical tests were used for continuous univariate analysis and are given as means ± standard deviation [SD].

Operative technique

In this study, we applied the new fortune cookie flap to cover the surgical defect following complete keloid resection or debridement of infected wounds. The defect was measured intraoperatively in two dimensions, with the longest dimension being the length and its perpendicular axis measurement, the width. We then proceeded with the flap design. As shown in Fig. 1b, the width of the wound "a" is equal to the width of the keystone arc. To effectively cover the defects, we began with complete excision including removal of proliferating core collagen (Fig. 1a, b). After complete resection, each patient underwent immediate reconstruction. The flap was incised along the entire design. The flap was fully elevated while preserving the central "hot spot" including the perforators. Then, the 2 limbs and margins adjacent to the wound were conjoined to cover the defect (Fig. 1c). As illustrated in Fig. 1d, the conjoined flap is a sector shape with a suture line from the centre, giving it the appearance of a fortune cookie.

Results

We identified and reviewed 3 patients (2 men and 1 woman; mean age, 27 years who underwent the fortune cookie flap procedure for chest keloid resection and reconstruction. The average wound dimensions were 5. 0 cm × 4.2 cm, and the average flap size was 7.7 cm × 5. 7 cm. Among them, 2 cases were referred from another hospital due to wound disruption with methicillin resistant *Staphylococcus aureus* (MRSA) infection after surgical resection followed by purse-string suture or primary closure (Additional file 1).

The mean operation time from surgical incision to total flap closure was 30 min. The postoperative courses were uneventful. No patient experienced partial or total flap loss or underwent any additional surgery. The representative cases are shown in Figs. 2 and 3.

Discussion

Once the surgical resection of keloids is indicated, the selected reconstruction method is dependent on the surgeon's preference and postoperative adjuvant therapy. If radiation therapy is scheduled postoperatively, flap surgery is better than skin grafting. This is because physicians can easily determine when to initiate radiation therapy when performing flap surgery. On the other hand, it is difficult to determine when to initiate radiation in the case of a skin graft because grafted, thin skin has a relatively weak vascularity during early wound

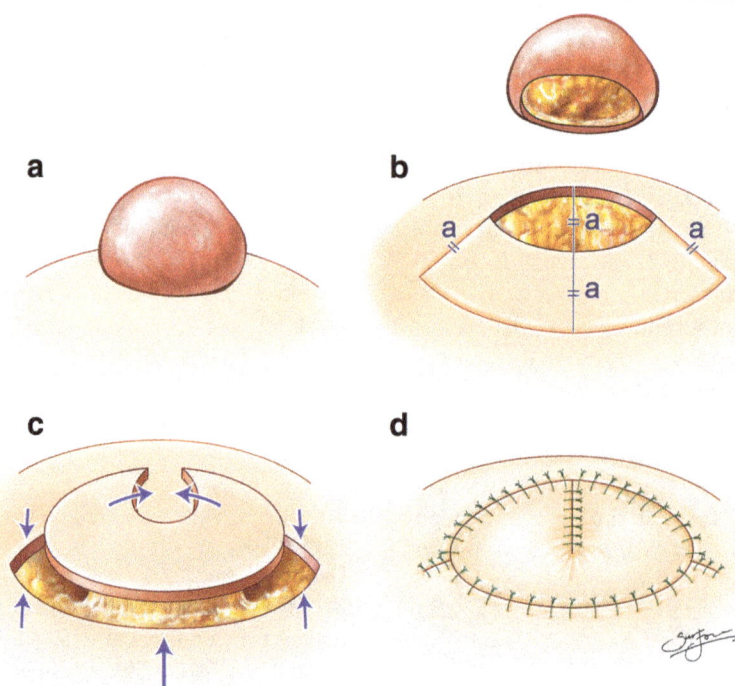

Fig. 1 Schematic illustration of a fortune cookie flap, modified from the keystone flap, to cover the surgical defect following complete keloid resection or debridement of infected wounds

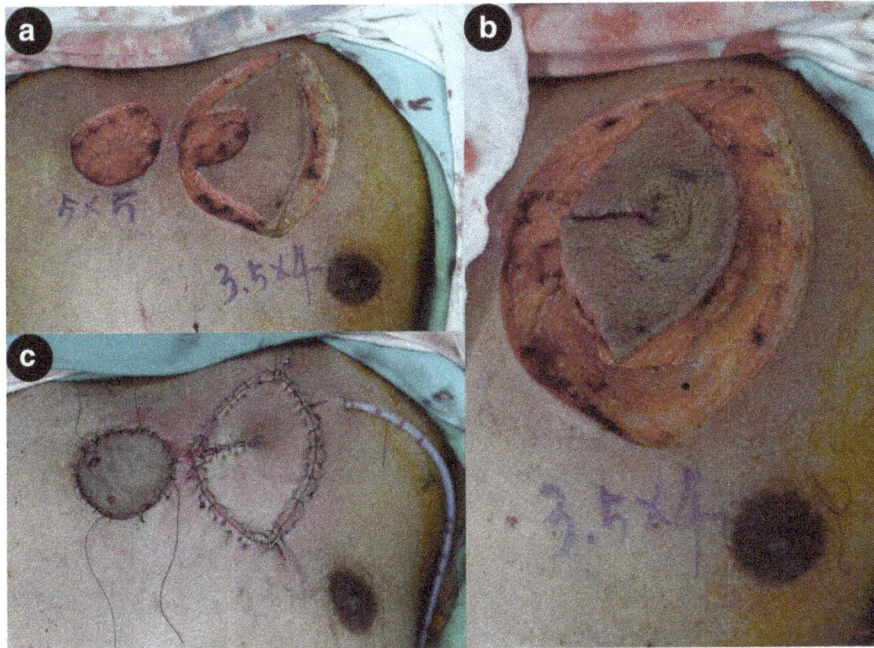

Fig. 2 a Intraoperative view of 2 defects, measuring 5.0 × 5.0 cm and 3.5 × 4.0 cm, after resection of an infected wound. **b** A 3.5 × 4.0 cm defect on the left side of the anterior chest wall was reconstructed using the fortune cookie design perforator island flap. **c** Final closure following inset of the perforator flap and split thickness skin graft

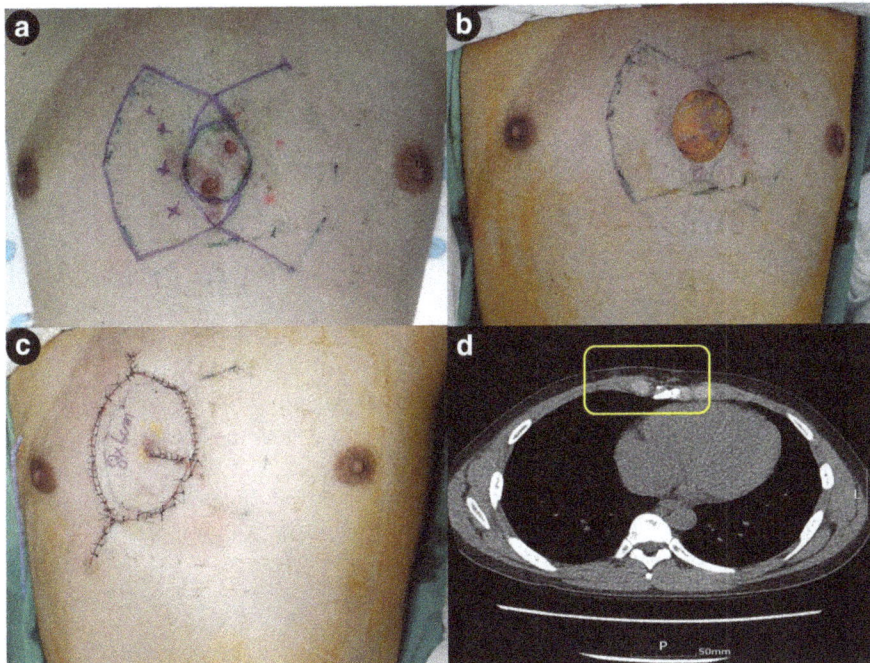

Fig. 3 a A 29-year-old man with wound dehiscence following a keloid excision with direct primary closure on the anterior chest wall, performed at another clinic. Marking of cutaneous perforators, identified using a handheld Doppler preoperatively, and design of the keystone flap. The wound was infected with methicillin resistant *Staphylococcus aureus* (MRSA). **b** Intraoperative view of a defect, measuring 5.5 × 5.0 cm, after resection of an infected wound. **c** Immediate postoperative result of the fortune cookie design perforator island flap and **d** Computed tomography scan in axial plane at 2 months' follow-up

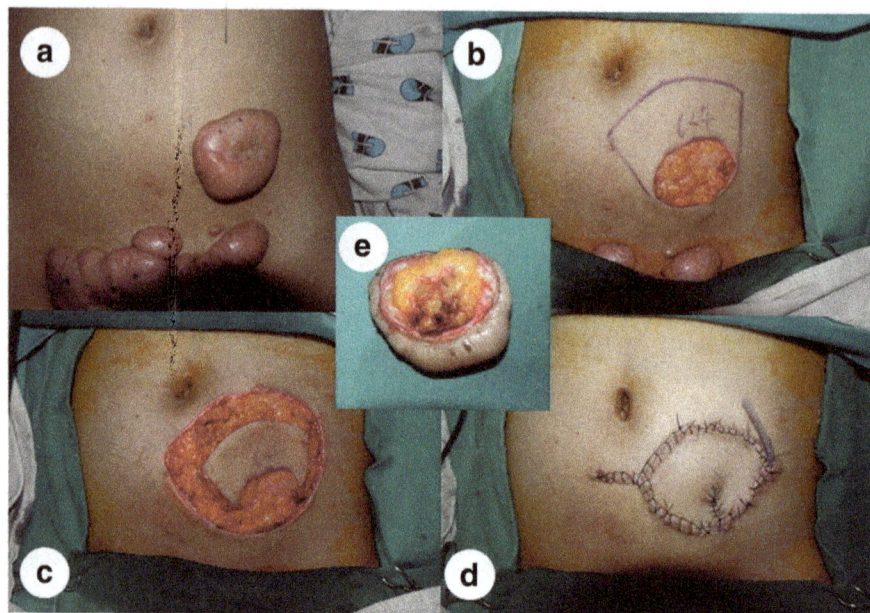

Fig. 4 a A 21-year-old woman with a large keloid on the lower abdomen, experiencing significant discomfort and severe pain caused by a belt. **b** A 6.0 × 4.0 cm defect following resection of the keloid. **c** A keystone flap designed for reconstruction on the upper side of the defect because of a lack of surrounding tissue laxity and quality, with other keloids on the lower side. **d** Immediate postoperative result of the fortune cookie design perforator island flap with V-Y closure of the donor site with a drain in situ. **e** No remnant proliferating collagen core on the surgical resection margin is shown, which is related to local recurrence

healing and early radiation therapy can cause secondary wound problems [4]. Therefore, flap surgery is considered better than skin grafting in many cases of keloid resection. Nevertheless, traditional perforator flap surgery requires tedious perforator dissection and inadvertent injury to perforators leading to flap congestion or necrosis can be encountered [5]. Minimising perforator dissection to prevent perforator injury causes venous congestion and uneven tension distribution, with especially high tension furthest away from the perforator.

Despite growing interest in the traditional keystone flap, the use of this flap for reconstruction after keloid resection is extremely rare. Recently, there have been geometric controversies over the tension distribution with skin paddle expansion of the traditional keystone flap. In using this flap, the possible expansion and advancement has limits and double, opposing keystone flaps are required to repair some large defects [6, 7].

Even though further follow-up is needed, our fortune cookie flap is also effective for MRSA infected open wounds following chest keloid resection. Moreover, the fortune cookie flap is more time-efficient than any other local or distant flaps and can be successfully used in other anatomical locations (Fig. 4). Our average operation time was 30 min, and the total time did not vary much depending on the location. Especially in a perforator-rich area such as the abdomen, re-elevation

of a previously-harvested fortune cookie flap, even after prior flap failure, or elevation of new fortune cookie flap using adjacent tissue is always a feasible and reliable option. Based on our experience of this flap in cases other than keloids, the failure rate is extremely low.

Our study has several limitations. This is a small retrospective case series having inherent limitations. Our sample size of 3 is relatively small, and further study of a greater number of cases will aid revealing other strengths or downsides of this technique. In addition, as we did not provide long-term follow up of these cases; further follow-up with the addition of more patients is required.

Conclusions
Our novel fortune cookie flap provides an excellent surgical option for reconstruction after chest keloid resection that maintains a natural look with minimal donor-site morbidities.

Abbreviations
MRSA: methicillin resistant *Staphylococcus aureus*; SD: standard deviation

Funding
This work was supported by the National Research Foundation of Korea (NRF) grant, funded by the Korean government (MSIP; Ministry of Science, ICT & Future Planning) (No. 2017R1C1B5017180 and 2017R1B5A2085456, TH Park).

Authors' contributions

PTH conceived and designed the study. He also performed all surgical procedures. PTH, LJW, and KCW analysed and interpreted the patient data. PTH supervised the entire study. All authors read and approved the final manuscript.

Competing interests

The authors declare that they have no competing interests.

References

1. Park TH, Seo SW, Kim JK, Chang CH. Management of chest keloids. J Cardiothorac Surg. 2011;6:49.
2. Chuang GS, Rogers GS, Zeltser R. Poiseuille's law and large-bore needles: insights into the delivery of corticosteroid injections in the treatment of keloids. J Am Acad Dermatol. 2008;59(1):167–8.
3. Park TH, Kim CW, Chang CH. Aesthetic reconstruction of retroauricular keloid: creating a keystone flap from the mastoid-helix area. J Dermatol. 2018; https://doi.org/10.1111/1346-8138.14223.
4. Ogawa R, Ono S, Akaishi S, Dohi T, Iimura T, Nakao J. Reconstruction after anterior Chest Wall keloid resection using internal mammary artery perforator propeller flaps. Plast Reconstr Surg Glob Open. 2016;4(9):e1049.
5. Park TH, Park JH, Chang CH. Clinical features and outcomes of foot keloids treated using complete surgical excision and full thickness skin grafting followed by corticosteroid injections. J Foot Ankle Res. 2013;6:(1)
6. Donovan LC, Douglas CD, Van Helden D. Wound tension and 'closability' with keystone flaps, V-Y flaps and primary closure: a study in fresh-frozen cadavers. ANZ J Surg. 2017; https://doi.org/10.1111/ans.14163.
7. Rao AL, Janna RK. Keystone flap: versatile flap for reconstruction of limb defects. J Clin Diagn Res. 2015;9(3):PC05–7.

16

Prognostic significance of preoperative plasma D-dimer level in patients with surgically resected clinical stage I non-small cell lung cancer: a retrospective cohort study

Kaoru Kaseda[1*], Keisuke Asakura[1], Akio Kazama[2] and Yukihiko Ozawa[3]

Abstract

Background: Plasma D-dimer level, a marker of hypercoagulation, has been reported to be associated with survival in several types of cancers. The present study aimed to evaluate the prognostic significance of preoperative D-dimer levels in patients with surgically resected clinical stage I non-small cell lung cancer (NSCLC).

Methods: Participants comprised 237 patients with surgically resected clinical stage I NSCLC. In addition to factors such as age, sex, and smoking status, the association between preoperative D-dimer level and survival was explored.

Results: Patients were divided into two groups according to D-dimer level: Group A, $\leq$ 1.0 µg/ml ($n = 170$); and Group B, > 1.0 µg/ml ($n = 67$). The 5-year recurrence-free survival rate was 81.6% for Group A and 66.6% for Group B ($p < 0.001$). The 5-year overall survival rate was 93.6% for Group A and 84.7% for Group B ($p = 0.002$). Multivariate survival analysis identified D-dimer level as an independent prognostic factor, along with age, maximum standardized uptake value of the primary tumor, and pathological stage.

Conclusions: Preoperative D-dimer level is an independent prognostic factor in patients with surgically resected clinical stage I NSCLC.

Keywords: D-dimer, Non-small cell lung cancer, Prognosis

Background

Patients with malignant tumors sometimes develop hypercoagulability, which can present as conditions like disseminated intravascular coagulation (DIC) and venous thromboembolism (VTE). Systemic hypercoagulability is frequently observed in patients with advanced-stage cancer, even if no thrombosis is present. One previous study expanded the definition of Trousseau's syndrome to include chronic disseminated intravascular coagulopathy associated with microangiopathy, verrucous endocarditis and arterial emboli in patients with cancer, and this syndrome is frequent among patients with mucin-positive carcinoma [1]. More recently, the term has been applied to a wide variety of clinical situations, from classic descriptions to any form of coagulopathy occurring against a background of malignancy [2].

Physiological degradation of fibrin results in plasma D-dimer (D-dimer), and levels of this stable end product are increased by significant fibrin formation and fibrinolysis. D-dimer level thus offers an indicator of the hypercoagulable state often evident in patients with thrombosis or DIC. As levels of D-dimer are increased following clotting, measurement of D-dimer concentration is a standard initial assessment for suspected cases of acute VTE [3]. Increased concentrations of D-dimer are also seen with other situations, including infection, pregnancy, and cancer, and after trauma or surgery.

* Correspondence: kaseda@wb4.so-net.ne.jp
[1]Department of Thoracic Surgery, Sagamihara Kyodo Hospital, 2-8-18 Hashimoto, Midori-ku, Sagamihara, Kanagawa 252-5188, Japan
Full list of author information is available at the end of the article

Tumor-induced coagulation and fibrin formation have been reported as prerequisite to tumor angiogenesis, metastasis and invasion, with cross-linked fibrin in the extracellular matrix providing the basis for endothelial cell and tumor cell migration during angiogenesis and invasion [4, 5]. Various investigations have reported that D-dimer levels, reflecting the degree of coagulation and fibrinolytic activation, correlate with tumor stage, response to chemotherapy and prognosis for several types of cancer [6–9], including non-small cell lung cancer (NSCLC) [9–11]. However, the relevance of D-dimer level for primary lung cancer has yet to be established. This study aimed to elucidate the prognostic significance of preoperative D-dimer levels after complete resection of clinical stage I NSCLC.

Methods
Patient eligibility
Between April 2007 and August 2013, a total of 306 consecutive patients with potentially resectable NSCLC underwent measurement of D-dimer levels at Sagamihara Kyodo Hospital, Kanagawa, Japan. D-dimer level was measured within 4 weeks of surgery. We reviewed the data from 237 of these patients who were diagnosed with clinical stage I NSCLC according to the seventh edition of the TNM Staging Classification for Lung Cancer [12]. Patients who underwent incomplete resection or neoadjuvant chemotherapy/radiotherapy were excluded.

In addition to the D-dimer level, we reviewed the medical records of each patient for the following clinicopathological information: age, sex, smoking habit, serum concentration of carcinoembryonic antigen (CEA), extent of pulmonary resection, tumor location, maximum standardized uptake value (SUVmax) of the primary tumor, maximum tumor diameter, histological type, grade, pleural invasion, and pathological stage. All clinical, intraoperative, radiological, and pathological findings from two hospitals in Kanagawa, Japan (Sagamihara Kyodo Hospital and Yuai Clinic) were reviewed. Histological classification of NSCLC was based on the criteria of the World Health Organization [13]. Pre- and postoperative staging was based on the TNM staging system. Data collection and analyses were approved, and the need to obtain written informed consent from each patient was waived by the first author's institutional review board, due to the retrospective nature of this investigation.

Computed tomography
Diagnostic-quality contrast-enhanced computed tomography (CT) of the chest with a slice thickness of 5 mm was performed for all patients. A tumor was deemed central if the center was located in the inner one-third of the lung parenchyma (adjacent to the mediastinum) on transverse CT. Peripherally located tumors were identified as those centered in the outer two-thirds of the lung parenchyma on transverse CT. The maximal diameter of lung nodules was measured on contrast-enhanced chest CT. All imaging was performed within 4 weeks of surgery.

Integrated ^{18}F–fluorodeoxyglucose positron emission tomography imaging
Each patient underwent integrated ^{18}F–fluorodeoxyglucose positron emission tomography/CT (FDG-PET/CT) imaging before surgical resection. All integrated FDG-PET/CT imaging was performed within 4 weeks of surgery. After fasting for 6 h, FDG (3.5 MBq/kg body weight) was intravenously injected if the blood sugar level was lower than 200 mg/dl. Image acquisition was started 60 min after the injection using a single PET/CT combined scanner (Eminence-SOPHIA; Shimadzu, Kyoto, Japan) [14]. Image emission data from the eyes to the mid-thigh area were continuously acquired over a period of approximately 20 min. After attenuation corrections were made for the resulting image data, reconstruction was performed using a dynamic row-action expectation maximization algorithm [15]. The reconstructed sectional images were then evaluated both visually and quantitatively using the SUV$_{max}$ inside a volume of interest (VOI) placed on the lesions. SUV$_{max}$ was calculated as follows: [(maximum activity in VOI) / (volume of VOI)] / [(injected FDG dose) / (patient weight)]. The quality of radiation measurements of the PET/CT scanner was assured by calibration in accordance with National Electrical Manufacturers Association NU-2 2001 standards [16].

Nodal uptake with an SUV$_{max}$ > 2.5 was considered positive. To determine the SUV, a cylindrical region of interest (ROI) was placed over the tumor site manually on the hottest trans-axial slice. Activity within the ROI was determined and expressed as the SUV, defined as the ratio of activity in the tissue to the decay-corrected activity injected into the patient. All SUV measurements were normalized for patient body weight. SUV$_{max}$ within an ROI was used as the reference measurement.

Three experienced radiologists individually analyzed the integrated FDG-PET/CT images, with the final assessment made by consensus if initial assessments differed.

Surgical resection
All patients underwent anatomical lung resection (lobectomy or greater and segmentectomy) and radical lymphadenectomy in our hospital. All surgical resections were performed by thoracic surgeons at Sagamihara Kyodo Hospital. All surgical resection techniques were standardized. Systematic lymph node dissection was performed in all patients according to the criteria of the

American Thoracic Society, removing at least three hilar and three mediastinal stations.

Pathological examination

All resected tumor specimens were examined by experienced pulmonary pathologists. Histological classification of NSCLC was based on WHO classifications. Dissected lymph nodes were histologically examined following hematoxylin and eosin staining.

Statistical analysis

Statistical analysis was performed using SPSS version 23.0 software (IBM Corporation, Armonk, NY). Survival curves were constructed using the Kaplan-Meier method. Recurrence-free survival (RFS) probabilities and overall survival (OS) rates were compared using the log-rank test. The Cox proportional hazard model was used to estimate hazard ratio (HR) with 95% confidence interval (CI) for uni- and multivariate analyses. All tests were two-sided, and values of $P < 0.05$ were considered statistically significant. Factors identified as significant in univariate analysis ($P < 0.05$) were entered into the multivariate analysis.

Results

Patient characteristics

Patients were divided into two groups according to the D-dimer level: Group A, ≤ 1.0 µg/ml ($n = 170$); and Group B, > 1.0 µg/ml ($n = 67$). Patient characteristics are shown in Table 1. Participants comprised 140 men and 97 women, ranging in age from 31 to 85 years (median, 69 years). Median observation period in the survivors was 60.0 months (range, 2–110 months). Associations between D-dimer level and clinicopathological characteristics are shown in Table 2. D-dimer level correlated with serum CEA ($p < 0.001$), SUVmax of the primary tumor ($p < 0.001$), tumor size ($p = 0.023$), and pathological stage ($p = 0.003$).

Survival analysis of patients with pathological stage I adenocarcinoma after surgical resection

The 5-year RFS rate was 81.6% for Group A, and 66.6% for Group B (p < 0.001) (Fig. 1a). The 5-year OS rate was 93.6% for Group A, and 84.7% for Group B ($p = 0.002$) (Fig. 1b).

Univariate survival analysis revealed age (<70 vs. ≥70, OS: HR 2.31; 95%CI 1.12–5.13), serum CEA (≤5 vs. >5, RFS: HR 2.11; 95%CI 1.03–4.12, OS: HR 2.42; 95%CI 1.31–5.46), SUVmax of the primary tumor (≤2.3 vs. >2.3, RFS: HR 5.89; 95%CI 3.45–14.2, OS: HR 3.89; 95%CI 1.64–9.01), D-dimer level (≤1.0 vs. >1.0, RFS: HR 2.62; 95%CI 1.41–5.61, OS: HR 2.67; 95%CI 1.23–5.12), pleural invasion (absent vs. present, OS: HR 2.42; 95%CI 1.06–5.52) and

Table 1 Clinicopathological characteristics of 237 patients with clinical stage I NSCLC

Variables	n (%) or mean ± SD
Age at operation, y	69.0 ± 9.7
Gender	
Female	97 (40.9%)
Male	140 (59.1%)
Smoking habit	
Never smoker	94 (39.7%)
Ever smoker	143 (60.3%)
Serum CEA, ng/ml	
≤ 5	178 (75.1%)
> 5	59 (24.9%)
Extent of pulmonary resection	
Segmentectomy	34 (14.3%)
Lobectomy or more	203 (85.7%)
Tumor location	
Central	24 (10.1%)
Non-central	213 (89.9%)
SUVmax of primary tumor	2.3 ± 2.8
D-dimer, µg/ml	
≤ 1.0	170 (71.7%)
> 1.0	67 (28.3%)
Tumor size, cm	2.7 ± 1.5
Histological type	
AD	188 (79.3%)
SQ	36 (15.3%)
Others	13 (5.4%)
Grade	
1	156 (65.8%)
2 / 3 / 4	81 (34.2%)
Pleural invasion	
Absent	209 (88.2%)
Present	28 (11.8%)
Pathological stage	
Stage I	205 (86.4%)
Stage II	19 (8.2%)
Stage III	13 (5.4%)

NSCLC non-small cell lung cancer, SD standard deviation, CEA carcinoembryonic antigen, AD adenocarcinoma, SQ squamous cell carcinoma, SUV$_{max}$ maximum standardized uptake value

pathological stage (Stage I vs. Stage II/III, RFS: HR 5.61; 95%CI 3.22–9.12, OS: HR 3.91; 95%CI 1.65–8.98) as significant prognostic factors (Table 3). Multivariate survival analysis identified age (<70 vs. ≥70, OS: HR 2.39; 95%CI 1.09–5.24), SUVmax of the primary tumor (≤2.3 vs. >2.3, RFS: HR 3.78; 95%CI

Table 2 Association between D-dimer level and clinicopathological characteristics in patients with clinical stage I NSCLC

Variables	GroupA:D-dimer, μg/ml ≤1.0 (n = 170) n (%)	GroupB:D-dimer, μg/ml >1.0 (n = 67) n (%)	P value
Age at operation, y			
< 70	82 (48.1%)	31 (46.3%)	0.785
≥ 70	88 (51.9%)	36 (53.7%)	
Gender			
Female	68 (40.0%)	29 (43.3%)	0.643
Male	102 (60.0%)	38 (56.7%)	
Smoking habit			
Never smoker	70 (41.2%)	24 (35.8%)	0.448
Ever smoker	100 (58.8%)	43 (64.2%)	
Serum CEA, ng/ml			
≤ 5	140 (82.3%)	38 (56.7%)	<0.001
> 5	30 (17.7%)	29 (43.3%)	
Extent of pulmonary resection			
Segmentectomy	24 (14.1%)	10 (14.9%)	0.873
Lobectomy or more	146 (85.9%)	57 (85.1%)	
Tumor location			
Central	16 (9.4%)	8 (12.0%)	0.561
Non-central	154 (90.6%)	59 (88.0%)	
SUV_{max} of primary tumor			
≤ 2.3	123 (72.4%)	28 (41.8%)	<0.001
> 2.3	47 (27.6%)	39 (58.2%)	
Tumor size, cm			
≤ 3	118 (69.4%)	36 (53.7%)	0.023
> 3	52 (30.6%)	31 (46.3%)	
Histological type			
AD	139 (81.7%)	49 (73.1%)	0.140
Others	31 (28.3%)	18 (26.9%)	
Grade			
1	113 (72.4%)	43 (64.2%)	0.738
2 / 3 / 4	57 (27.6%)	24 (35.8%)	
Pleural invasion			
Absent	154 (90.6%)	55 (82.0%)	0.068
Present	16 (9.4%)	12 (18.0%)	
Pathological stage			
Stage I	154 (90.6%)	51 (76.1%)	0.003
Stage II / III	16 (9.4%)	16 (23.9%)	

NSCLC non-small cell lung cancer, *CEA* carcinoembryonic antigen, *AD* adenocarcinoma, *SUVmax* maximum standardized uptake value

1.61–8.72, OS: HR 3.43; 95%CI 1.36–8.61), D-dimer level (≤1.0 vs. >1.0, RFS: HR 1.92; 95%CI 1.33–2.91, OS: HR 2.24; 95%CI 1.05–4.69), and pathological stage (Stage I vs. Stage II/III, RFS: HR 4.01; 95%CI 1.64–9.91, OS: HR 4.11; 95%CI 1.65–9.98) as significant prognostic factors (Table 4).

Discussion

This retrospective investigation examined the prognostic significance of preoperative D-dimer concentrations in patients after surgical resection of clinical stage I NSCLC. Factors affecting the prognosis of surgically resected NSCLC have not yet been characterized in

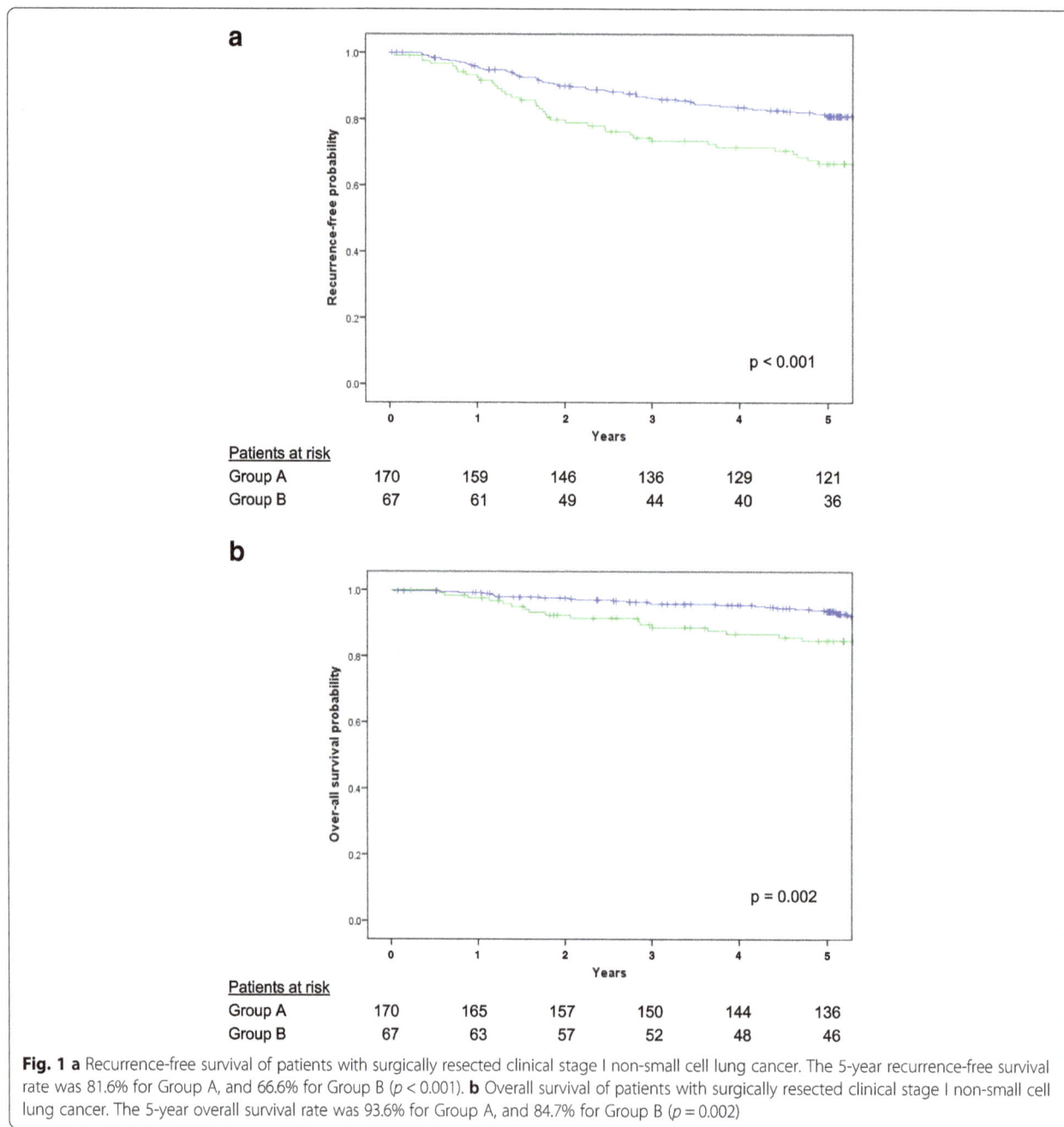

Fig. 1 a Recurrence-free survival of patients with surgically resected clinical stage I non-small cell lung cancer. The 5-year recurrence-free survival rate was 81.6% for Group A, and 66.6% for Group B ($p < 0.001$). **b** Overall survival of patients with surgically resected clinical stage I non-small cell lung cancer. The 5-year overall survival rate was 93.6% for Group A, and 84.7% for Group B ($p = 0.002$)

detail. However, clinicopathological factors such as positive cytological findings from pleural lavage, high preoperative concentrations of CEA, high tumor SUVmax and presence of lymphovascular invasion have been reported as associated with recurrence or decreased survival after surgery for NSCLC [17–19]. As a product of fibrin degradation, D-dimer is produced when cross-linked fibrin is broken down by plasmin-induced fibrinolysis. Concentrations of D-dimer are considered to represent a global biomarker of hemostasis and fibrinolysis. The processes of metastasis and tumor growth involve various interactions between the tumor and host.

Metastatic cancer cells must separate from the primary tumor, enter the circulation, attach to the vasculature of the destination, invade the tissue at this new site and establish neovasculature [20, 21]. Following initial cancer cell arrest in the vasculature of the destination organ, clotted plasma and platelets act in concert to stabilize circulating cancer cells by generating a thrombus that facilitates the attachment of cancer cells and allows invasion into the vessel wall [22]. Fibrin remodeling is involved in almost all the steps of metastasis, and plays a central role in neovascularization [20, 21]. Within the tumor extracellular matrix, cross-linked fibrin offers a

Table 3 Univariate analyses for recurrence-free and overall survival in patients with clinical stage I NSCLC

Variables	RFS HR (95% CI)	P value	OS HR (95% CI)	P value
Age at operation, y				
<70	1		1	
≥70	1.12 (0.56–2.14)	0.762	2.31 (1.12–5.13)	0.031
Gender				
Female	1		1	
Male	1.13 (0.54–2.28)	0.668	1.02 (0.78–1.52)	0.869
Smoking habit				
Never smoker	1		1	
Ever smoker	1.22 (0.88–1.72)	0.281	1.21 (0.86–1.82)	0.225
Serum CEA, ng/ml				
≤5	1		1	
>5	2.11 (1.03–4.12)	0.049	2.42 (1.31–5.46)	0.019
Extent of pulmonary resection				
Segmentectomy	1		1	
Lobectomy or more	0.75 (0.56–1.21)	0.221	0.81 (0.55–1.26)	0.231
Tumor location				
Central	1		1	
Non-central	0.94 (0.44–1.86)	0.852	0.58 (0.79–4.22)	0.586
SUV$_{max}$ of primary tumor				
≤2.3	1		1	
>2.3	5.89 (3.45–14.2)	<0.001	3.89 (1.64–9.01)	0.001
D-dimer, μg/ml				
≤1.0	1		1	
>1.0	2.62 (1.41–5.61)	0.019	2.67 (1.23–5.12)	0.021
Tumor size, cm				
<3	1		1	
>3	1.32 (0.64–2.72)	0.483	1.16 (0.54–2.76)	0.688
Histological type				
AD	1		1	
Others	1.33 (0.64–2.76)	0.486	1.35 (0.64–2.81)	0.479
Grade				
1	1		1	
2 / 3 / 4	1.33 (0.61–2.79)	0.438	1.41 (0.68–2.82)	0.439
Pleural invasion				
Absent	1		1	
Present	2.42 (1.06–5.52)	0.038	1.95 (0.76–5.01)	0.181
Pathological stage				
Stage I	1		1	
Stage II/III	5.61 (3.22–9.12)	<0.001	3.91 (1.65–8.98)	0.001

NSCLC non-small cell lung cancer, CEA carcinoembryonic antigen, AD adenocarcinoma, SUVmax maximum standardized uptake value, RFS recurrence-free survival, OS overall survival, HR hazard ratio, CI confidence interval

Table 4 Multivariate analyses for recurrence-free and overall survival in patients with clinical stage I NSCLC

Variables	RFS HR (95% CI)	P value	OS HR (95% CI)	P value
Age at operation, y				
< 70			1	
≥ 70	–	–	2.39 (1.09–5.24)	0.029
Serum CEA, ng/ml				
≤ 5	1		1	
> 5	1.03 (0.98–1.05)	0.061	1.74 (0.79–3.81)	0.163
SUV$_{max}$ of primary tumor				
≤ 2.3	1		1	
> 2.3	3.78 (1.61–8.72)	0.002	3.43 (1.36–8.61)	0.008
D-dimer, μg/ml				
≤ 1.0	1		1	
> 1.0	1.92 (1.33–2.91)	0.041	2.24 (1.05–4.69)	0.032
Pleural invasion				
Absent	1			
Present	1.05 (0.98–1.09)	0.071	–	–
Pathological stage				
Stage I	1		1	
Stage II/III	4.01 (1.64–9.91)	0.003	4.11 (1.65–9.98)	0.003

NSCLC non-small cell lung cancer, CEA carcinoembryonic antigen, SUV$_{max}$ maximum standardized uptake value, RFS recurrence-free survival, OS overall survival, HR hazard ratio, CI confidence interval

stable platform for endothelial cell migration during angiogenesis and for cancer cell migration during invasion. Even the early stages of tumor development show local fibrin deposition and initiation of angiogenesis [22]. Moreover, fibrin deposits around cancer cells in the circulation helps these cells avoid destruction by natural-killer cells [23]. A comparison of tumor dissemination in control and fibrinogen-deficient mice revealed that the absence of circulating fibrinogen markedly reduced the formation of pulmonary metastases after intravenous injection of cancer cells [24]. Similar results were described in another study of mice tumor model, with fibrinogen-deficiency markedly reducing spontaneous macroscopic metastasis in the lungs and regional lymph nodes. In addition, quantities of pulmonary micrometastases were significantly reduced among fibrinogen-deficient mice after intravenous injection of lung carcinoma cells [25]. Several reports in patients with malignancy have examined the prognostic significance of D-dimer concentrations. Ay et al. prospectively analyzed 1178 cancer patients without VTE over a period of 2 years until VTE or death. Study participants comprised 829 patients (70.4%) with solid tumors, 148 (12.6%) with brain tumors and 201 (17%) with hematological malignancies [26]. Patients were divided into quartiles according to D-dimer concentrations, revealing that high concentrations of D-dimer were associated with significantly poorer survival among patients with any type of malignancy. Other reports have examined the prognostic relevance of D-dimer among patients with primary lung cancer. Taguchi et al. measured D-dimer concentrations in 70 patients with lung carcinoma, finding that low levels of D-dimer were predictive of longer survival [27]. Buccheri et al. demonstrated a correlation between prognosis and D-dimer concentration. For 826 patients with lung carcinoma, median survival times were 154 days for patients with above-normal concentrations of D-dimer, and 308 days for patients with normal concentrations [28].

Altiay et al. investigated the relationship between D-dimer level and prognosis in a study of 78 patients with non-surgically treated primary lung cancer [29]. Zhang et al. investigated 232 patients with resected NSCLC, including 17 patients who developed VTE postoperatively, and confirmed the prognostic relevance of D-dimer concentrations [30]. Although the aim and results of that study showed some overlap with our own, our multivariate survival analysis also adjusted for additional factors strongly associated with prognosis, including CEA, smoking, and SUVmax of the tumor. Moreover, our study population was considered more homogeneous, given the lack of postoperative VTE events.

Uni- and multivariate analyses in this study revealed that increased D-dimer levels were predictive of worsened outcomes. Our findings support previous experimental and clinical findings of enhanced tumor progression and unfavorable outcomes in patients showing up-regulated coagulation and fibrinolytic activities. Such results strongly suggest that interactions between angiogenesis and hemostasis facilitate metastasis in patients with NSCLC. In general, the development of postoperative recurrence is likely due to the establishment of micrometastases or the presence of circulating tumor cells (CTCs) prior to treatment. Such cells appear undetectable with current diagnostic modalities, such as CT and FDG-PET/CT [31]. Given our findings, we speculate that high preoperative levels of D-dimer may be indicative of micrometastasis or CTCs, and thus in turn postoperative recurrence of NSCLC. D-dimer concentrations could therefore offer a predictor of NSCLC recurrence, even though D-dimer is not released by the tumor itself, unlike CEA.

Some limitations must be considered when interpreting the results of this retrospective analysis. The retrospective evaluation of D-dimer levels represents one clear problem. In addition, the study cohort was small, despite being relatively large compared to other such investigations of NSCLC patients.

Given our results and the data from previous basic studies, increased coagulation and fibrinolytic activities appear to be associated with increased risks of tumor progression and metastasis among patients with NSCLC. Concentrations of D-dimer before surgery may also offer a useful marker of recurrence and metastasis in NSCLC patients following radical resection. Furthermore, functional inhibition of fibrinogen and other coagulation factors might represent novel strategies for treating NSCLC. Further investigations are needed to clarify the relationships among circulating coagulation and angiogenic factors in neoplastic tissues.

Conclusions

The findings of this study suggest that preoperative D-dimer concentration offers an independent predictor of prognosis for completely resected clinical stage I NSCLC, along with age, SUVmax of the primary tumor, and pathological stage. The clinical implications of this finding remain to be determined.

Abbreviations
CEA: carcinoembryonic antigen; CI: confidence interval; CT: computed tomography; CTCs: circulating tumor cells; D-dimer: plasma D-dimer; DIC: disseminated intravascular coagulation; FDG-PET/CT: integrated 18F–fluorodeoxyglucose positron emission tomography/computed tomography; HR: hazard ratio; NSCLC: non-small cell lung cancer; OS: overall survival; RFS: recurrence-free survival; SUVmax: maximum standardized uptake value; VTE: venous thromboembolism

Acknowledgements
We acknowledge the assistance of Mr. Tomoyuki Kanno, Yuai Clinic, in the acquisition of study data.

Funding
No funding body provided support for the design of the study, the collection, analysis, or interpretation of data, or the writing of the manuscript.

Authors' contributions
KK wrote the manuscript. KK and KA performed surgery. AK carried out pathological examinations. All authors approved the final manuscript.

Competing interests
The authors declare that they have no competing interests.

Author details
[1]Department of Thoracic Surgery, Sagamihara Kyodo Hospital, 2-8-18 Hashimoto, Midori-ku, Sagamihara, Kanagawa 252-5188, Japan. [2]Department of Pathology, Sagamihara Kyodo Hospital, 2-8-18 Hashimoto, Midori-ku, Sagamihara, Kanagawa 252-5188, Japan. [3]Yuai Clinic, 1-6-2 Kitashinyokohama, Kohoku-Ku, Yokohama, Kanagawa 223-0059, Japan.

References

1. Sack GH, Levin J, Bell WR. Trousseau's syndrome and other manifestations of chronic disseminated coagulopathy in patients with neoplasms: clinical, pathophysiologic, and therapeutic features. Medicine. 1977;56:1–37.
2. Varki A. Trousseau's syndrome: multiple definitions and multiple mechanisms. Blood. 2007;110:1723–9.
3. Pabinger I, Ay C. Biomarkers and venous thromboembolism. Arterioscler Thromb Vasc Biol. 2009;29:332–6.
4. Pantel K, Alix-Panabieres C, Riethdorf S. Cancer micrometastases. Nat Rev Clin Oncol. 2009;6:339–51.
5. Rut W, Mueller BM. Thrombin generation and the pathogenesis of cancer. Semin Thromb Hemost. 2006;32(Supp1 1):61–8.
6. Batschauer APB, Figueiredo CP, Bueno EC, Ribeiro MA, Dusse LM, Fernandes AP, et al. D-dimer as a possible prognostic marker of operable hormone receptor-negative breast cancer. Ann Oncol. 2010;21:1267–72.
7. Blackwell K, Hurwitz H, Lieberman G, Novotny W, Snyder S, Dewhirst M, et al. Circulating D-dimer levels are better predictors of overall survival and disease progression than carcinoembryonic antigen levels in patients with metastasis colorectal carcinoma. Cancer. 2004;101:77–82.
8. Diao D, Zhu K, Wang Z, Cheng Y, Li K, Pei L, et al. Prognostic value of the D-dimer test in esophageal cancer during the perioperative period. J Surg Oncol. 2013;108:34–41.
9. Antonion D, Pavlakou G, Stathopoulos GP, Karydis I, Chondrou E, Papageorgiou C, et al. Predictive value of D-dimer plasma levels in response and progressive disease in patients with lung cancer. Lung Cancer. 2006;53:205–10.
10. Sheng L, Luo M, Sun X, Lin N, Mao W, Serum SD. Fibrinogen is an independent prognostic factor in operable non-small cell lung cancer. Int J Cancer. 2013;133:2720–5.
11. Zhao J, Zhao M, Jin B, Yu P, Hu X, Teng Y, et al. Tumor response and survival in patients with advanced non-small-cell lung cancer: the predictive value of chemotherapy-induced changes in fibrinogen. BMC Cancer. 2012;12:330.
12. Goldstraw P, Crowley J, Chansky K. International Association for the Study of Lung Cancer International Staging Committee, Participating Institutions, et al. The IASLC Lung Cancer Staging Project: Proposals for the revision of the TNM stage groupings in the forthcoming (seventh) edition of the TNM classification of malignant tumours. J Thorac Oncol. 2007;2:706–14.
13. World Health Organization. Histological typing of lung and pleural tumours, 4th edn. 2004; IARC Press, Lyon.
14. Matsumoto K, Kitamura K, Mizuta T, Tanaka K, Yamamoto S, Sakamoto S, et al. Performance characteristics of a new 3-dimensional continuous-emission and spiral-transmission high-sensitivity and high-resolution PET camera evaluated with the NEMA NU 2-2001 standard. J Nucl Med. 2006;47:83–90.
15. Kitamura K, Ishikawa A, Mizuta T, Yamaya T, Yoshida E, Murayama H. 3D continuous emission and spiral transmission scanning for high- throughput whole-body PET. Nuclear Science Symposium Conference Record, 2004; IEEE 2004, Rome, Italy; Vol 5: 2801–2805.
16. The Association of Electrical Equipment and Medical Imaging Manufacturers. Performance Measurements of Positron Emission Tomographs. NEMA Standards .Publication NU 2–2001. NEMA, Rosslyn, VA 2001.
17. Matsuguma H, Nakahara R, Igarashi S, Ishikawa Y, Suzuki H, Miyazawa N, et al. Pathologic stage I non-small cell lung cancer with high levels of preoperative serum carcinoembryonic antigen: clinicopathologic characteristics and prognosis. J Thorac Cardiovasc Surg. 2008;135:44–9.
18. Lim E, Clough R, Goldstraw P, Edmonds L, Aokage K, Yoshida J, et al. Impact of positive pleural lavage cytology on survival in patients having lung resection for non-small-cell lung cancer: an international individual patient data meta-analysis. J Thorac Cardiovasc Surg. 2010;139:1441–6.
19. Shiono S, Abiko M, Sato T. Positron emission tomography/computed tomography and lymphovascular invasion predict recurrence in stage I lung cancers. J Thorac Oncol. 2011;6:43–7.
20. Wojtukiewicz MZ, Sierko E, Klemont P, Rak J. The hemostatic system and angiogenesis in malignancy. Neoplasia. 2001;3:371–84.
21. Chiarug V, Ruggiero M, Magnelli L. Angiogenesis and the unique nature of tumor matrix. Mol Biotechnol. 2002;21:85–90.
22. Im JH, Fu W, Wang H, Bhatia SK, Hammer DA, Kowalska MA, et al. Coagulation facilitates tumor cell spreading in the pulmonary vasculature during early metastatic colony formation. Cancer Res. 2004;64:8613–9.
23. Palumbo JS, Talmage KE, Massari JV, La Jeunesse CM, Flick MJ, Kombrinck KW, et al. Platelets and fibrin (ogen) increase metastatic potential by impeding natured killer cell-mediated elimination of tumor cells. Blood. 2005;105:178–85.
24. Palumbo JS, Kombrinck KW, Drew AF, Grimes TS, Kiser JH, Degen JL, et al. Fibrinogen is an important determinant of the metastatic potential of circulation tumor cells. Blood. 2000;96:3302–9.
25. Palumbo JS, Potter JM, Kaplan LS, Talmage K, Jackson DG, Degen JL. Spontaneous hematogenous and lymphatic metastasis, but not primary tumor growth or angiogenesis, is diminish in fibrinogen-deficient mice. Cancer Res. 2002;62:6966–72.
26. Ay C, Dunkler D, Pirker R, Thaler J, Quehenberger P, Wagner O, et al. High D-dimer levels are associated with poor prognosis in cancer patients. Haematologica. 2012;97:1158–64.
27. Taguchi O, Gabazza EC, Yasui H, Kobayashi T, Yoshida M, Kobayashi H. Prognostic significance of plasma D-dimer levels in patients with lung cancer. Thorax. 1997;52:563–5.
28. Buccheri G, Torchio P, Ferrigno D. Plasma levels of D-dimer in lung carcinoma: clinical and prognostic significance. Cancer. 2003;97:3044–52.
29. Altiay G, Ciftci A, Demir M, Kocak Z, Sut N, Tabakoglu E, et al. High plasma D-dimer levels is associated with decreased survival in patients with lung cancer. Clin Oncol. 2007;19:494–8.
30. Zhang PP, Sun JW, Wang XY, Liu XM, Li K. Preoperative plasma D-dimer levels predict survival in patients with operable non-small cell lung cancer independently of venous thromboembolism. Eur J Surg Oncol. 2013;39:951–6.
31. Tanaka F, Yoneda K, Kondo N, Hashimoto M, Takuwa T, Matsumoto S, et al. Circulating tumor cell as a diagnostic marker in primary lung cancer. Clin Cancer Res. 2009;15:6980–6.

17

Surgical repair via submammary thoracotomy, right axillary thoracotomy and median sternotomy for ventricular septal defects

Zhi-Nuan Hong[†], Qiang Chen[†], Ze-Wei Lin, Gui-Can Zhang, Liang-Wan Chen, Qi-Liang Zhang and Hua Cao[*]

Abstract

Background: Right submammary thoracotomy and right vertical infra-axillary thoracotomy are performed for ventricular septal defect (VSD) to reduce the invasiveness of the conventional surgical repair through median sternotomy approach. No comparative studies have been conducted among these three procedures.

Methods: From January 2016 to December 2016, 182 patients with isolated VSD who underwent surgical repair via one of these 3 approaches were reviewed to compare these three procedures.

Results: The procedure success rates were similar in these three groups. There was no statistically significant difference in operative time, aortic cross-clamping time, the duration of CPB, blood transfusion amount and medical cost. However, postoperative mechanical ventilation time, the duration of intensive care and postoperative length of hospital stay were longer in median sternotomy group than the other two groups. ($P < 0.05$) The median sternotomy group required the longest incision. No significant difference was noted in major adverse events. There were different advantages and disadvantages in the three kinds of operative procedures.

Conclusions: Regarding conventional surgical repair VSD, right submammary thoracotomy and right vertical infra-axillary thoracotomy both delivered better cosmetic results for patients with isolated VSD, while all the three procedures could obtain satisfactory clinical effect.

Keywords: Congenital heart diseases, Ventricular septal defect, Surgery, Submammary thoracotomy, Right axillary thoracotomy, Median sternotomy

Background

Median sternotomy is still considered the gold standard surgical repair approach for ventricular septal defect(VSD) for its high success rate. However, conventional surgical repair can't avoid long midline scar, long postoperative hospital stay and thoracic deformation. With the development of surgical technique and accumulation of experience, the mortality rate of surgical closure isolated VSD is down to nearly 0 % in recent years. Cosmetic result has become an important factor to evaluate surgical procedures. Thoracoscopic assisted surgery, robotic assisted surgery and different approaches including lower ministernotomy, right submammary thoracotomy, right axillary thoracotomy and right posterolateral thoracotomy have been developed to achieve better cosmetic results. In our institution, we apply right submammary thoracotomy and right subaxillary thoracotomy in patients with isolated VSD, and by document retrieval we found that comparative studies on these three procedures were scarce. In this article, we compare the early and mid-term results of these three procedures.

* Correspondence: caohua0791@163.com
[†]Equal contributors
Department of Cardiovascular Surgery, Union Hospital, Fujian Medical University, Fuzhou 350001, People's Republic of China

Methods

In this study, we reviewed the medical records of 182 patients who underwent VSD closure at our cardiac center between January and December 2016. There were 56 patients in group A (via median sternotomy), 62 patients in group B (via right submammary thoracotomy) and 64 patients in group C (via right vertical infra-axillary thoracotomy). All the patients' clinical data are shown in Table 1. There were no statistically significant differences in gender, age (median and range, group A: 1.3 years, 2 months-2.5 years, group B: 1.4 years, 6 months-3.0 years, group C: 1.3 years, 6 months-2.8 years), body weight(group A: 6.0 kg, 5.0-12.6 kg, group B: 7.2 kg, 6.2-13.2 kg, group C: 7.3 kg, 5.9-13.0 kg) or VSD size(group A: 6.0 mm, 3.0-8.2 mm, group B: 5.4 mm, 3.1-7.8 mm, group C: 5.2 mm, 3.0-7.6 mm) distribution among these three groups. Routine clinical examinations were performed, which included a standard lead electrocardiogram, a chest X-ray examination, and routine blood and biochemical tests. All the patients had a confirmed diagnosis of VSD and were sufficiently assessed by transthoracic echocardiography(TTE). Pulmonary hypertension (which was accessed by TTE) (group A: 60 mmHg, 30-82 mmHg, group B: 54 mmHg, 32-78 mmHg, group C: 52 mmHg, 30-76 mmHg) and cardiothoracic ratio (group A: 0.58, 0.40-0.72, group B: 0.56, 0.42-0.61, group C: 0.57, 0.47–0.61) were similar among these three groups. The inclusion criteria: isolated VSD and no other intracardiac malformation. The exclusion criteria: respiratory diseases, history of thorax procedure, history of failed attempt of transcatheter closure, severe valvular regurgitation, and right to left shunt caused by severe pulmonary hypertension. The successful VSD closure were defined as no large residual shunt (< 2 mm) assessed by postoperative TTE.

Operative technique

VSD surgical repair via median sternotomy (group A)

Conventional surgical closure was conducted through median sternotomy approach under cardiopulmonary bypass. Pericardial patch was conducted in all patients.

VSD surgical repair via right submammary thoracotomy (group B)

The patients were canted to the right at an angle of 20° to 30°, with the right arm positioned beside the body. Under general anesthesia, we performed the incision in the right submammary groove, while with the cases of undeveloped breasts we made the incision in the fourth intercostal space to avoid deformity of the breast and the pectoral muscle. Then we spread muscle softly to avoid causing trauma to the rib periosteum and try to preserve the right internal mammary vessels [1]. The incision was about 4-5 cm based on the patient's height and weight. To provide a better operation field, we used a small rib spreader. The pericardium was opened in the site 1 cm anterior to the phrenic nerve and suspended to expose the right atrium and the aortic root.

Then we performed cannulations of the ascending aorta, the superior vena cava and the inferior vena cava to setup a standard CPB after systemic heparin administration. Aortic cross-clamp was performed in the same incision, then isothermal blood cardioplegia was provided to achieve adequate myocardial protection. To get enough exposure of the intracardiac anatomy, we performed a standard oblique right atriotomy, and did the procedures for VSD surgical closure as used in the median sternotomy approach. Finally, we gradually discontinued the CPB and partially closed the pericardium. We closed the chest in a routine fashion with an intradermal continuous suture for the skin after placement of chest drainage.

Table 1 Preoperative data comparison among three groups of patients

Item	Group A	Group B	Group C	P
N	56	62	64	
Age (year)	1.1 ± 1.4	1.3 ± 1.2	1.3 ± 1.5	$P > 0.05$
Gender (M/F)	26/30	31/31	30/34	$P > 0.05$
Weight (kg)	6.1 ± 3.2	8.3 ± 2.3	8.4 ± 2.5	$P > 0.05$
Size of VSD (mm)	6.2 ± 1.05	5.3 ± 1.12	5.1 ± 1.04	$P > 0.05$
Perimembrous VSD	48	60	63	
Muscular VSD	1	0	0	
Subatrial VSD	7	2	1	
Pulmonary hypertension (mmhg)	45.2 ± 11.7	42.1 ± 8.2	40.5 ± 9.2	$P > 0.05$
Cardiothoracic ratio	0.61 ± 0.10	0.56 ± 0.08	0.57 ± 0.06	$P > 0.05$

VSD surgical repair via right vertical infra-axillary thoracotomy (group C)

The patient was canted to the right at an angle of 90° with the right arm placed on the head and the shoulder-joint abducted at approximately 120°. The right vertical infra-axillary skin incision was done from the second intercostal space along the right midaxillary line to the fifth intercostal space along the preaxillary line. The incision was about 4-5 cm, adjusted to patient's weight and height. We entered the right thoracic cavity through the third or fourth intercostal space after muscle sparing and retracted the lung posteriorly with a wet gauge to expose the pericardium. The pericardium, opened from 2 cm superior to the phrenic nerve, was then suspended with sling sutures at the superior, middle, and inferior aspects of the pericardium to expose the right atrium and the aortic root.

We placed standard purse sutures in right side of the ascending aorta, the superior vena cava, and the right atriocaval junction. After heparinization, we cannulated the ascending aorta, the superior vena cava and the inferior vena cava. Then, a standard CPB were started and aortic cross-clamp was performed in the same incision. The same VSD closure was done as used in other procedures. Finally, we closed the pericardium partially and place a chest drainage in the right thorax.

All patients were given TTE, electrocardiogram, physical examinations 3 months, 6 months and 1 year after their operations.

Statistical analysis

Continuous variables were expressed as x ± s in table, t-test or analysis of variances were applied to continuous variables and the χ^2 or Fisher's test to categorical variables. P value< 0.05 were defined as statistical significance.

Results

The procedures were successful in the patients of these three groups. No perioperative death, low cardiac output syndrome, malignant arrhythmia, delayed recovery, reoperation for VSD, complete atrioventricular block (AVB), or cerebrovascular events were recorded in any group. Comparison among these three groups, shows that there were no statistically significant differences in operative time, aortic cross-clamping time, duration of CPB, or blood transfusion amount. ($P > 0.05$).

However, postoperative mechanical ventilation time (group A: 16.0 h, 8.8-22.0 h, group B: 8.0 h, 6.3-17.2 h, group C: 7.8 h, 5.0-16.4 h), duration of intensive care (group A: 20.0 h, 16.5-24.3 h, group B: 13. 6 h, 10.0-16.2 h, group C: 13.5 h, 9.8-17.6 h), postoperative length of hospital stay (group A: 9.0 days, 6.2-15.3 days, group B: 6.5 days, 3.2-9.0 days, group C: 6.4 days, 3.4-11.0 days), and pleural fluid drainage (group A: 50.0 ml, 20.0-100.5 ml, group B: 22.0 ml, 10.5-45.5 ml, group C: 20.5 ml, 8.5-47.5 ml) in group A was larger than that in group B and C ($P < 0.05$). Medical cost was similar among the three groups ($P > 0.05$). (Table 2) Group A required the longest incision (13.0 cm, 11.2-15.0 cm). The incidence rates of postoperative pulmonary infection were not significantly different, but the incidence rates of postoperative pneumothorax and subcutaneous emphysema were significantly higher in group B and C ($P < 0.05$). (Table 3).

During postoperative follow-ups, no serious complications or malignant arrhythmia occurred in any of these patients. Through physical examinations, we found 7 cases with thoracic deformity in group A. Then, these 7 patients were given thoracic CT scan and the results showed 5 cases with pectus carinatum and 2 cases with funnel chest. The above 7 patients were asymptomatic during the follow-up period. So close medical observation were given to these 7 patients without any intervention. No chest deformity were found in the other two

Table 2 Peri-operative and post-operative data comparison among three groups of patients

Item	Group A	Group B	Group C	P
Operative time (min)	110.4 ± 22.3	105.2 ± 25.4	103.6 ± 18.5	P > 0.05
Aortic occlusion clamping time (min)	38.3 ± 11.5	36.4 ± 12.8	37.1 ± 9.9	P > 0.05
Cardiopulmonary bypassing time (min)	60.5 ± 12.3	62.5 ± 10.2	63.2 ± 13.6	P > 0.05
Mechanical ventilation time (h)	16.6 ± 4.4	10.4 ± 3.1*	9.8 ± 2.5*	P < 0.05
Intensive care unit time (h)	21.7 ± 5.2	14.5 ± 2.3*	13.8 ± 2.6*	P < 0.05
Drainage (ml)	50.5 ± 21.5	24.4 ± 15.6*	20.5 ± 18.6*	P < 0.05
Blood transfusion volume (ml)	320.5 ± 80.4	338.3 ± 96.7	340.5 ± 86.5	P > 0.05
The incision length (cm)	13.7 ± 1.1	10.2 ± 2.3*	8.5 ± 2.4*	P < 0.05
Postoperative hospital stay (d)	9.2 ± 3.2	6.8 ± 2.1*	6.9 ± 3.2*	P < 0.05
Hospital costs (10000RMB)	5.85 ± 0.63	5.45 ± 0.83	5.25 ± 0.92	P > 0.05

Table 3 Post-operative complications comparison between two group of patients(%)

Item	Group A	Group B	Group C	P
Cerebrovascular accident	0	0	0	
Small residual shunt	5	3	4	
Large residual shunt requiring reoperation	0	0	0	
Severe Arrhythmia				
Complete AVB	0	0	0	
Mobitz type II AVB	0	0	0	
Low cardiac output syndrome	0	0	0	
Pulmonary infection	5	7	9	P > 0.05
Surgical wound bad healing	4	0	1	
Pneumothorax	0	3	4	P < 0.05
Subcutaneous emphysema	0	2	3	P < 0.05
Thoracic deformity	7	0	0	
Pericardial effusion	2	0	0	
Pleural effusion	0	2	2	
Transient Arrhythmia	5	6	5	

groups. CT Haller index changes in the above 7 patients were shown in Table 4. No significant progress of these patients was found in the follow-up period.

Discussion

Ventricular septal defect is one of the most common congenital cardiac defects [1, 2]. Although the transcatheter techniques have been widely used and performed and delivered promising early and midterm results in recent years, the X-ray exposure and potential vascular injury limited the promotion of this approach [3–5].And the median sternotomy approach was limited by its visible mid-sternotomy scar, which should be taken into consideration. Surgeons then developed other approaches to reduce the invasiveness of complete median sternotomy and pursue better cosmetic results, especially in children, teenager and female patients [6]. These alternatives included lower mini-sternotomy incision [7, 8], right submammary incision [9, 10], right posterolateral thoracotomy incision [11] and right vertical infra-axillary incision [12–14].

In our institution, we applied right submammary thoracotomy and right vertical infra-axillary thoracotomy in VSD repair. The advantages of the right submammary thoracotomy and right vertical infra-axillary

Table 4 CT Haller Index change in 7 patients with thoracic deformity

CT Haller Index	3-month	6-month	12-month	P
Pectus Carinatum (n = 5)	2.30 ± 0.19	2.31 ± 0.20	2.31 ± 0.18	P > 0.05
Funnel Chest (n = 2)	3.00 ± 0.03	3.00 ± 0.03	3.00 ± 0.03	P > 0.05

thoracotomy have been previously described. These two thoracotomies are similar to median sternotomy in having enough exposure, no need for special instrument, no difficulty in CPB establishment, and no increased medical cost in most reports. And their advantages have been described, such as faster recovery and better cosmetic results. However, technical complexity including satisfactory exposure, invisible site and the length of incision remained the focus of exploration. As no comparative study has been conducted among right submammary thoracotomy, right vertical infra-axillary thoracotomy and median sternotomy, our study aims to compare these three approaches in repairing VSD under CPB.

Compared with group A, there was no significant difference in CPB time, aortic cross-clap time or operative time in group B and C. We contributed these to those right submammary thoracotomy and right vertical infra-axillary thoracotomy could provide enough good exposure of the inferior vena cava and the ascending aorta without increasing the technical difficulty. However, according to our experience, it's difficult to setup CPB in female patients with large breast and in patients with a BMI > 28 kg/m [2] in group B and C. The chest incision in these two groups were also significantly shorter than the median sternotomy group. Meanwhile, there was no need for sternum split or wire fixation, which may lead to negative post-operative X-ray chest examination. But the incidence rates of postoperative pneumothorax and subcutaneous emphysema were significantly higher in group B and C. With strengthened operative technique and management, however, such complications can be well controlled. The surgical success rate of VSD repair via right submammary thoracotomy and right vertical infra-axillary thoracotomy were similar to median sternotomy in this study, which means all the three methods can achieve satisfactory clinical results. Based on these findings, we recommend that right submammary thoracotomy and right vertical infra-axillary thoracotomy be used as effective and safe alternatives in VSD surgical repair.

Cosmetic results should be taken into consideration in such operations, which include incision length, visible or invisible and whether this incision causes thoracic deformity. We found that the incidence of thoracic deformity was higher in median sternotomy group, although 7 patients suffered from pectus carinatum or funnel chest. No significant progress was found in the follow-up period. Close medical observation were given to these 7 patients without any other intervention. In most medical centers, the right submammary thoracotomy was made through the fourth or fifth intercostal space. Compared to the median sternotomy group, the incision caused can't be seen from the collar, which may be more acceptable to women patients. However, this incision may dissect the breast tissue and result in asymmetrical development and a decrease in sensitivity of the nipple [15, 16]. We contributed these side effects to the difference in incision choice in our institution, where the incision was in the fourth intercostal space for children. In addition, we also obey the rule that the incision should be at least 1.5 cm away from the mammary areola in patients with undeveloped breasts [17]. For female patients the incision was in the submammary groove so that when the operation via the incision would be covered by breast. In addition, during the procedure, we did our best to preserve the right internal mammary vessels.

In our institution, we also repaired VSD via right vertical infra-axillary thoracotomy. Wang et al. reported 274 patients with ventricular septal defects went through repair via a minimal right vertical infra-axillary thoracotomy [14]. In their study there were no deaths or complications from the infection of incisional wound and arrhythmia, and no significant differences in CPB time or postoperative ventilator time. However, the length of incision, postoperative volume drainage and ICU stay, minimal right vertical infra-axillary thoracotomy was significantly shorter than median sternotomy. These results were consistent with the results of our study. First, unlike some other new technology, this incision didn't require special instruments and most part of the procedure is similar to conventional surgical repair, which means no increase in hospital cost and short learning cure for experienced surgeons. Second, it could provide enough surgical field. Based on these two reasons, the CPB time and the aortic clamping time of this procedure were also similar to those of median sternotomy. And we also found that the hospital stay and the time needed to recover to normal activities in the right vertical infra-axillary thoracotomy group

were superior to those of the median sternotomy group, which also suggested faster recovery. Although in most patients this procedure didn't increase the technical difficulty, it's still difficult, even for experienced surgeons, to close subarterial VSDs through such procedure. In repairing such kind of VSD, we preferred the right submammary thoracotomy to right vertical infra-axillary thoracotomy, which also provide enough surgical field if placing a wet sponge under pericardial cavity beneath the heart.

For female patients with developed breast, if we chose right submammary thoracotomy, the incision would be covered by breast. However, when operating on children, right vertical infra-axillary thoracotomy may be a better choice. The reasons are listed below: First, this short incision is located under the armpit, which makes it almost invisible; Second, the incision of right submammary thoracotomy never surpasses the preaxillary line and thus will not cause dysplasia. Finally, the incision site is in the chest wall and far from the costochondral junction. Thus, it does not interfere with the development of the chest wall.

The incidence of arrhythmia was similar in all groups. According to previous report, surgical approach (right atrium or right ventricle) did not influence the arrhythmia rate [18, 19], which was the reason why we didn't conduct subgroup analysis of arrhythmia. According to above-mentioned comparisons, we could conclude that right submammary thoracotomy and right vertical infra-axillary thoracotomy are both safer and more efficient approaches for VSD closure than median sternotomy. We then further compared right submammary thoracotomy and right vertical infra-axillary thoracotomy. We found that there weren't significant differences in procedure success rate, operation time, ICU stay, postoperative hospital stay or volume of transfusion in these two groups. And the rate of complications were also similar in right submammary thoracotomy and right vertical infra-axillary thoracotomy.

This study was a retrospective study and was limited by the number of cases and the fact that it was done in a single center. Prospective randomized controlled studies with a larger sample size, even multi-center cooperation, must be conducted to confirm the results. In addition, a longer follow-up is essential, especially for those patients with thoracic deformity.

Conclusion

All the three procedures can obtain satisfactory clinical effects. Regarding surgical repair VSD, right submammary thoracotomy and right vertical infra-axillary thoracotomy both deliver good cosmetic results for patients with isolated VSD, while the latter may be a better choice to pursue better cosmetic results for children.

Surgical repair via submammary thoracotomy, right axillary thoracotomy and median sternotomy...

117

Abbreviations

AVB: atrioventricular block; CHD: congenital heart disease; ICU: intensive care unit; TTE: transthoracic echocardiography; VSD: ventricular septal defect

Acknowledgements

We highly acknowledge the contribution by the participating doctors: Dao-zhong Chen, Feng Lin, QI-min Wang, Zhong-yao Huang, Han-fan Qiu, Xue-shan Huang, Dong-shan Liao, Xiao-fu Dai, Xi-jie Wu, Hui Zhang, Zeng-chun Wang.

Funding

This research was sponsored by Chinese national and Fujian provincial key clinical specialty construction programs.

Authors' contributions

Zhi-Nuan Hong, Qiang Chen and Hua Cao designed the study, collected the clinical data, performed the statistical analysis, participated in the operation, and drafted the manuscript. Ze-Wei Lin, Gui-Can Zhang, Liang-Wan Chen and Qi-Liang Zhang participated in the operation and revised the article. All authors read and approved the final manuscript.

Competing interests

The authors declare that they have no competing interests.

References

1. Cherup LL, Siewers RD, Futrell JW. Breast and pectoral muscle maldevelopment after anterolateral and posterolateral thoracotomies in children. Ann Thorac Surg. 1986;41:492–7.
2. Tynan M, Anderson RH. Ventricular septal defects. In: Anderson RH, Baker EJ, Maccartney FJ, Rigby ML, Shinebourne EA, Tynan M,editors. Paediatric cardiology, 2nd ed. London: Churchill Livingstone;2002;983-1014.
3. Chessa M, Butera G, Negura D. Transcatheter closure of congenital ventricular septal defects in adult: mid-term results and complications. Int J Cardiol. 2009;133:70–3.
4. Odemis E, Saygi M, Guzeltas A, Tanidir IC, Ergul Y, Ozyilmaz I, Bakir I. Transcatheter closure of perimembranous ventricular septal defects using nit-Occlud(®) Lê VSD coil: early and mid-term results. Pediatr Cardiol 2014; 35(5):817–23.
5. Yang J, Yang L, Wan Y, Zuo J, Zhang J, Chen W, Li J, Sun L, Yu S, Liu J, Chen T, Duan W, Xiong L, Yi D. Transcatheter device closure of perimembranous ventricularseptal defects: mid-term outcomes. Eur Heart J. 2010;31(18):2238–45.
6. Cingoz F, Tavlasoglu M, Sahin MA, Kurkluoglu M, Guler A, Günay C, Arslan M. Minimally invasive pediatric surgery in uncomplicated congenital heart disease. Asian Cardiovasc Thorac Ann. 2013;21(4):414–7.
7. Bichell DP, Geva T, Bacha EA, Mayer JE, Jonas RA, del Nido PJ. Minimal access approach for the repair of atrial septal defect: the initial 135 patients. Ann Thorac Surg. 2000;70:115–8.
8. Nicholson IA, Bichell DP, Bacha EA, del Nido PJ. Minimal sternotomy approach for congenital heart operations. Ann Thorac Surg. 2001;71:469–72.
9. De Mulder W, Vanermen H. Repair of atrial septal defects via limited right anterolateral thoracotomy. Acta Chir Belg. 2002;102:450–4.
10. Mishaly D, Ghosh P, Preisman S. Minimally invasive congenital cardiac surgery through right anterior minithoracotomy approach. Ann Thorac Surg. 2008;85:831–5.
11. Vida VL, Padalino MA, Bhattaral A, Stellin G. Right posteriorlateral minithoracotomy access for treating congenital heart disease. Ann Thorac Surg. 2011;92:2278–80.
12. Mishaly D, Ghosh P, Preisman S. Minimally invasive congenital cardiac surgery through right anterior minithoracotomy approach. Annals Thoracic Surg. 2008;85(3):831–5.
13. Lei H, Yan ZY, Yan Y, Zhang QC. Comparison of right axillary straight incision and median sternotomy in mitral valve replacement. Anhui Med J. 2013;34(9):1287–9.
14. Wang Q, Li Q, Zhang J, Wu Z, Zhou Q, Wang DJ. Ventricular septal defects closure using a minimal right vertical infraaxillary thoracotomy: seven-year experience in 274 patients. Ann Thoracic Surg. 2010;89(2):552–5.
15. Cherup LL, Siewers RD, Futrell JW. Breast and pectoral muscle maldevelopment after anterolateral and posterolateralthoracotomies in children. Ann Thorac Surg. 1986;41(5):492–7.
16. Fisher JC, Rudolph R. Augmentation mammaplasty. In: Fisher JC, Guerrerosantos J, Gleason M, eds. Manual of aesthetic surgery. 1 st ed. New York: Springer; 1985:13-23.
17. Massimo M, Gerard B, Antom R, et al. Operation for atrial septal defect through a right anterolateral thoracotomy: current outcome. Ann Thorac Surg. 1966;62(4):110–2.
18. Shirasawa B, Hamano K, Katoh T, Fujimura Y, Tsuboi H, Esato K. A case report of open heart surgery in an infant with MNMS caused by femoral arterial cannulation during cardiopulmonary bypass. J Jpn Assoc Thorac Surg. 1996;44:1902–6.
19. Houyel L, Vaksmann G, Fournier A, Davignon A. Ventricular arrhythmias after correction of ventricular septal defects: importance of surgical approach. J Am Coll Cardiol. 1990;16:1224–8.

18

Reoperation for isolated rheumatic tricuspid regurgitation

Younes Moutakiallah[1,4]*, Mahdi Aithoussa[1,4], Noureddine Atmani[1,4], Aniss Seghrouchni[1,4], Azeddine Moujahid[2,4], Abdedaïm Hatim[2,4], Iliyasse Asfalou[3,4], Zouhair Lakhal[3,4] and Abdelatif Boulahya[1,4]

Abstract

Background: The reoperation for isolated tricuspid regurgitation in rheumatic population is rare and still unclear and controversial because of the rarity of publications. The aim of this study was to analyze short and long-term results and outcome of tricuspid valve surgery after left-sided valve surgery in rheumatic patients.

Methods: Twenty six consecutive rheumatic patients who underwent isolated tricuspid valve surgery after left-sided valve surgery between January 2000 and January2017 were retrospectively registered in the study. The mean age was 48. 2 ± 8.6 years with 8.3% as sex-ratio (M/F). EuroSCORE was 6.1 ± 5 (range 2.5 to 24.1). The mechanism of tricuspid regurgitation was functional and organic in respectively 14 (53.8%) and 12 cases (46.2%). Ten patients (38.5%) had previous tricuspid valve repair. Surgery consisted of 15 ring annuloplasty and 11 tricuspid valve replacement (5 bioprostheses and 6 mechanical prostheses). Follow-up was 96.1% complete, with a mean follow-up of 55. 6 ± 38.8 months (range 1 to 165).

Results: The operative mortality rate was 15.4% ($n = 4$) and the cumulative survival at 1, 5 and 10 years was respectively 80% ± 8%, 75.6% ± 8.7% and 67.2% ± 11.1% with no significant difference at 8 years between tricuspid valve replacement (80% ± 12.6%) and repair (57.6% ± 16.1%) ($p = 0.5$). Multivariable Cox regression analysis revealed that ascites (HR, 5.8; $p = 0.01$), and right ventricular dysfunction (HR, 0.94; $p = 0.001$) were predictors of major adverse cardiac events. There were no recurrence of tricuspid regurgitation and no structural or non-structural deterioration of valvular prostheses.

Conclusion: The reoperation of rheumatic tricuspid regurgitation should be considered before the installation of complications such as right ventricular dysfunction and major signs of right heart failure. Despite the superiority of repair techniques, tricuspid valve replacement should not be banished.

Keywords: Isolated tricuspid regurgitation, Reoperation, Rheumatic

Background

Rheumatic heart disease (RHD) is still a serious problem of national health in our country with a significant cost and an enormous social and economic impact. This cost is widely expressed by redo valve surgery that usually requires several human and material resources, which is not easily available in underdeveloped areas like African countries. The reoperation for tricuspid regurgitation (TR) is the typical example of this redo valve heart surgery so much apprehended because of its operating risks related to the pathology itself, the surgical technique and the patient's condition. In addition, this entity remains uncommon with many dark areas because of the rarity of publications in this field.

Methods

After approval of our institutional review board, we retrospectively collected and analyzed the data of 26 consecutive patients who underwent isolated tricuspid valve surgery for neglected late TR appearing at distance of left-sided heart valve surgery (LSHVS) without tricuspid procedure or recurrent TR reappearing after tricuspid valve repair (TVrp) concomitantly performed with

* Correspondence: dryouns@hotmail.com
[1]Cardiac surgery department, Mohammed V teaching military hospital, Hay Riyad, PB 10100, Rabat, Morocco
[4]Faculty of medicine and pharmacy, Mohammed V university, Rabat, Morocco
Full list of author information is available at the end of the article

LSHVS. Data were extracted from preoperative and postoperative clinical notes, anaesthesia and operating data records, intensive care unit progress notes and laboratory data.

We used the term "redo" to describe the recurrent TR reappeared after tricuspid valve repair and the term "late" for the neglected TR appeared after LSHVS without tricuspid procedure. The term "functional" means TR secondary to the annular dilatation without involvement of the tricuspid leaflets as a result of increased pulmonary and right ventricular pressures consequently to mitro-aortic pathology. In opposition, the term "organic" describes the direct involvement of the tricuspid valve (TV) by the RHD [1, 2].

Patients

The study included all patients ($n = 26$) operated in our institution for isolated "late" or "redo" rheumatic TR on a 17-year period between January 2000 and January 2017. Patients operated for non-rheumatic TR and patients operated for TR and any other concomitant valvular or bypass surgery were excluded from the study. Table 1 shows preoperative data. The average age at operation was 48.1 ± 8.6 years (range 29 to 63 years). Fifteen patients (57.7%) underwent tricuspid valve repair and 11 patients (42.3%) underwent tricuspid valve replacement (TVR) with 6 mechanical prostheses (32.1%) and 5 bioprostheses (19.2%). The New York Heart Association (NYHA) functional class was respectively 1, 2, 3 and 4 in 1 patients (3.8%), 4 patients (15.4%), 15 patients (57.7%) and 6 patients (23.1%). The mean interval from previous LSHVS and the current surgery was 164.1 ± 49.8 months (range 59 to 240 months) in the tricuspid valve repair group and 111.5 ± 72.1 months (range 6 to 241 months) in the replacement group ($p = 0.04$). Patients of repair group were significantly older than replacement group (51.2 ± 9.1 years vs 44 ± 0.9 years, $p = 0.03$); they had a longer delay between the two last surgeries (164.1 ± 49.8 months vs 111.5 ± 72.1 months, $p = 0.04$); they had also a larger tricuspid annulus (45 ± 3 mm vs 39.7 ± 7 mm, $p = 0.02$). In addition, there was significantly more likely to find a history of previous TV surgery in the replacement group (8 vs 2, $p = 0.004$), with a high proportion of organic TR with thickened leaflets and rheumatic lesions in the replacement group (10 vs 2, $p < 0.001$) and subsequently high percentage of tricuspid commissurotomy with or without Devega procedure (7 vs 1, $p = 0.001$).

Operative technique and data

All patients were electively operated under general anesthesia made by Cisatracurium besylate, Midazolam, Thiopental and Propofol. Twenty four patients (92.3%) were approached by median sternotomy and 2 patients (7.7%) by right anterolateral thoracotomy (4th intercostal space). Cardiopulmonary bypass was established in a conventional manner by central cannulation (ascending aorta and both vena cavae) and performed under moderate systemic hypothermia (32 °C). The tricuspid procedure was performed on arrested heart in 17 patients (65.4%) and on beating heart in 9 patients (34.6%) ($p = 0.02$), depending on surgical preference. Myocardial protection was achieved with antegrade cold (4 °C) crystalloid St. Thomas cardioplegia in 9 patients (34.6%) or antegrade cold (4 °C) blood high potassium cardioplegia in 8 patients (30.8%) ($p = 0.05$). The choice between tricuspid valve repair and replacement was made according to anatomical conditions with a preference for plasty techniques if suitable. Otherwise, we performed a tricuspid valve replacement by mechanical or biological prosthesis, which was inserted into the annulus with interrupted pledgeted mattress sutures using an everting suture technique. The native TV leaflets were left in place, preserving the subvalvular apparatus. In the septal area, the sutures were placed at the level of the leaflets avoiding the atrioventricular node injury. Conventional ultrafiltration was performed in 6 cases (23.1%). Fifteen patients (57.7%) underwent tricuspid valve repair, all by a Carpentier-Edwards (C-E) Semi-rigid Ring (Edwards Lifesciences, Irvine, CA), and 11 patients (42.3%) underwent tricuspid valve replacement. The mechanical prostheses used were 3 ATS Valve (ATS Medical Inc., Minneapolis, MN), 1 Sorin Bicarbon Slimline (Sorin Biomedica, Saluggia, Italy), 1 St. Jude Medical (St. Jude Medical, Inc) and 1 Carbo-Medics Valve (CarboMedics, Inc., Austin, TX). The biological prostheses used were 2 St. Jude Epic Biocor Valve (St. Jude Medical Inc), 2 Medtronic Hancock II Tissue Valve (Medtronic Inc., Minneapolis, MN) and 1 Sorin Pericarbon More (Sorin Biomedica, Saluggia, Italy). Table 2 summarizes operative data.

Follow-up

Data was obtained from our local database. After discharge, all patients were included in our scheduled follow-up protocol with routine clinical controls at 1, 3, 6, and 12 months and annually afterwards. Follow-up data were provided either routinely by our outpatient clinic evaluation and telephone interviews with patients, relatives or referring physicians. The control was based on clinical examination, electrocardiogram, chest X-ray and echocardiography. The postoperative events and results were described according to the guidelines for reporting mortality and morbidity after cardiac valve interventions, approved by The Society of Thoracic Surgeons [3]. Follow-up was closed on September 30, 2017 and was 96.1% complete, with a cumulative duration of follow-up of 1746 patient-years and a mean follow-up period of 67.2 ± 46.7 months (range 1 to 165 months).

Table 1 Preoperative characteristics of patients undergoing tricuspid valve surgery for isolated rheumatic tricuspid regurgitation ($n = 26$). Data are Presented as Mean ± SD, Median (Range), or n (%)

Characteristics	All patients $n = 26$	Functional TR $n = 14$	Organic TR $n = 12$	p-Value
Age (year)	48.2 ± 8.6	51.4 ± 9.3	44.4 ± 5.9	0.04
Sex (female)	24 (92.3%)	12 (85.7%)	12 (100%)	0.28
Symptoms duration (month)	29.5 ± 23.1	23.6 ± 16.5	36.3 ± 28.2	0.17
EuroSCORE	4.2 (2.5–24.1)	12.2 (2.5–24.1)	15 (3–16.2)	0.3
NYHA class 3–4	21 (80.8%)	11 (78.6%)	10 (83.3%)	0.58
Lower extremities edema	16 (61.5%)	9 (64.3%)	7 (58.3%)	0.54
Ascites	7 (26.9%)	4 (28.6%)	3 (25%)	0.60
Diabetes mellitus	3 (11.5%)	2 (14.3%)	1 (8.3%)	0.56
Gastro-duodenal ulcer	2 (7.7%)	2 (14.3%)	0 (0%)	0.28
History of stroke	3 (11.5%)	0 (0%)	3 (25%)	0.09
Haemoglobin < 12 g/dl	6 (23.1%)	3 (21.4%)	3 (25%)	0.60
Creatinine ≥2 mg/dl	2 (7.7%)	1 (7.1%)	1 (8.3%)	0.72
Atrial fibrillation	26 (100%)	14 (100%)	12 (100%)	1
Cardio-thoracic ratio	0.63 ± 0.09	0.62 ± 0.09	0.65 ± 0.09	0.4
Nature of tricuspid regurgitation				
- Late	16 (61.5%)	13 (92.9%)	3 (25%)	0.001
- Redo	10 (38.5%)	1 (7.1%)	9 (75%)	0.001
Tricuspid annulus diameter (mm)	42.8 ± 5.6	45.2 ± 3.1	40 ± 6.7	0.02
Tricuspid regurgitation severity	3.8 ± 0.4	3.7 ± 0.5	3.8 ± 0.4	0.5
- Grade 3	6 (23.1%)	4 (28.6%)	2 (16.7%)	0.65
- Grade 4	20 (76.9%)	10 (71.4%)	10 (83.3%)	0.40
Right ventricular dysfunction	12 (46.2%)	7 (50%)	5 (41.7%)	0.49
Systolic pulmonary arterial pressure (mmHg)	47 ± 16.4	41.7 ± 11.6	53.2 ± 19.3	0.09
Left ventricular ejection fraction (%)	57.1 ± 9.4	57.9 ± 6.7	56.1 ± 12.4	0.64
Left ventricular ejection fraction < 40%	1 (3.8%)	0 (0%)	1 (8.3%)	0.46
Left atrium diameter (mm)	55.9 ± 13.9	56.4 ± 17.1	55.4 ± 10.8	0.88
Number of previous heart operations	1.4 ± 0.6	1.2 ± 0.4	1.6 ± 0.8	0.2
- 1	18 (69.2%)	11 (78.6%)	7 (58.3%)	0.4
- 2	6 (23.1%)	3 (21.4%)	3 (25%)	1
- 3	2 (7.7%)	0 (0%)	2 (16.7%)	0.2
Previous left side valve surgery				
- Mitral valve replacement	16 (61.5%)	10 (71.4%)	6 (50%)	0.42
- Mitral and aortic valve replacement	10 (38.5%)	4 (28.6%)	6 (50%)	0.24
Previous tricuspid procedure				
- No tricuspid procedure	16 (61.5%)	13 (92.9%)	3 (25%)	0.001
- Devega technique	2 (7.7%)	1 (7.1%)	1 (8.3%)	1
- Devega + Commissurotomy	7 (26.9%)	0 (0%)	7 (58.3%)	0.001
- Commissurotomy	1 (3.8%)	0 (0%)	1 (8.3%)	0.5

TR: tricuspid regurgitation, *EuroSCORE*: European System for Cardiac Operative Risk Evaluation, *NYHA*: New York Heart Association

Statistical analysis

The statistical analysis was performed using the IBM statistical package software for social sciences 19.0 (SPSS, Chicago, Illinois, USA). Data was presented as mean ± standard deviation (SD) or median (range) for continuous variables and n (%) for categorical variables. For the two group comparisons, chi-square test or Fisher's exact test were used for categorical variables and

Table 2 Operative characteristics of patients undergoing tricuspid valve surgery for isolated rheumatic tricuspid regurgitation (n = 26). Data are Presented as Mean ± SD, Median (Range), or n (%)

Characteristics	All patients n = 26	Functional TR n = 14	Organic TR n = 12	p-Value
Median sternotomy	24 (92.3%)	14 (100%)	10 (83.3%)	0.20
Right thoracotomy	2 (7.7%)	0 (0%)	2 (16.7%)	0.11
Beating heart	9 (34.6%)	2 (14.3%)	7 (58.3%)	0.02
Cardioplegia	17 (65.4%)	12 (85.7%)	5 (41.7%)	0.02
- Cold crystalloid St Thomas cardioplegia	9 (52.9%)	7 (77.8%)	2 (22.2%)	0.62
- Cold blood high potassium cardioplegia	8 (47.1%)	5 (35.7%)	3 (25%)	0.62
Cardio-pulmonary bypass time (minute)	95.4 ± 39.7	87.9 ± 19.7	104.1 ± 54.4	0.35
Cross aortic clamping time (minute)	60 (35–170)	60 (38–170)	52 (35–103)	0.60
Hemofiltration (n, %)	6 (23.1%)	4 (28.6%)	2 (16.7%)	0.21
Mean ± SD (ml/Kg)	78.7 ± 34.6	89.7 ± 16.4	56.8 ± 16.2	0.58
Difficult weaning from cardio-pulmonary bypass	9 (34.6%)	3 (21.4%)	6 (50%)	0.22
Tricuspid valve repair:	15 (57.7%)	13 (92.9%)	2 (16.7%)	< 0.001
- Carpentier Edwards ring n°30	1 (3.8%)	1 (7.1%)	0 (0%)	0.9
- Carpentier Edwards ring n°32	11 (42.3%)	9 (64.3%)	2 (16.7%)	< 0.001
- Carpentier Edwards ring n°34	3 (11.5%)	3 (21.4%)	0 (0%)	0.03
Tricuspid valve replacement:	11 (42.3%)	1 (7.1%)	10 (83.3%)	< 0.001
- Mechanical prosthesis:	6 (23.1%)	0 (0%)	6 (50%)	< 0.001
- SJM n°27	1 (3.8%)	0 (0%)	1 (8.3)	0.87
- Sorin Bicarbon n°27	1 (3.8%)	0 (0%)	1 (8.3)	0.87
- ATS n°29	2 (7.7%)	0 (0%)	2 (16.7%)	0.7
- ATS n°31	1 (3.8%)	0 (0%)	1 (8.3)	0.87
- Carbomedics Valve n°31	1 (3.8%)	0 (0%)	1 (8.3)	0.87
- Biological prosthesis:	5 (19.2%)	1 (7.1%)	4 (33.3%)	< 0.001
- Sorin Pericarbon More n°27	1 (3.8%)	0 (0%)	1 (8.3%)	0.87
- SJM Epic Biocor Valve n°27	1 (3.8%)	0 (0%)	1 (8.3%)	0.87
- Medtronic Hancock Tissue Valve II n°29	2 (7.7%)	1 (7.1%)	1 (8.3%)	0.95
- SJM Epic Biocor Valve n°31	1 (3.8%)	0 (0%)	1 (8.3%)	0.87

TR: tricuspid regurgitation, SJM: St Jude Medical, SD: standard deviation

either Student's t-test or non-parametric Wilcoxon rank-sums test for continuous variables. Survival curves were constructed with the Kaplan-Meier method, and the Log-rank test was used for intergroup comparisons. Independent predictors of 30-day mortality and clinical outcomes were identified by Cox proportional hazard analysis. Predictors associated with a p-value of less than 0.2 on univariate analysis were considered in the multivariate analysis using stepwise selection. Results are expressed using hazard ratios (HRs). For all analyses, p-values < 0.05 were considered statistically significant.

Results

Immediate postoperative outcome

Postoperative events and results are described according to the guidelines for reporting morbidity and mortality after cardiac valve operations, approved by the Society of Thoracic Surgeons and The American Association for Thoracic Surgery. An early complication was defined as an event occurring after surgery during hospitalization, and a late complication as an event occurring after discharge. Reoperation is any operation that repairs, alters, or replaces a previously operated valve. A neurologic event includes any new, temporary, or permanent focal or global neurologic deficit. A bleeding event is any episode of major internal or external bleeding that causes death, hospitalization, or permanent injury or required transfusion. Cardiac complication was defined by the presence of one of the following: more than 72 h requiring an inotrope, return to operating room for bleeding or tamponade, new onset of atrial fibrillation, permanent pacemaker placement or in-hospital cardiac arrest. Respiratory complication was defined by the presence of one of the followings: duration of mechanical ventilation

≥24 h, re-intubation or tracheostomy. Infective complication was defined by the presence of one of the followings: pneumonia, sternal wound infection, mediastinitis or sepsis. Renal complication was defined by new onset renal failure, new onset renal replacement therapy [3].

The 30-day mortality was 15.4% with 4 early deaths. There was no significant difference between replacement group ($n = 1$; 9.1%) and repair group ($n = 3$; 20%) ($p = 0.61$). The causes of death were low cardiac output syndrome and multiorgan failure in 3 patients and a massive stroke in 1 patient. The early outcome and incidence of major postoperative complications are summarized in Table 3. There was no statistically difference between tricuspid valve repair and replacement concerning immediate outcome, with the same finding in the comparison between functional and organic TR.

Long-term outcomes
Late mortality

There were 3 late deaths (13.6%) at 6, 24 and 96 months. The causes of death were global cardiac failure and multiorgan failure. Two of the three deceased patients had a long history with RHD over more than three decades of disease progression with at least three cardiac surgeries; and all patients had a poor right ventricular function. The cumulative survival (calculated by Kaplan-Meier method) at 1, 5 and 10 years was respectively $80 \pm 8\%$, $75.6 \pm 8.7\%$ and $67.2 \pm 11.1\%$, with no significant difference at 10 years

between tricuspid valve replacement ($80\% \pm 12.6\%$) and tricuspid valve repair ($60\% \pm 14.8\%$) ($p = 0.52$). Similarly, there was no significant difference between functional TR ($77.1\% \pm 11.7\%$) and organic TR ($48.5\% \pm 21.7\%$) ($p = 0.41$), and, on the other hand, between redo TR ($55.6\% \pm 16.6\%$) and late TR ($75 \pm 13.6\%$) ($p = 0.16$).

Univariate analysis identified the nature organic of the TR, NYHA class, EuroSCORE > 8, anemia, ascites, systolic pulmonary artery pressure > 60 mmHg, right ventricular dysfunction, postoperative bleeding, blood transfusion and cardiac complications as significant predictors of overall mortality. On multivariable Cox regression analysis, ascites (HR, 5.8; $p = 0.01$) and right ventricular dysfunction (HR, 0.94; $p = 0.001$) were independent predictors of overall mortality (Figs. 1, 2, 3 and Table 4).

Late reoperation

Of the 19 patients who survived the surgery, no patient needed a reoperation for TV disease or any other cardiac condition. There were no recurrence of TR and no structural or non-structural deterioration of valvular prosthesis. The 10-year event-free survival rate was $36.5\% \pm 18.2\%$ and was significantly higher in repair group ($50\% \pm 23\%$) in comparison with replacement group (0%) ($p = 0.04$).

All patients had mechanical mitral valve prostheses and, consequently, received oral anticoagulation by

Table 3 In-hospital outcomes of patients undergoing tricuspid valve surgery for isolated rheumatic tricuspid regurgitation ($n = 26$) with comparison between tricuspid valve repair group and tricuspid valve replacement group. Data are Presented as Mean ± SD, Median (Range), or n (%)

Characteristics	All patients $n = 26$	TV repair $n = 15$	TV replacement $n = 11$	p-Value
Ventilator support (hours)	12.5 (3–120)	9 (3–96)	17 (4–120)	0.47
ICU stay (hours)	71.4 ± 38.8	73.1 ± 44.4	69 ± 31.6	0.79
Postoperative stay (days)	16.9 ± 10.1	14.7 ± 10.8	19.8 ± 8.7	0.21
30-day mortality	4 (15.4%)	3 (20%)	1 (9.1%)	0.61
Low cardiac output syndrome	7 (26.9%)	4 (26.7%)	3 (27.3%)	1
Transitory renal failure	8 (30.8%)	5 (33.3%)	3 (27.3%)	0.54
Pneumonia	6 (23.1%)	4 (26.7%)	2 (18.2%)	1
Red Blood Cells transfusion > 1 unit	10 (55.6%)	5 (41.7%)	5 (83.3%)	0.15
Bleeding	6 (23.1%)	4 (26.7%)	2 (18.2%)	1
Reexploration for bleeding	3 (11.5%)	2 (13.3%)	1 (9.1%)	0.62
Sternal wound infection	1 (3.8%)	1 (6.7%)	0 (0%)	0.58
Sepsis	2 (7.7%)	1 (6.7%)	1 (9.1%)	1
Cardiac complication	11 (42.3%)	6 (40%)	5 (45.5%)	1
Respiratory complication	7 (26.9%)	4 (26.7%)	3 (27.3%)	0.66
Infective complication	7 (26.9%)	4 (26.7%)	3 (27.3%)	1
Renal complication	8 (30.8%)	5 (33.3%)	3 (27.3%)	1
Neurologic complications	1 (3.8%)	1 (6.7%)	0 (0%)	1

TV: tricuspid valve, *TVrp*: tricuspid valve repair, *TVR*: tricuspid valve replacement, *ICU*: intensive care unit

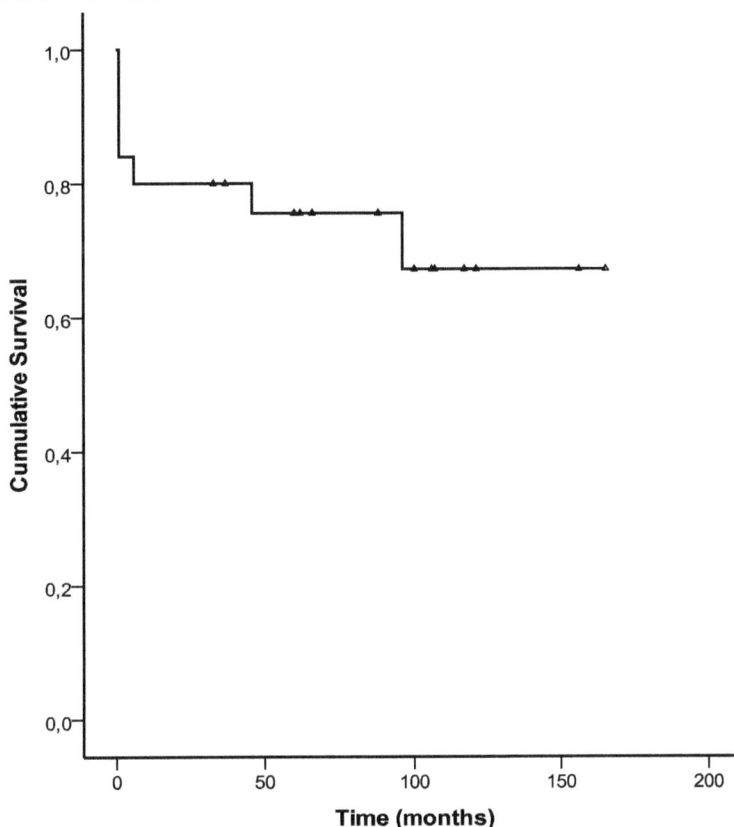

Fig. 1 Kaplan-Meier curve of survival in patients who underwent reoperation for isolated rheumatic TR

acenocoumarol without systematic use of platelet aggregation inhibitors. The target International Normalized Ratio (INR) ranged between 3 and 4. We recorded no thromboembolic events and 2 patients had hemorrhagic episodes related to over-anticoagulation (recurrent epistaxis and spontaneously resolving psoas hematoma).

Of the 18 controlled survivors, 16 patients (88.9%) were in NYHA class 1–2 and 2 patients (11.1%) were in class 3. All patients expressed an improvement of their functional status. Two patients (11.8%) had signs of right heart failure requiring enhanced medical treatment. All patients maintained atrial fibrillation as cardiac rhythm, and no patient experienced conductive disorder or needed a permanent pacemaker insertion in early or long-term period. The mean cardio-thoracic ratio on the chest x-ray was 0.63 ± 0.1 (range 0.59 to 0.7).

The assessment of TR was done only by echocardiography and no patients had cardiac catheterization. According to the most recent echocardiography, no controlled patient had moderate or severe TR. There was no case of structural or non-structural dysfunction of implanted tricuspid valvular prostheses or rings. However, 1 patient had elevated mean gradient of aortic valvular prosthesis above 35 mmHg.

Discussion

The TR appearing after LSHVS should be considered differently depending on whether it is a repeat TV operation (redo TR) or not (late TR). In our experience, late TR is dominated by functional mechanism with normal leaflets and dilated tricuspid annulus; whereas, redo TR is dominated by the organic rheumatic origin with direct involvement of the TV components by abnormal thickening of the leaflets, adhesion of the commissures and shortness of chordae. This concept influenced significantly the type of tricuspid valve surgery with significant dominance of tricuspid valve repair for "late" and "functional" TR, and high proportion of replacement for "redo" and "organic" TR.

The management of TR in rheumatic patients remains controversial with many shadows. If the severe TR rises no doubt about the need of surgical correction concomitantly with LSHVS, the decision for moderate and mild TR remains uncertain and not unanimous. Some authors suggest no treatment, hoping the return of pulmonary pressures to acceptable levels making the TR "spontaneously" disappear, or at least stabilize at a non-significant level; believing the dogma that "functional" TR will subside after appropriate LSHVS [4]. However, the annular dilatation is a progressive process and may not be

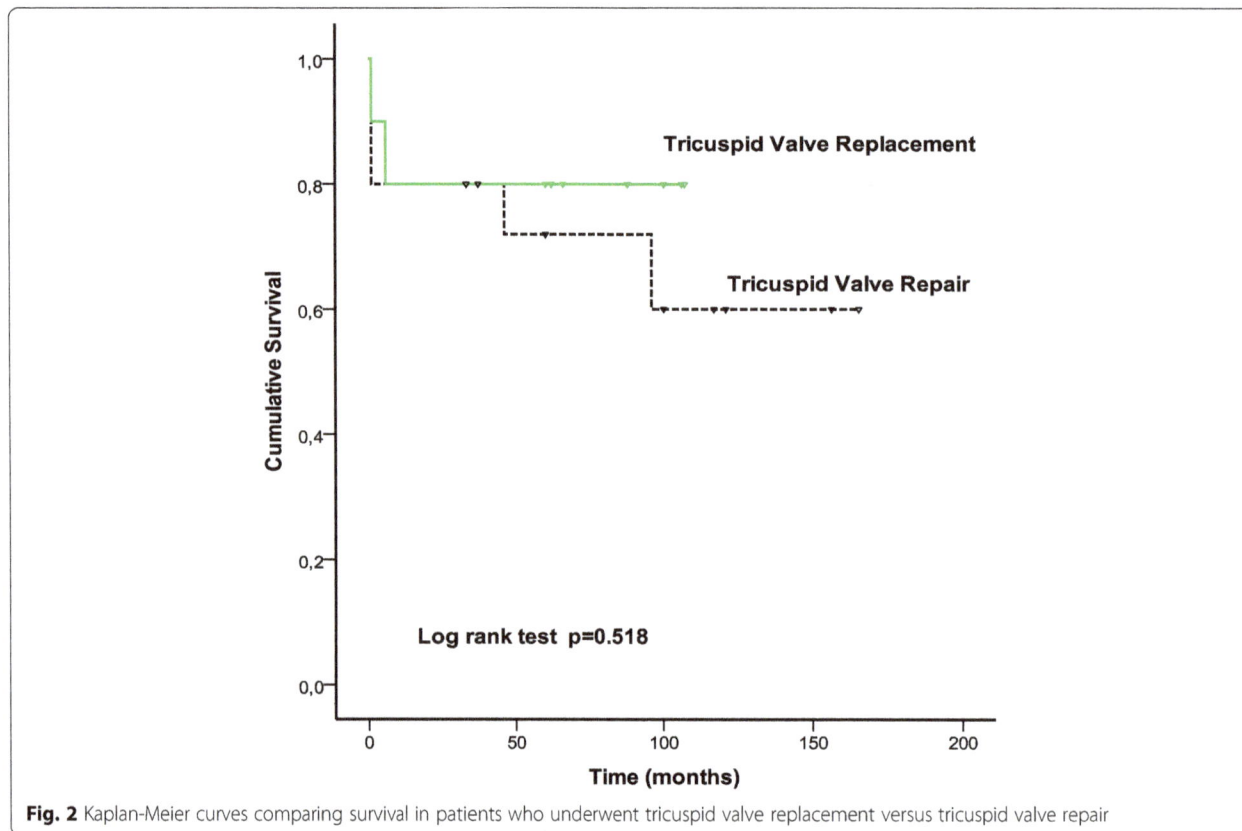

Fig. 2 Kaplan-Meier curves comparing survival in patients who underwent tricuspid valve replacement versus tricuspid valve repair

accompanied by TR initially, but eventually leads to it [4]. In our study, all patients with functional TR had at the time of the initial operation at most a mild TR with normal or non significant dilated annulus at the preoperative echocardiography; and the TR appeared or worsted progressively with significant annular dilatation. Antunes suggested as risk factors for persisting or worsening TR after a mitral valve procedure without TV surgery, the persistence or recurrence of mitral valve disease, longstanding right ventricular dilatation [4]. Xiao mentioned five main factors of the Late TR progression after LHVS: the persistence of pulmonary hypertension, the right ventricle tricuspid valvular disproportion, the atrial fibrillation, the progression or development of rheumatic lesions and DeVega's suture annuloplasty technique [5]. In our experience, we found other risk factors: female sex, major left atrium dilatation, pulmonary hypertension and organic TR.

For patients with previous tricuspid valve repair (redo TR), the failure of the primary plasty were mainly due to direct rheumatic involvement of the TV where the progressive worsening of the TR is more evident and faster. Additionally, in this case, TR was usually associated with some degree of stenosis where the leaflets were thick, immobile and rigid; the commissures were fused, the chordea were short and agglutinated and the annulus was deformed. On 10 patients of Redo TR, 90% had

organic rheumatic TV disease with 8 cases of combined Devega procedure and tricuspid commissurotomy, 1 case of Devega procedure alone, 1 case of tricuspid commissurotomy alone and no case of ring annuloplasty. Then, we think a posteriori that Devega procedure was wrongly used in this group of severe patients with organic TR where an aggressive attitude with rigid ring annuloplasty to remodel the deformed tricuspid annulus was probably more appropriate and accurate. Actually, we changed our policy towards organic TR and we performed since 2005 systematically a rigid ring annuloplasty with tricuspid commissurotomy if needed. Devega procedure is reserved to moderate functional TR with mildly dilated annulus.

It is true that since its first description in 1969, the tricuspid valve replacement has acquired the reputation of bad operation with increased incidence of thromboembolic event for the mechanical prostheses and degeneration problems of bioprostheses. However, it must be said that the prostheses used in this setting were of the older generations with many problems even in mitro-aortic position.

Generally, in valve heart surgery, valve repair techniques had shown their superiority to valve replacements. This concept is more patent in TV surgery for several reasons: first of all, TV surgery is usually done in multivalvular patients with mitro-aortic prosthesis;

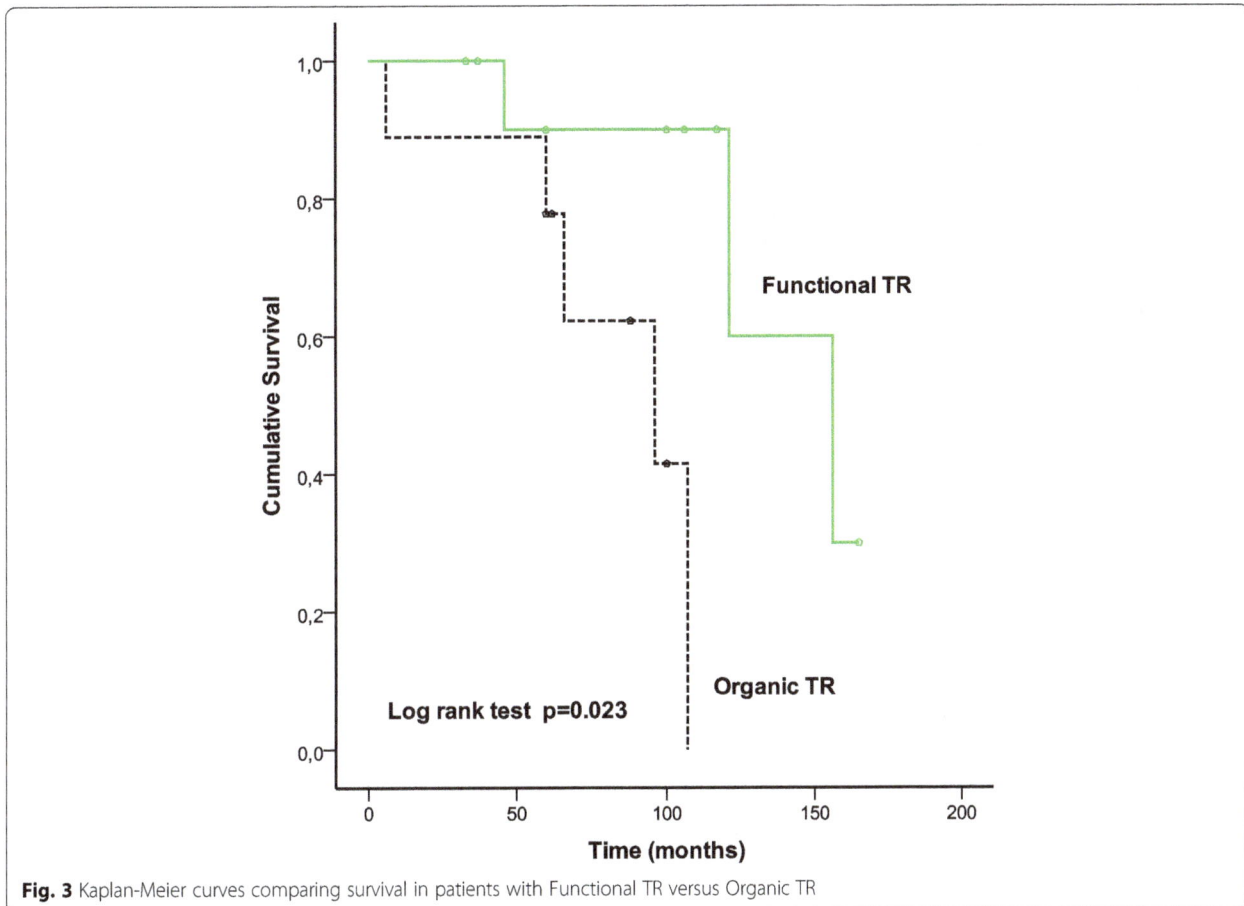

Fig. 3 Kaplan-Meier curves comparing survival in patients with Functional TR versus Organic TR

secondly, prosthesis in tricuspid position had shown their limits in many studies with high risk of complications and, finally, the TV tolerates well a less than perfect repair contrasting with mitro-aortic position [4].

However, repairing an organic rheumatic TV disease with abnormal leaflet, commissures and chordae, is not

always possible. In some cases, we insist to repair a deeply pathological valve at the expense of a significant risk of plasty failure and recurrence of TR while a valve replacement could solve the problem effectively with relatively acceptable risk of related-valves complications especially with the new generation of prosthesis. We

Table 4 Independent predictors of overall mortality after reoperation for isolated rheumatic tricuspid regurgitation

Characteristics	Univariate Analysis			Multivariate Analysis		
	HR	95% CI	p-Value	HR	95% CI	p-Value
EuroSCORE > 8	0.03	0.001–0.68	0.03[a]	0.6	0.33-1.11	0.1
NYHA class	0.25	0.05–1.24	0.09[a]	0.28	0.01-9.16	0.48
Anemia	0.27	0.04–1.86	0.18[a]			
Organic TR	7	0.5–98.6	0.15[a]			
Ascites	0.06	0.004–1.04	0.05[a]	5.8	1.25-9.26	0.01[b]
SPAP > 60 mmHg	0.95	0.88–1.03	0.19[a]			
RV dysfunction	0.2	0.03–1.35	0.09[a]	0.94	0.004-1.43	0.001[b]
Postoperative bleeding	0.21	0.03–1.95	0.18[a]			
Blood transfusion	0.14	0.013–1.63	0.12[a]			
Cardiac complications	0.14	0.01–2.01	0.15[a]			

HR: hazard ratio, CI: confidence interval, TR: tricuspid regurgitation, SPAP: systolic pulmonary arterial pressure, RV: right ventricle
[a]: p-Value < 0.2 (for univariate analysis);
[b]: p-Value < 0.05 (for multivariate analysis)

should define objectively good candidates either for tricuspid valve repair or replacement in rheumatic population. In addition, repair techniques of deeply affected rheumatic valves require much more dexterity and surgical experience, which is not easily available for all, especially young surgeons and low volume centers.

For tricuspid valve replacement, bioprostheses were initially considered ideal because they would not require anticoagulation and were expected to have a slower degeneration than in the mitral or aortic position [6]. However, a Nakano review of the Carpentier-Edwards pericardial bioprosthesis reported non-structural dysfunction in 72.8% of patients by pannus formation on the ventricular side of the cusps. Control echocardiography revealed an incidence of pannus in 35% of patients with at least 5 years of follow-up [7]. Guerra reported similar changes on explanted porcine Hancock valves with the presence of a pannus on the ventricular side of the cusps limiting their flexibility and function [8]. The same finding was supported by Carrier's work [9]. Rizzoli in his meta-analysis suggested that mechanical prostheses should be preferred in young patients and in patients with left sided mechanical prostheses [6]. A meta-analyse of Kunadian, involving 561 articles and more than 1000 mechanical and biological tricuspid prostheses, confirmed that there is no significant difference in survival and the re-operation for bioprosthetic degeneration remains equivalent to the re-operation for thrombosis of mechanical prostheses. In addition, the study showed that 95% of patients with bioprostheses continue to receive anticoagulation [10].

In rheumatic condition, we believe that new generation of mechanical prostheses are at least non inferior to bioprostheses in tricuspid position, because patients need effective oral anticoagulation for mechanical prostheses on the mitro-aortic position with enlarged cardiac chambers and atrial fibrillation. So, the main indication and the principal benefit of bioprostheses is absent with additional risk of structural deterioration and re-operation, which is not negligible for multi-operated patients and in low income population like in African countries. Recently, we have changed our therapeutic strategy regarding the choice of TV prosthesis; when it is about isolated TR without involvement of mitro-aortic valves (like traumatic, infectious and congenital TR ...etc), we follow the usual guidelines concerning heart valves replacement policy. However; in case of rheumatic polyvalvulopathy, we prefer now new generation of mechanical prosthesis for several raisons: our patients are mostly young, with mitral or mitro-aortic mechanical prostheses, dilated left atrium and atrial fibrillation.

Reoperation for TR is associated with high operative risk because of its high operative risk related to the pathology itself, the condition of the patient and the risk of thoracic re-entry [11]. The results of this surgery were poor with high rates of mortality, which might reach 10–20% [4]. However, the mortality had dropped to acceptable levels in the recent reports [12–14] thanks to preoperative preparation, medical therapy, physiotherapy, myocardial protection, anesthetic and surgical techniques [4]. Major signs of right heart failure, such as ascites and right ventricular dysfunction, were significant predictors of morbid-mortality in our study. We can add other risk factors like high functional class and pulmonary hypertension.

Limitations

This study is mainly limited by its retrospective design and relatively small cohort size. In addition, it is limited by the heterogeneity of mechanical and biological prostheses. Consequently, we cannot draw strong conclusions about this subject especially in absence of control group. However, in many ways our study is original, because, at the expense of a limited number of patients, we focused on the reoperation for isolated rheumatic TR which constitutes a homogeneous group, with particularities that differentiate it from other etiologies of TR and the relative rarity of articles that treat the subject.

Conclusion

The reoperation of rheumatic TR should be considered before the installation of complications such right ventricular dysfunction and major signs of right heart failure. Despite the superiority of repair techniques, tricuspid valve replacement should not be banished.

Abbreviations

LSHVS: Left-sided heart valve surgery; RHD: Rheumatic heart disease; TR: Tricuspid regurgitation; TV: Tricuspid valve; TVR: Tricuspid valve replacement; TVrp: Tricuspid valve repair

Acknowledgements

We thank Mr. Fadl Abdeljabbar for correcting the English version of the manuscript.

Author's contributions

YM and MA collected data. YM and NA performed the statistical analysis and analyzed data. YM and ZL designed and drafted the manuscript. MA and AB did most operations and helped to draft the manuscript. AS, AM, AH and IA participated to the operations and the management of patients and revised the paper. All authors read and approved the final manuscript.

Competing interests

The authors declare that they have no competing interest.

Author details
[1]Cardiac surgery department, Mohammed V teaching military hospital, Hay Riyad, PB 10100, Rabat, Morocco. [2]Intensive care of cardiac surgery, Mohammed V teaching military hospital, Rabat, Morocco. [3]Cardiology department, Mohammed V teaching military hospital, Rabat, Morocco. [4]Faculty of medicine and pharmacy, Mohammed V university, Rabat, Morocco.

References
1. Simon R, Oelert H, Borst HG, Lichtlen PR. Influence of mitral valve surgery on tricuspid incompetence concomitant with mitral valve disease. Circulation. 1980;62(suppl I):S152–7.
2. King RM, Schaff HV, Danielson GK, Gersh BJ, Orszulak TA, Piehler JM, Puga FJ, Pluth JR. Surgery for TR late after mitral valve replacement. Circulation. 1984;70(suppl I):S193–7.
3. Akins CW, Miller DC, Turina MI, Kouchoukos NT, Blackstone EH, Grunkemeier GL, Takkenberg JJ, David TE, Butchart EG, Adams DH, Shahian DM, Hagl S, Mayer JE, Lytle BW, STS, ATS, EACTS. Guidelines for reporting mortality and morbidity after cardiac valve interventions. Ann Thorac Surg. 2008;85:1490–5.
4. Antunes MJ, Barlow JB. Management of tricuspid valve regurgitation. Heart. 2007;93:271–6.
5. Xiao XJ, Huang HL, Zhang JF, Wu RB, He JG, Lu C, Li ZM. Surgical treatment of late tricuspid regurgitation after left cardiac valve replacement. Heart Lung Circ. 2004;13:65–9.
6. Rizzoli G, Vendramin I, Nesseris G, Bottio T, Guglielmi C, Schiavon L. Biological or mechanical prostheses in tricuspid position? A meta-analysis of intra-institutional results. Ann Thorac Surg. 2004 May;77(5):1607–14.
7. Nakano K, Eishi K, Kosakai Y, Isobe F, Sasako Y, Nagata S, Ueda H, Kito Y, Kawashima Y. Ten-year experience with the Carpentier-Edwards pericardial xenograft in the tricuspid position. J Thorac Cardiovasc Surg. 1996 Mar; 111(3):605–12.
8. Guerra F, Bortolotti U, Thiene G, Milano A, Mazzucco A, Talenti E, Stellin G, Gallucci V. Long-term performance of the Hancock porcine bioprosthesis in the tricuspid position. A review of forty-five patients with fourteen-year follow-up. J Thorac Cardiovasc Surg. 1990 May;99(5):838–45.
9. Carrier M, Hébert Y, Pellerin M, Bouchard D, Perrault LP, Cartier R, Basmajian A, Pagé P, Poirier NC. Tricuspid valve replacement: an analysis of 25 years of experience at a single center. Ann Thorac Surg. 2003;75:47–50.
10. Kunadian B, Vijayalakshmi K, Balasubramanian S, Dunning J. Should the tricuspid valve be replaced with a mechanical or biological valve? Interact Cardiovasc Thorac Surg. 2007;6:551–7.
11. Li ZX, Guo ZP, Liu XC, Kong XR, Jing WB, Chen TN, Lu WL, He GW. Surgical treatment of tricuspid regurgitation after mitral valve surgery: a retrospective study in China. J Cardiothorac Surg. 2012;7:30.
12. Xiao XJ, Huang HL, Zhang JF, Wu RB, He JG, Lu C, Li ZM. Surgical treatment of late tricuspid regurgitation after left cardiac valve replacement. J Cardiothorac Surg. 2012;7:30.
13. Jeong DS, Park PW, Mwambu TP, Sung K, Kim WS, Lee YT, Park SJ, Park SW. Tricuspid reoperation after left-sided rheumatic valve operations. Ann Thorac Surg. 2013;95:2007–14.
14. Park CK, Park PW, Sung K, Lee YT, Kim WS, Jun TG. Early and midterm outcomes for tricuspid valve surgery after left-sided valve surgery. Ann Thorac Surg. 2009;88:1216–23.

19

Stanford type B aortic dissection is more frequently associated with coronary artery atherosclerosis than type A

Naoki Hashiyama[1], Motohiko Goda[2*], Keiji Uchida[3], Yukihisa Isomatsu[2], Shinichi Suzuki[2], Makoto Mo[1], Takahiro Nishida[4] and Munetaka Masuda[2,3]

Abstract

Background: The relationship between aortic dissection and coronary artery disease is not clear. The purpose of this study was to clarify the difference in the rate of coronary artery atherosclerosis between Stanford type A and type B aortic dissection by reviewing our institutional database.

Methods: One hundred and forty-five patients (78 males, 67 females; mean age: 60 ± 12 years) admitted to our hospital with acute aortic dissection who underwent coronary angiography during hospitalization from 2000 through 2002 were enrolled in this study. The background characteristics, coronary risk factors, and coronary angiography findings (number of significant stenoses, stenoses according to Bogaty standards, extent index) of patients were compared between type A (Group A; $n = 71$) and type B dissection (Group B; $N = 74$).

Results: Significantly more patients had prior histories of complications from ischemic heart disease in Group B than in Group A ($P = 0.04$), with no significant differences in comparison to other risk factors observed except for hypertension. Significantly ($p = 0.005$) more stenoses were observed in Group B (1.54 ± 0.04) than in Group A (0.38 ± 0.1). A significantly higher ($P < 0.05$) index score indicating the severity of coronary atherosclerosis was observed in Group B (1.49 ± 0.09) than in Group A (0.72 ± 0.07).

Conclusions: Stanford type B acute aortic dissection was significantly more frequently associated with coronary artery atherosclerosis than type A.

Keywords: Acute aortic dissection, Stanford classification, Coronary artery, Athroscrelosis, Coronary angiography

Background

While the survival rate of surgical patients with acute aortic dissection (AAD) has been improving recently, it remains over 10% in Asian and Western developed countries [1–3]. We previously reported that the ST-T abnormality on admission electrocardiograms in AAD patients was a significant risk factor of in-hospital mortality [4, 5]. The prevalence of coronary artery disease due to not only dissection involved but also atherosclerotic stenosis must therefore be taken into account in the treatment of AAD. However, the relationship between coronary artery diseases and AAD remains unclear.

Recently, coronary artery computed tomography (CT) has been used widely because of its convenience and low invasiveness [6]. However, an angiographic evaluation of coronary arteries is still clinically important and reliable because coronary CT cannot evaluate coronary lesions adequately in cases of severe coronary artery calcification.

The purpose of this study was to clarify the relationship between coronary artery disease and AAD in accordance with Stanford type A and B based on coronary angiogrphy (CAG) by reviewing our local AAD database during a time when we routinely performed CAG in AAD patients.

* Correspondence: gogomotto@gmail.com
[2]Department of Cardiovascular Surgery, Yokohama City University Hospital, Fukuura 3-9, Kanazawaku, Yokohama 236-0004, Japan
Full list of author information is available at the end of the article

Methods

Study design and patient population

This retrospective cohort study was performed at a single Japanese center in human subjects and was reviewed and approved by the Institutional Review Board at Yokohama City University Medical Center. Informed consent for this study was waived because no individual patients were identified.

We identified 145 patients (78 males, 67 females; mean age: 60 ± 12 years) who had undergone coronary angiography, among 221 patients hospitalized at our center from January 2000 to December 2002, when we routinely performed CAG in AAD patients. Seventy-six patients in whom CAG was not performed were excluded (49 with type A and 27 with type B). Patients presenting with traumatic aortic dissection or Marfan syndrome were also excluded. The remaining 145 patients who underwent coronary angiography were included in this study and divided into 2 groups based on the type of AAD: Stanford type A acute aortic dissection (A; $n = 71$) and Stanford type B (Group B; $n = 74$) aortic dissection.

Clinical evaluation

The baseline clinical data of the enrolled patients, including the patient demographics, medical history, clinical findings at presentation, imaging study results and preoperative complications, were collected by a retrospective chart review. Type A aortic dissection was defined as observing an intimal flap separating 2 lumina in the ascending aorta with a presentation within 14 days of its onset [7].

Angiographic analyses of the coronary artery (Fig. 1)

We performed CAG within three weeks after emergency aortic surgery in Group A or admission in Group B.

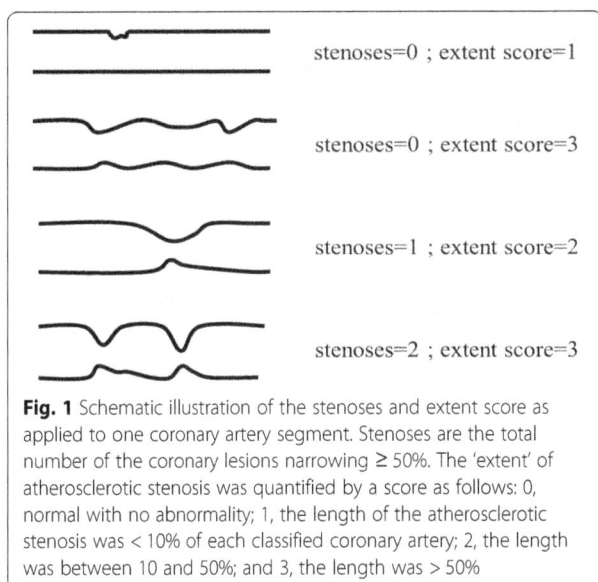

Fig. 1 Schematic illustration of the stenoses and extent score as applied to one coronary artery segment. Stenoses are the total number of the coronary lesions narrowing $\geq 50\%$. The 'extent' of atherosclerotic stenosis was quantified by a score as follows: 0, normal with no abnormality; 1, the length of the atherosclerotic stenosis was $< 10\%$ of each classified coronary artery; 2, the length was between 10 and 50%; and 3, the length was $> 50\%$

The angiograms were comprehensively analyzed based on the descriptive concepts developed and described by Bogaty et al.: severity, stenosis and extent [8]. In brief, 'severity' was defined as the number of major epicardial vessels with stenosis $\geq 75\%$. A left main trunk with stenosis $\geq 50\%$ was defined as 2 vessels. 'Stenoses' were defined as the total number of stenosis $\geq 50\%$. The 'extent' of atherosclerotic stenosis was quantified by a score as follows: 0, normal: 1, the length of the atherosclerotic stenosis was $\leq 10\%$ of each classified coronary artery: 2, the length was between 10 and 50%: and 3, the length was $\geq 50\%$. The extent index was the extent score divided by the number of coronary arteries with a proper antegrade flow, allowing a range from 0 to 3 (extent score 0–45 divide by the classical 15 segments of the coronary artery).

Statistical analyses

All statistical analyses were performed using the IBM SPSS statics software program, ver. 20 (IBM Corporation, Armonk, NY, USA). All continuous variables are presented as the means ± standard error. Fisher's exact test and Student's t-tests were used for the univariate analyses. Categorical variables are expressed as absolute numbers or percentages and were compared using chi-squared testing. $P < 0.05$ was considered to be significant.

Results

Patient's characteristics and coronary risk factors

All variables are listed in Tables 1 and 2. The proportion of women was significantly higher in Group A than in Group B (56.3% vs. 36.5%; $p = 0.02$). Ischemic heart disease (3% vs 12%; $P = 0.04$) and arterial hypertension (55% vs. 80%; $p = 0.003$) were observed significantly more frequently in Group B than in Group A. No significant differences were observed between the two groups in the age, height, body weight or other coronary

Table 1 Clinical characteristics of the patients

Variables	Group A (n = 71)	Group B (n = 74)	p value
Gender (Men/Women)	31/40	47/27	0.02
Age (years)	60 ± 1.4	60 ± 1.3	0.725
Height (cm)	160 ± 1.2	163 ± 0.9	0.052
Weight	62 ± 1.7	65 ± 2	0.21
History of coronary artery disease	2 (3%)	9 (12%)	0.042
Angina pectoris	1	6	
Myocardial infarction	0	1	
Previous coronary surgery	1	2	

A: Stanford type A dissection; B: Stanford type B dissection
Continuous variables are expressed as the mean ± standard error and categorical variables as the number (%) or as indicated

Table 2 Coronary risk factors

Variables	Group A (n = 71)	Group B (n = 74)	p value
Hypertension	39 (55%)	59 (80%)	0.003
Hyperlipidemia	11 (15%)	15 (20%)	0.594
Diabetes Mellitus	5 (7%)	11 (15%)	0.216
Smoking habit	30 (42%)	37(50%)	0.406
Family history	28 (39%)	30 (41%)	0.865

A: Stanford type A dissection; B: Stanford type B dissection
Continuous variables are expressed as the mean ± standard error and
categorical variables as the number (%) or as indicated

risk factors, including hyperlipidemia, diabetes mellitus, smoking habit and a family history of coronary disease.

Coronary artery analyses

- Severity:

Only 3 patients in Group A (4.2%) had a single-vessel coronary disease detected by CAG, while 16 patients in Group B (21.6%) had significant coronary disease, including 8 patients with single-vessel disease, 4 with double-vessel disease and 4 with triple-vessel disease. (p = 0.04: Fig. 2).

- Stenoses

Significantly fewer (p = 0.005) total numbers of stenoses (≥ 50%) were observed in Group A (26 lesions, 0.38 lesions per patient) than in Group B (114 lesions, 1.54 lesions per patient: Fig. 3).

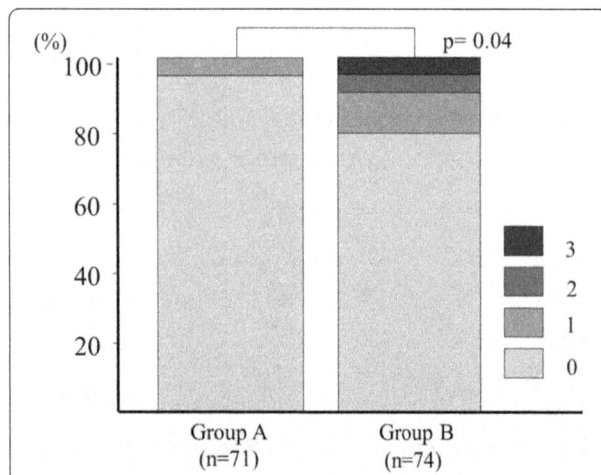

Fig. 2 Number of coronary artery diseases defined as ≥ 75% stenosis. Significantly fewer coronary artery diseases were observed in Group A than in Group B (P = 0.05)

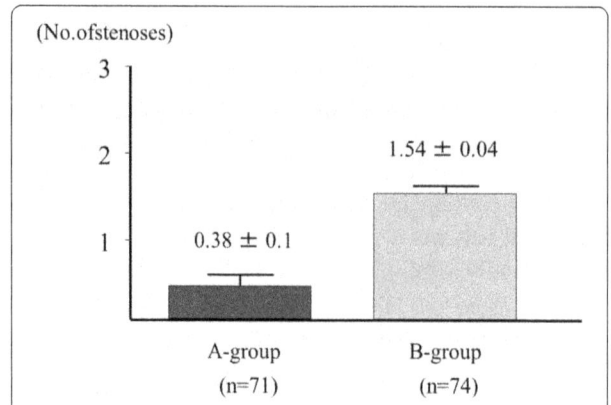

Fig. 3 Number of significant stenoses (≥ 50%). Significantly fewer (p = 0.005) total numbers of stenoses (≥ 50%) were observed in Group A (26 lesions, 0.38 lesions per patient) than in Group B (114 lesions, 1.54 lesions per patient)

- Extent

There was also a significant difference in the extent index, representing the longitudinal extension of atherosclerotic stenosis between Group A (0.72) and Group B (1.49, p = 0.005: Fig. 4).

Discussion

AAD naturally has an extremely poor prognosis, and it has been noted that many cases prove fatal shortly after the onset with emergency operation normally required to rescue patients suffering from type A aortic dissection [1–3]. Exclusion of the entry by replacing the dissected ascending aorta and/or aortic arch to the artificial graft is the standard technique for Stanford A dissection; however, surgeons generally do not recognize asymptomatic coronary artery disease without ST-T changes in the electrocardiogram because CAG or coronary CT are not routinely performed before emergent operation. Therefore, treating AAD still carries a potential risk for

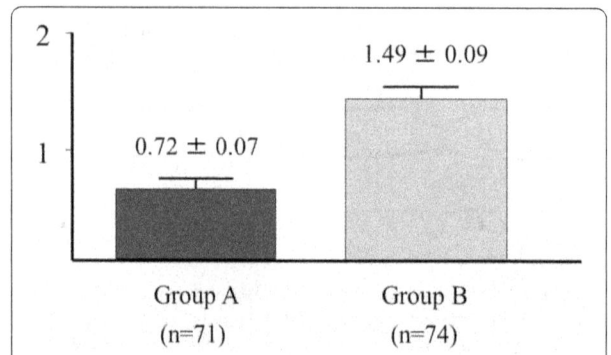

Fig. 4 Extent of coronary lesions. There was also a significant difference in the extent index, representing the longitudinal extension of atherosclerotic stenosis between Group A (0.72) and Group B (1.49, p = 0.005)

severe coronary stenosis leading to perioperative myocardial infarction [9, 10].

Only a few reports exist concerning cases of AAD complicated by organic coronary artery atherosclerosis, but in general, complications due to coronary atherosclerosis are still believed to occur with a low frequency [11–13]. Furthermore, there has never been a report describing the relationship between significant atherosclerotic coronary artery stenosis and the Stanford classification. To prevent perioperative myocardial infarction, it is desirable to confirm the presence or absence of significant coronary stenosis during treatment for AAD, especially before emergent operation for type A dissection. Because it is not always possible to examine coronary arteries before emergent operation, it is important to clarify the underlying relationship between atherosclerotic coronary artery stenosis and AAD. Therefore, we examined AAD cases associated with coronary artery atherosclerosis based on coronary angiographical analyses to clarify the incidence of atherosclerotic coronary artery stenosis in these patients.

The present results showed that the number of significant stenoses, overall number of stenoses and extent index indicating the severity of coronary lesions were significantly higher in Group B than in Group A and only 3 of the 71 patients in Group A (4.2%) had single-vessel coronary disease with no patients undergoing CABG in this group. These data suggest that it is not always neccessary to perform a precise coronary artery examination befroe emergent operation for type A dissection, especially in cases with no significant ST-T changes before surgery. In contrast, 16 of the 74 patients in Group B (22%) had coronary artery disease. Thus, in cases of type B dissection, CAG is required to rule out coronary artery disease after the medical treatment of type B dissection.

Why significant differences in the coronary artery lesions were observed between type A and B dissection in our current study in unclear. Some studies have reported that atherosclerosis does not significantly contribute to AAD development [14–16]. However, recent reports from IRAD investigators [17, 18] have shown that the prevalence of coexisting atherosclerosis, aortic aneurysm and even hypertension was significantly higher in type B dissection than in type A dissection, which certainly supports the results of this current study. Indeed, Group B had more atherosclerotic risk factors than Group A in the present study, including proportions of male gender, hypertension and a history of coronary disease. Based on these present and previous findings, we hypothesize that the development of type A dissection is less attributable to atherosclerosis than type B dissection, leading to fewer atherosclerotic coronary lesions.

In addition, several striking reports have described a negative association between atherosclerosis and type A

aortic dissection [19], ascending aortic aneurysm [20] and thoracic aortic aneurysm [21]. Although the mechanisms underlying these observations were unclear, those authors hypothesized that the same genetic mutations were responsible for (1) the progressive loss and destruction of elastic fibers or smooth muscle cells in the ascending aortic media leading to aortic dissection and (2) a protective effect against atherosclerosis.

Conclusions

Stanford type B acute aortic dissection was significantly more frequently associated with coronary artery atherosclerosis than type A. These data suggest that a precise coronary examination is not required before emergent operation for type A dissection, while CAG or coronary CT is required to rule out coronary artery disease in patients with type B dissection.

Study limitation

This study was based on old data derived from a single center. Furthermore, the small number of subjects did not give the study adequate power to reach robust conclusions.

Abbreviations

AAD: Acute aortic dissection; CAG: Coronary angiography; CT: Computed tomography

Authors' contributions

Concept/design: NH, Data collection: NH, MG, KU, SS, Data analysis/interpretation: NH, Drafting article: NH, MG, TN, Critical revision of the article: MG, KU, YI, SS, MMo, MMasuda, Approval of the article: MMasuda. NH and MG contributed equally to this work. All authors read and approved the final manuscript.

Competing interests

The authors declare that they have no competing interests.

Author details

[1]Department of Cardiovascular Surgery, Yokohama Minami-kyosai Hospital, Mutsuurahigashi 1-21-1, Kanazawa-ku, Yokohama 236-0037, Japan. [2]Department of Cardiovascular Surgery, Yokohama City University Hospital, Fukuura 3-9, Kanazawaku, Yokohama 236-0004, Japan. [3]Cardiovascular Center, Yokohama City University Medical Center, Yokohama, Japan. [4]Department of Cardiovascular Surgery, Yokohama Citizen's Municipal Hospital, Yokohama, Japan.

References

1. Committee for scientific affairs, the Japanese associasion for thoracic surgery, Masuda M, Okumura M, Doki Y, Endo S, Hirata Y et al. Thoracic and cardiovascular surgery in Japan during 2014: Annual report by The Japanese Association for Thoracic Surgery. Gen Thorac Carduovasc Surg. 2016;64:665–97.

2. Goda M, Imoto K, Suzuki S, Uchida K, Yanagi H, Yasuda S, et al. Risk analysis for hospital mortality in patients with acute type a aortic dissection. Ann Thorac Surg. 2010;90:1246–50.

3. Raghupathy A, Nienaber CA, Harris KM, Myrmel T, Fattori R, Sechtem U, et al. Geographic differences in clinical presentation, treatment, and outcome in acute type a aortic dissection (from the international registry of acute aortic dissection). Am J Cardiol. 2008;102:1562–6.

4. Kosuge M, Uchida K, Imoto K, Hashiyama N, Ebina T, Hibi K, et al. Frequency and implication of ST-T abnormalities on hospital admission electrocardiogram in patients with type a acute aortic dissection. Am J Cardiol. 2013;112:424–9.

5. Kosuge M, Kimura K, Uchida K, Masuda M, Tamura K. Clinical implication of electrocardiogram for patients with type A acute aortic dissection. Circ J. 2017; https://doi.org/10.1253/circ.CJ-17-0309.

6. Raman SV, Zareba KM. Coronary artery disease testing: past, present and future. JACC Cardiovascular imaging. 2017; https://doi.org/10.1016/j.jcmg.2016.11.023.

7. Evangelista A, Mukherjee D, Mehta RH, et al. Acute intramural hematoma of the aorta: a mystery in evolusion. Circulation. 2005;111:1063–70.

8. Bogaty P, Brecker SJ, White SE, Stevenson RN, El-Tamimi H, Balcon R, et al. Comparison of coronary angiographic findings in acute and chronic first presentation of ischemic heart disease. Circulation. 1993;87:1938–46.

9. Guenther SPW, Peterss S, Reichelt A, Born F, Fischer M, Pichlmaier M, et al. Diagnosis of coronary affection in patients with AADA and treatment of postcardiotomy myocardial failure using extracorporeal life support (ECLS). Heart Surg Forum. 2014;17(5):E253–7.

10. Waterford SD, Di Eusanio M, Ehrlich MP, Reece TB, Desai ND, Sundt TM, Myrmel T, Gleason TG, Forteza A, de Vincentiis C, DiScipio AW, Montgomery DG, Eagle KA, Isselbacher EM, et al. Postoperative myocardial infarction in acute type A aortic dissection: A report fron the international registry of acute aortic dissection. J Thorac Cardiovasc Surg. 2017;153(3):521–7.

11. Creswell LL, Kouchoukos NT, Cox JL, Rosenbloom M. Coronary artery disease in patients with type a aortic dissection. Ann Thorac Surg. 1995;59:585–90.

12. Rizzo RJ, Aranki SF, Aklog L, Couper GS, Adams DH, Collins JJ, et al. Rapid non-invasive diagnosis and surgical repair of acute ascending aortic dissection: improved survival with less angiography. J Thorac Cardiovasc Surg. 1994;108:567–75.

13. Kojima S, Suwa T, Fujiwara Y, Inoue K, Mineda Y, Ohta H, et al. Incidence and severity of coronary artery disease in patients with acute aortic dissection : comparison with abdominal aortic aneurysm and arteriosclerosis obliterans. J Cardiol. 2001;37:165–71.

14. Tamura K, Sugizaki Y, Kumazaki T, Tanaka S. Atherosclerosis-related aortic dissection. Jpn J Thorac Surg. 2000;53:194–201.

15. Christoph AN, Yskert VK, Volkmar N, Volker SAP, Carsten B, Dietmar HK, et al. The diagnosis of thoracic aortic dissection by noninvasive imaging procedures. NEJM. 1993;328:1–9.

16. Mark AC, Daniel WJ, J.Donald E, Jonathan LH, Alan TH, Alan HM et al. Atherosclerotic vascular disease conference : writing group V:medical decision making and therapy. Circulation 2004;109:2634–3642.

17. Tsai T, Trimarchi S, Nienaber CA. Acuteaortic dissection: perspectives from the international registry of acute aortic dissection (IRAD). Eur J Vasc Endvasc Surg. 2009;37:149–59.

18. Pepe LA, Awais M, Woznicki EW, Suzuki T, Trimarchi S, Evangelista A, et al. Presentation, diagnosis, and outcomes of acute aortic dissection. 17-year trends from the international registry of acute aortic dissection. J Am Coll Cardiol. 2015;66:350–8.

19. Achneck H, Modi B, Shaw C, Rizzo J, Albomoz G, Fusco D, et al. Ascending thoracic aneurysm are associated with decreased systemic atherosclerosis. Chest. 2005;128(3):1580–6.

20. Chau K, Elefteriades JA. Ascending thoracic aortic aneurysm protect against myocardial infarctions. Int J Angiol. 2014;23(3):177–82.

21. Ito S, Akutsu K, Tamori Y, Sakamoto S, Yoshimura T, Hashimoto H, Takeshita S. Differences in atherosclerotic profiles between patients with thoracic and abdominal aortic aneurysm. Am J Cardiol. 2008;101:696–9.

20

Microbiological and clinical profile of infective endocarditis patients: an observational study experience from tertiary care center Karachi Pakistan

Uzma Shahid[1], Hasanat Sharif[2], Joveria Farooqi[1], Bushra Jamil[3] and Erum Khan[1*]

Abstract

Background: The study analyzed microbiological and antimicrobial susceptibility profile of organisms isolated from patients with infective endocarditis (2015–17) and compared disease outcomes in cohorts of endocarditis patient with history of prior invasive vascular intervention (high risk group) vs those without (native valve group). We hypothesized that high risk group would be more likely to have severe disease outcomes.

Methods: This was a prospective cohort study (2015–17). All blood and cardiac tissue samples of enrolled patients suspected of endocarditis according to modified Duke's criteria were followed for microbiological and antimicrobial susceptibility profile. The high risk group was compared with the native valve group with 90 day follow up to determine difference in clinical course and outcome in terms of disease severity (defined as any patient with endocarditis undergoing surgical management, readmission or dying). The data was analyzed using SPSS 21.0 software and chi-square test. 90 day mortality was calculated using Kaplan Meier survival curves.

Results: Total 104 patients with endocarditis were enrolled. Overall culture positivity rate was 71.2%. *Streptococcus* species were the most common isolate (36.7%), followed by *S. aureus* (17.3%) cases. In *Streptococcus* species, 14.2% showed intermediate susceptibility to penicillin. Thirty six patients were included in the cohort analysis. A poor outcome was seen in 85.7% high risk group as compared to 50% of native valve group. The overall mortality rate was 19.4%.

Conclusions: We found *Streptococcus* species to be the predominant pathogen for endocarditis overall. However *Staphylococcus aureus* predominated native valve group. High risk group showed more complicated clinical course.

Keywords: Infective endocarditis, Surgical intervention, Microbiological profile, Clinical features, Pakistan

Background

Infective Endocarditis (IE) is associated with significant disease burden, globally. In 2010, IE was associated with 1.58 million disability-adjusted life-years or years of healthy life lost as a result of death and nonfatal illness or impairment [1]. In past few decades the epidemiology, microbiologic profile and treatment outcomes of patients with IE in developed countries have changed significantly. Rheumatic heart disease (RHD) which was

once considered the main risk factor for IE is now being superseded by other factors such as invasive vascular interventions (IVI), prosthetic cardiac devices, implants and correction procedures for congenital cardiac defects [1]. Up to 30% of all IE cases have been associated with such factors in developed countries [2]. In Pakistan, there is a mix of population of various socioeconomic strata. While high infant mortality and burden of common infectious diseases including RHD is common in lower strata, there is an expanding population on the other end of the spectrum that is able to afford recent advances in medical care. They have risk factors of IE similar to modern world, such as cardiac implants,

* Correspondence: erum.khan@aku.edu
[1]Section of Microbiology, Department of Pathology and Laboratory Medicine, Aga Khan University, Karachi, Pakistan
Full list of author information is available at the end of the article

invasive vascular interventions and correction of congenital defects. Thus, it is important to study the changing epidemiology and microbiologic profile of patients with endocarditis that may provide better treatment / management strategies in local scenario.

IE studies conducted in Pakistan mainly retrospectively designed; have highlighted younger population being affected more frequently than those reported in the western world [3–6]. As regards etiologic agents, most published studies have limitations in terms of poor sensitivity of bacterial culture methods utilized, such as conventional in-house blood culture methods.; as a result up to 50% of IE cases are reported as culture negative [7, 8]. Lack of authentic data of the common etiologic agents and their susceptibility pattern seriously hampers the choice of empirical antibiotic treatment. Moreover, there is a complete dearth of information that correlates use of vascular / cardiac procedure and implants with IE, disease severity and treatment outcomes in Pakistan.

IE patients with cardiac interventions / prosthetic valves have worse outcomes or complicated disease course compared to patients with native valves. A study in Cleveland compared long term post-surgery survival amongst patient with endocarditis having native valve endocarditis (NVE) and prosthetic valve disease (PVE) and reported improved survival in patients with NVE [9]. This may possibly be due to increased disease severity in patients with PVE. Brenan et al. in their study at 605 centers within the Society of Thoracic Surgeons Adult Cardiac Surgery Database showed an elevated 12-year risk of reoperation and endocarditis amongst bio prosthesis patients [10]. In this study we analyzed the frequency of common etiological agents of IE using the highly sensitive standard automated system of blood culture methods (Bactec 9240). In addition, we assessed patient characteristics along with management outcomes amongst those with history of prior IVI labeled as high risk group (HRG) vs those without such risk factors termed as native valve group (NVG) and performed survival analysis for 90-day mortality. We hypothesized that HRG would be more likely to have severe disease outcomes, require further surgical interventions or readmissions, or die as opposed to conservative medical treatment.

Methods

This was a prospective cohort study performed at the Clinical Laboratory (microbiology section) and cardiothoracic surgery of the Aga Khan University Hospital (AKUH), Karachi, Pakistan 2015–17. This is the biggest diagnostic laboratory set-up in Pakistan. We receive average of 1200–1500 blood culture samples per week from more than 200 outreach blood sample collection units in all major cities of Pakistan: hence the data represents country wide distribution.

We identified suspected IE patients from samples submitted at the clinical lab: all blood and relevant tissue samples (cardiac vegetation, cardiac valves, valvular abscess etc.) that were received with history suggestive of endocarditis were enrolled and verbal consent obtained for it. We followed blood / tissue culture to determine the microbiological and antimicrobial susceptibility profile of all recruited patients. The study was exempted from ethical approval by the research ethics committee under study number 3721-Pat-ERC-15 of the Aga Khan University hospital.

In addition, we closely followed patients treated at AKUH; these patients were divided into two groups. A cohort of IE patients with prior history of prosthetic heart implants /prior cardiac intervention, valve repair/ replacements, Coronary artery bypass (CABG), angiography or angioplasty, correction of congenital cardiac vascular and valvular defects, pacemaker insertions within the last 12 years from time of enrollment in this study were classified as HRG and those without were labeled as NVG (see Fig. 1). To illustrate clinical characteristics and outcomes with respect to medical and surgical management, these two cohorts of patients were followed up till 90 days.

All suspected patients admitted under the service of internal medicine and cardio thoracic surgery fulfilling the modified Duke's criteria (MoDC) for IE [2] were considered eligible and were enrolled. Eligible patients who could not be contacted for history were excluded. Any samples with damaged blood culture bottles or tissue in unsterile container were rejected and not included in the study. Details of patient's clinical and microbiological profile were collected prospectively and entered in the predefined data collection form. Confidentiality was maintained by giving unique research identification number, and forms were kept under lock and key. Details included patient demographics, clinical presentation, duration of illness, use of prior antibiotics for the illness, predisposing cardiac condition, history of invasive cardiac procedures, microbiological and radiological findings along with echocardiography results; medical and surgical management details were recorded along with treatment outcome. Outcome in terms of disease severity was defined as any patient with IE undergoing surgical management, readmission or dying.

For microbiological profile, specimens were processed according to the standard techniques. Bactec 9240 automated system was used for blood culture as per Clinical & Laboratory Standards Institute (CLSI) protocol [11]. Tissue cultures were incubated for 21 days, antibiotic susceptibility testing was performed by disc diffusion method or Minimal inhibitory concentration

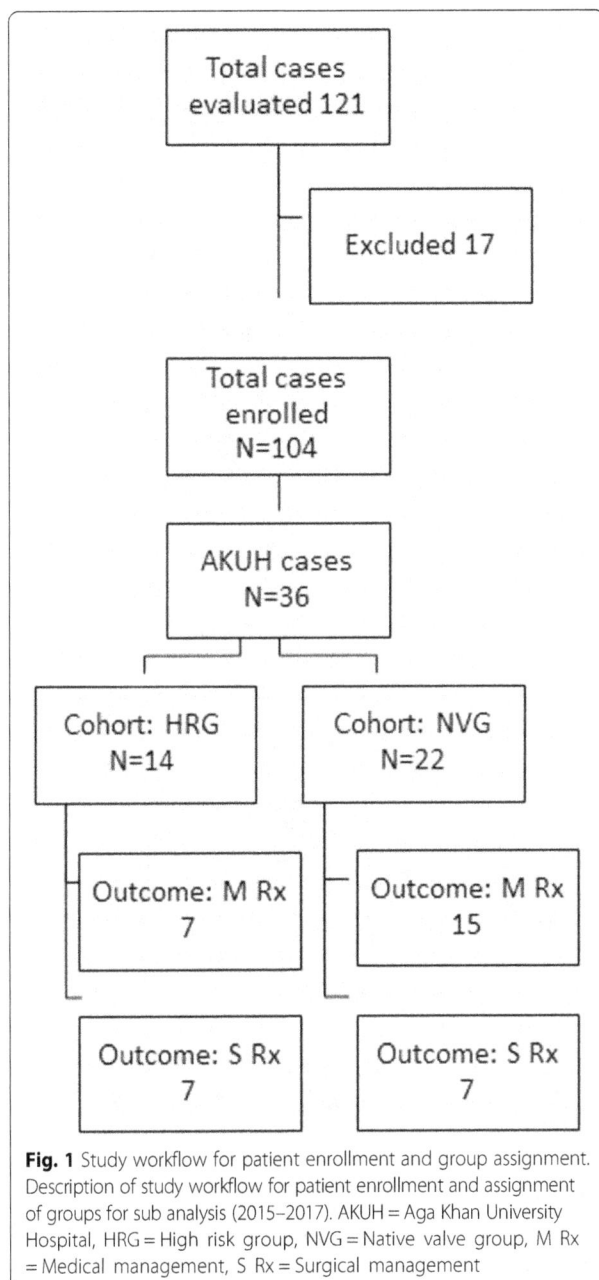

Fig. 1 Study workflow for patient enrollment and group assignment. Description of study workflow for patient enrollment and assignment of groups for sub analysis (2015–2017). AKUH = Aga Khan University Hospital, HRG = High risk group, NVG = Native valve group, M Rx = Medical management, S Rx = Surgical management

(MIC) methods as recommended by CLSI and British Society for Antimicrobial Chemotherapy (BSAC) protocols, whichever was applicable. MIC was performed using Vitek2 system or E-strips as recommended. Microbiological outcome was determined as type / frequency of microorganisms isolated, antimicrobial susceptibility pattern of those isolates. All negative cases were reported "no growth" after incubation of 21 days.

Statistical analysis

The data was analyzed using SPSS 21.0 software. In descriptive analysis mean and standard deviation of the continuous variables i.e. age, antibiotic MICs, duration of hospital stay etc. were calculated. Frequency and percentage of the categorical variables i.e. gender, etiological agent, antibiotic susceptibility pattern, clinical characteristics and surgical outcome were calculated. Risk of poor outcome was compared between HRG and NVG using chi-square test and difference was significant if p-value was ≤0.05. Kaplan Meier curves were generated to compare survival of HRG and NVG patients.

Results

During the study period, 104 patients with clinical diagnosis of IE were prospectively enrolled (Fig. 1). Mean age of patients was 34.84 years with 72.1% being males. Adult representation was 84.6% and 15.4% were below 16 years. Using the MoDC 65.4% ($n = 68$) were identified as "definite cases of infective endocarditis" rest fell in the "possible case". Cultures were sent on all 104 enrolled patients. Approximately 35% ($n = 36$) of patients were admitted at AKUH and were followed up for clinical outcomes.

Microbiological profile: Blood culture samples for laboratory diagnosis only, were received for 82.7% of the enrolled cases. Of these, 47.6% cases had 3 sets, while 14.6% had 2 sets of blood culture samples. For 10.6% cases both blood culture and cardiac tissues were received, while cardiac tissue or abscess pus aspirate samples without concomitant blood cultures were received in 6.7% of cases. Overall culture positivity rate was 71.2% ($n = 74$).

Among Gram positive organisms, *Streptococcus* species were the most common isolate (36.7%), predominantly *S. mitis*, followed by *Staphylococcus* species (23.1%). In *Streptococcus* species, 14.2% showed intermediate susceptibility to penicillin, (MIC50 = 0.12 µg/ml, MIC90 = 0.25 µg/ml); *S. oralis* being the species with the highest MIC range (0.06 µg/ml – 0.5 µg/ml). Half of the enterococcus isolates in the study were resistant to ampicillin, while all were sensitive to Vancomycin. *S. aureus* was isolated in 17.3% cases. Vancomycin MICs were performed only on Methicillin resistant strains of *S. aureus* (MIC range 0.5–1 µg/ml) and coagulase negative staphylococci (MIC 1 µg/ml). All MRSA strains were sensitive to Vancomycin. *Haemophilus actinomycetemcomitans*, *Klebsiella pneumoniae*, *Acinetobacter* species were isolated in 2.9% samples as primary pathogen and were found sensitive to third generation cephalosporin and carbapenem groups of antibiotics. Three patients had fungal endocarditis with *Candida albicans*, *Aspergillus niger*, *Fusarium* species, each. Table 1 shows details of frequency, type and antibiotic susceptibility of etiologic agents detected from blood and tissue cultures.

Table 1 Microbiological profile and antibiotic resistance pattern of isolates from patient with infective endocarditis received at the AKUH clinical laboratory (n = 104)

Microorganism	Total number cases n = 104(%)	Percent resistance of antibiotic for the species									
		CN	CI	ER	PE	VA	CH	OX	CP	AM	CR
Gram positive organism	**68 (65.4)**										
Staphylococcus species	**24 (23.1)**										
•*S. aureus*	18 (17.3)	27.0	22.2	50.0	100	00	00	77.	44.4	–	–
MSSA	4 (3.8)										
MRSA	14 (13.5)										
•CONS	6 (5.8)	16.6	16.6	33.3	100	00	00	83.3	60.0	–	–
Streptococcus species	**36 (34.7)**	NP	20.0	40.0	14.2	00	–	–	–	–	02.8
•*S. pneumoniae*	2 (1.9)										
•*S. mitis*	8 (7.7)										
•*S. oralis*	5 (4.8)										
•*S. sanguis*	3 (2.9)										
•*S. viridans*	3 (2.9)										
•*S. milleri*	1 (1.0)										
•*S. bovis*	3 (2.9)										
•*Streptococcus species*	5 (4.8)										
•*Granulicatella adiacens*	1 (1.0)										
•*Aerococcus viridans*	2 (1.9)										
•*Gemella haemolysan*	1 (1.0)										
Enterococcus species	**4 (3.8)**	25.0	–	50.0	50.0	00	25.0	–	–	50.0	–
Corynebaterium species	**4 (3.8)**	25	00	00	–	00	25.0	–	00		–
Gram negative organism	3 (2.9)	00	–	–	–	–	–	–	33.3	–	00
Haemophilus actinomycetemcomitans, Klebsiella pneumoniae, Acinetobacter species.											
Fungus	3 (2.9)	No resistance to azoles and Amphotericin									
Candida albicans, Aspergillus niger, Fusarium species											
Culture negative cases	30 (28.8)	–									

CN Gentamicin, *CI* Clindamycin, *ER* Erythromycin, *PE* Penicillin, *VA* Vancomycin, *CH* Chloramphenicol, *OX* Oxacillin, *CP* Ciprofloxacin *CR* Ceftriaxone, *MRSA* Methicillin resistant *Staphylococcus aureus*, *MSSA* Methicillin-Sensitive *Staphylococcus aureus*

AKUH patient cohort analysis

Table 2 shows the frequency and association of patient demographics and clinical characteristics with HRG at the time of presentation. Table 3 presents the frequencies and risk of clinical outcomes with the HRG. Thirty six patients were included in the cohort analysis. The HRG included 14 patients whereas 22 were included in the NVG. Mean age of patients in HRG was 45 years and 38 years in NVG. Male predominance was seen in both groups. Eighty five percent cases in HRG were diagnosed as definite IE, 41.6% presenting with acute symptoms. In the NVG, 72.2% were diagnosed as definite IE with acute symptoms in 54.4% patients. Culture positivity rate was 71.4% in HRG and 90.9% in NVG. RHD was seen in 18.1% cases of NVG only. In the HRG, prosthetic cardiac valve and implants (stents, pacemakers) were seen in 78.5% cases. A high proportion of

HRG patients had congenital heart disease (42.8%), who underwent invasive intervention in the past. Most patients presented with fever. Breathlessness was seen in 35.7% HRG and 54.5% NVG. Edema was present in 18% NVG patients. Signs of sepsis were more frequent in NVG (27.2% vs. 7.1% in HRG). Multi organ dysfunction including acute renal injury (AKI), splenomegaly, hepatomegaly, lymphadenopathy, pulmonary symptoms were seen in 31.81% of NVG vs 28.58% in HRG. Murmur was present in 36.6% NVG patients. Presence of vegetation was seen in almost all patients in HRG (92.8%) as shown in Table 2. Although too small a number to be significant, mitral valve prolapse was seen only in the NVG (13.6%) and pulmonary regurgitation only in HRG (14.2%).

Regarding clinical outcomes, the risk of disease severity was higher amongst the HRG than NVG (Table 3), with 85.7% HRG patients having poorer outcome compared to

Table 2 Frequency and association of patient demographics, clinical characteristics and underlying disease severity with HRG at the time of presentation of IE patients admitted at AKUH 2015–2017 (n = 36)

PATIENT CHARACTERISTICS	HRG N = 14	NVG N = 22	p-value	Odds Ratio (Confidence interval)
Mean Age	45	38	–	–
Gender: Male	8	15	0.501	0.838 (0.490–1.432)
MoDC				
•Definite	12	16	0.361	1.179 (0.844–1.645)
•Probable	2	6	0.361	0.524 (0.122–2.240)
Acute clinical presentation	5	12	0.270	0.655 (0.294–1.457)
Sub-acute presentation	9	10	0.270	1.414 (0.775–2.581)
Positive culture	10	20	0.126	0.786 (0.550–1.122)
Pure culture growth	14	18	0.091	1.222 (1.004–1.488)
Rheumatic heart disease	0	4	0.090	
Prosthetic heart valve / cardiac implants	11	0	–	–
Congenital heart disease	6	5	0.201	1.886 (0.708–5.022)
Severity at presentation				
Signs of thromboembolism[a]	2	7	0.236	0.449(0.108–1.860)
Sepsis	1	6	0.137	0.262 (0.951–1.714)
Multi organ dysfunction	4	7	0.837	0.898 (0.321–2.514)
Rash /splinter hemorrhage	0	4	0.091	–
•Previous history of infective endocarditis	1	0	0.204	–
•Murmur	2	8	0.149	0.393 (0.920–1.972)
•Raised infectious markers	1	2	0.837	0.786 (0.078–7.876)
Radiologic evidence on Echocardiography				
•Vegetation	13	14	*0.048*	*1.45 (1.03–2.066)*
•Mitral valve prolapse	0	3	0.149	–
•Peri-annular abscess	2	3	0.956	1.048 (0.199–5.504)
•Valve perforation / dehiscence	1	1	0.740	1.571 (0.107–23.140)
•Portal hypertension	8	11	0.826	–
•Aortic regurgitation	6	10	0.878	0.943 (0.442–2.013)
•Mitral regurgitation	4	7	0.837	0.898 (0.321–2.514)
•Pulmonary regurgitation	2	0	0.068[a]	–

HRG High risk group, NVG Native valve group, MoDC Modified Dukes Criteria
[a]= gangrene, unilateral weakness, slurring of speech, loss of consciousness

50% of NVG. However, more deaths were seen in the native valve group (22.72%), despite not achieving statistical significance probably due to small number of events. The Kaplan Meier curve is shown in Fig. 2. The risk of embolism or infarct was higher with NVG (45.5%); the involvement of central nervous system seen exclusively in this group (27.7%). Thirty six percent cases of the HRG had complications during hospital stay (NVG = 27.2%). Large vegetation was the most common indication for surgery in both groups (HRG = 64.2%, NVG = 22.7%), but significantly associated with HRG.

Additional file 1: Table S4 shows clinical presentations and outcomes specific to the organisms isolated amongst Infective Endocarditis patients admitted at AKUH 2015–

2017. *Streptococcus* spp. was equally prevalent in both groups (22.7% in NVG vs 21.4% in HRG). In the NVG, cases presented with murmur, thromboembolic (TE) event, rash, cardiac tamponade and abscess (*S. oralis*) on echocardiograph at presentation. All these cases were treated medically and had Penicillin MIC range of 0.03–0.5 μg/ml. There was one death; the patient's isolate had intermediate susceptibility to Penicillin with MIC of 0.12 μg/ml. In the HRG, 3 cases of *Streptococcus* species were seen; Penicillin MIC range was 0.015–0.012 μg/ml. Only one presented with an abscess and the infecting organism in this case was *S. sanguis*. *S.aureus* was seen more in the NVG compared to HRG. MRSA endocarditis cases presented with TE event, AKI, raised infectious

Table 3 Clinical outcome characteristics of IE patients admitted at AKUH 2015–2017 ($n = 36$)

CLINICAL OUTCOME	HRG $N = 14$	NVG $N = 22$	p-value	RISK
Disease severity	12	11	**0.030**	**1.714 (1.072–2.741)**
•Surgical management	7	15	0.275	1.571 (0.702–3516)
•Readmission	5	2	0.143	–
•Death	2	5	0.533	0.629 (.0141–2.808)
Presence of embolism / infarct	2	10	**0.05**	**0.314 (0.080–1.227)**
•Infarct	0	4	0.091	–
•Embolism	2	6	0.361	0.524 (0.122–2.240)
oBrain	0	6	**0.032**	–
oLung	1	4	0.350	0.393 (0.049–3.165)
olimbs	1	0	0.204	–
Complication during hospital stay	5	6	0.592	1.310 (0.492–3.488)
Sepsis	1	1	0.740	1.571 (0.107–23.140)
•Coagulation / Hematological issue	2	2	0.629	1.571 (0.249–9.913)
•Multi-organ dysfunction[a]	2	1	0.303	3.143 (0.314–31.506)
•Re- exploration	1	2	0.837	0.786 (0.078–7.876)
•Cardiac conduction defects	1	1	0.740	1.571 (0.107–23.140)
Indication for Surgical Intervention				
•Sepsis	2	2	0.629	1.571 (0.249–9.913)
•Embolism	0	2	0.246	–
•Large vegetation	9	5	**0.013**	**2.829 (1.192–6.710)**
•Cardiac failure	0	4	0.091	–
Valve replacement	**6**	**8**	**0.048**	
Cause of Death	–	–	0.852	–
•Cardiac arrest	1	2	0.852	–
•Cerebral bleed	0	1	0.143	–
•Sepsis	1	2	0.533	0.629 (.0141–2.808)

HRG High risk group, *NVG* Native valve group
[a]= acute renal injury (AKI), splenomegaly, hepatomegaly, lymphadenopathy, pulmonary symptoms

markers, murmur, splenomegaly, rash, sepsis and splinter hemorrhages and only two were treated surgically. Amongst the 3 mortalities, 2 received medical treatment only while one died at day 11 of hospital admission 24 h post valvuloplasty. The patient presented with signs of acute IE with MRSA (vancomycin MIC 1 µg/ml) and developed multiorgan dysfunction and pulmonary embolism. This patient had multiple vegetations (11x11mm, 9x7mm) on Tricuspid valve and underwent valve replacement due to heart failure and sepsis. Infections with coagulase negative staphylococcal species was seen exclusively in the HRG ($n = 3$), presenting with TE event, AKI, raised infectious markers, splenomegaly and abscess on echocardiograph. Two of these patients were treated surgically and 1 medically, who later expired.

Discussion

In the 2-year study period, we enrolled 104 patients of IE, of which 65.4% were definite cases based on MoDC.

Of enrolled cases 28.8% were culture negative as compared with 50% previously reported in studies from Pakistan [7, 8]. The most plausible explanation for this difference is the sensitivity of blood and tissue culture methods used in this study. Most etiological agents of IE are fastidious and require highly nutrient culture medium and controlled incubation conditions. BACTEC 9240 system of blood culture is known to have better culture yield [12] as compared to conventional blood culture method used in previous studies from Pakistan. However when compared with data from western studies reporting blood culture yield of 90% [13] our culture yield of 74.2% is much lower. The most compelling reason for this low yield are the pre-analytical factors, such as use of antibiotics prior to blood culture collection. This was noticeable in 71% of all enrolled cases in current study. Another important factor is the adequate volume of blood cultured. Since density of microorganisms in blood is often very low, adequate volume and

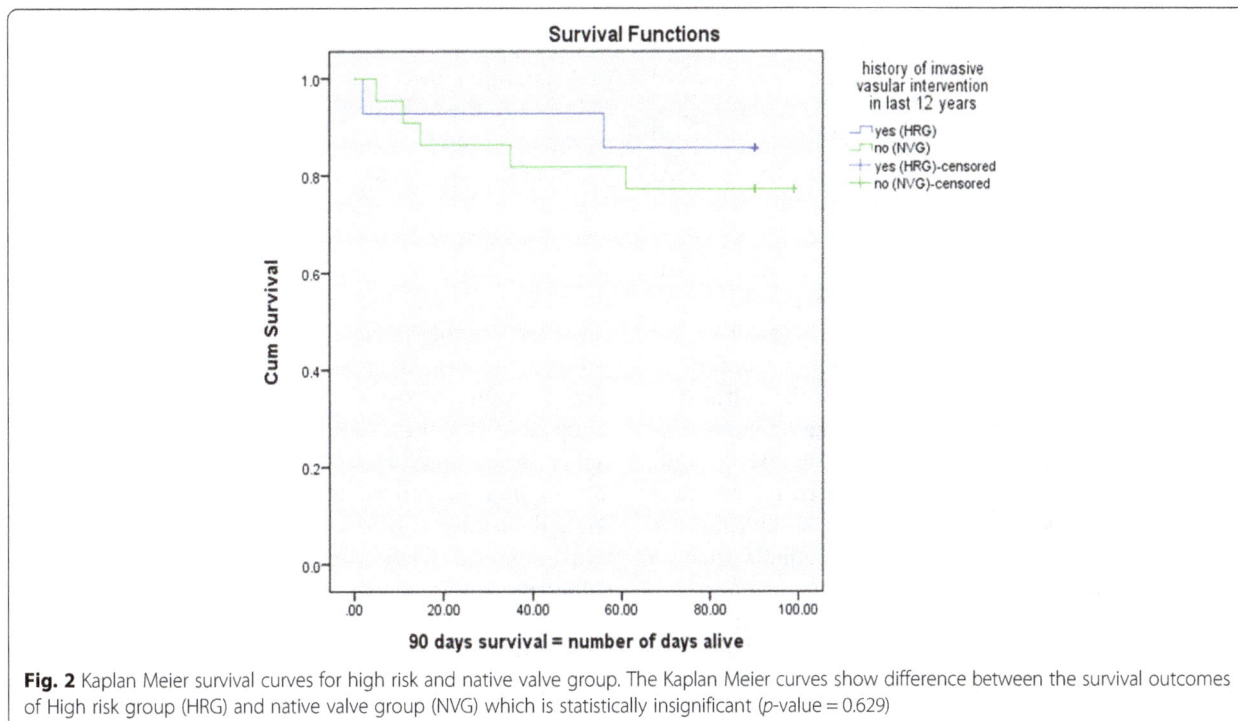

Fig. 2 Kaplan Meier survival curves for high risk and native valve group. The Kaplan Meier curves show difference between the survival outcomes of High risk group (HRG) and native valve group (NVG) which is statistically insignificant (*p*-value = 0.629)

multiple sampling is considered to be an important parameter for improved blood culture yield. Guidelines from most professional societies, such as American Society for Microbiology (ASM) and Infectious Disease Society of America (IDSA), recommend that adult patient with suspected IE must be investigated by drawing at least 3 blood culture sets with appropriate volume [1]. In our study population only 47.3% of total patients recruited had 3 sets of blood culture. Inaccessibility to health facilities, increasing diagnostic cost and lack of awareness are factors that often contribute to poor compliance to these essential pre-analytical components of blood culture analysis in Pakistan.

Contrary to previous reports of predominantly younger age group [3, 7] we found 15.4% of enrolled patients being below age of 16 years. Tariq et al. in his study conducted in 2004 reported mean age of 24 years [3], same group in 2015 has reported a shift in mean age 42 years [4], close to the mean age of patients in this study (34.5 years). This progressive increase perhaps reflects the shift in the underlying risk factors. During the last two decades reports from Pakistan are showing a gradual shift from communicable to non-communicable diseases (NCDs) such as cardiovascular diseases (including stroke and heart disease), diabetes, mental health disorders, cancers, and chronic airway diseases [14]. Management of most of these diseases often requires advanced medical care such as use of cardiac implants, invasive vascular interventions etc., predisposing patients to risk factors of endocarditis similar to those of the modern world –however more data is required to verify this change.

We found *Streptococcus* group of bacteria to be the most frequently isolated organisms from blood and tissue cultures in both groups. These findings are similar to those published by other groups nationally and from neighboring countries like China, India [3, 5, 7, 15–17] as well as internationally [2, 18]. Although *Streptococci* seem to predominate in developing regions, most western and developed parts of the world report *S. aureus* as the predominant causative agent of IE [19, 20]. *S. mitis* was the most common species isolated similar to a recent survey involving 118 hospitals in Japan reporting *S.viridians* as the predominant species in NVE [21]. Penicillin remains drug of choice against this group of bacteria however we found 14.2% of our isolates to be intermediately resistant with MIC as high as 1 µg/ml. No particular species of *S.viridans* predominantly showed higher MIC. The numbers of isolates in our study were too few to establish such association. A study in USA reported high-level penicillin resistance among 13.4% and intermediate resistance in 42.9% strains of *S. viridans* [22].To the best of our knowledge no prospective study in Pakistan relates pathogens and their respective MICs with disease severity in IE, a finding unique to our study.

Of the 18 *S. aureus* isolated, 77.7% were MRSA and were more frequent in the NVG. MRSA infections showed increase disease severity at time of presentation such as TE events, AKI, raised infectious markers, murmur splenomegaly, rash, sepsis and splinter hemorrhages. It was the commonest pathogen found amongst expired patients in both cohorts. A study in Turkey reported 18% of IE deaths due to endocarditis, a number higher than any other pathogen isolated [23]. This could be due to the high prevalence of MRSA in the region. Asia has higher prevalence of both healthcare-associated methicillin-resistant *Staphylococcus aureus* (HA-MRSA) and community-acquired methicillin-resistant *S. aureus* (CA-MRSA) [24].

Human brucellosis is common in Pakistan in patients with risk factors such as animal exposure, use of unpasteurized milk etc. Blood cultures positive for patients suffering from Brucella infections are often reported from this lab, however none of the cultures in this study yielded Brucella sp., as a cause of endocarditis. This could be because of selection bias of our patients as most of the samples recruited in the study were from patients under cardiac care. In addition, we had limitation of non-availability of methods such as PCR and serological analysis.

Embolism is not uncommon and risk is seen in 22–57% cases of IE: the risk progressively increased with the size of vegetation [25] . Amongst our patients 12 presented with evidence of embolism or infarct. Of these 6 were cerebral, 5 pulmonary and 1 with peripheral involvement. A prospective multicenter European study presented 34.1% cases with true embolic events [20]. Most were involving the CNS similar to our findings. Statistically significant difference was seen between the 2 cohorts with more embolic events in the NVG. A retrospective study in France presented embolism in 62% of PVE vs. 35% of NVE patients [25]. Although this contradicts our findings, this could be due to delay in diagnosis as patients with prior invasive intervention or cardiac anomalies tend to access tertiary care earlier. Embolism is directly related to the size of vegetations, therefore late presentations are likely to have larger vegetations.

The mortality rate in our study was 19.4% and we saw more deaths and more severe case presentations in NVG as opposed to HRG (Table 3). This is most likely due to inaccessibility to health facilities, increasing diagnostic cost leading to delay in diagnosis. HRG was associated with severe disease outcomes, a statistically significant finding despite a small sample size. These were mainly due to higher rates of surgical intervention and readmission due to complications. In a retrospective review of surgical patients with NVE and PVE, Manne et al. described a severe clinical course amongst those with PVE, with 23% 1 year mortality rate, higher risk of post-operative complication like cerebrovascular accident (3.3%), renal failure (11%), reoperation (9.4%) [9].

Our study had some limitations which included a small sample size and convenient sampling. Ideally, an additional control group comprising of uninfected surgical cases should have been included to remove confounding by surgical complications from those of complicated IE. The sample size was small to establish statistically significant findings. However, a larger sample size was not possible due to the low prevalence and short duration of this prospective study.

Secondly, we could not ascertain culture negative cases as we did not perform additional testing for organisms like *Bartonella* spp., *Coxiella burnetti* and *Tropheryma whipplei* due to lack of technical facilities and availability of reagents and positive control strains.. However for *Mycobacterium tuberculosis* culture was performed in selected patients; cardiac tissue and pus aspirates when requested by the clinicians, and in this study all MTb cultures remained negative. Being a single center study, unrecognized confounding factors and selection bias may have affected results. This study is strengthened by its prospective nature as well as description of clinical details and disease outcomes relating to pathogens in IE patients.

Conclusion

In conclusion our findings support the hypothesis that HRG can encounter a more complicated clinical course requiring further surgical interventions, readmissions or death as opposed to native valve endocarditis patients therefore we recommend close follow up of high risk population.

Abbreviations

AKI: Acute renal injury; AKUH: Aga Khan University Hospital; ASM: American Society for Microbiology; BSAC: British Society for Antimicrobial Chemotherapy; CABG: Coronary artery bypass; CA-MRSA: Community-acquired methicillin-resistant *S. aureus*; CH: Chloramphenicol; CI: Clindamycin; CLSI: Clinical & Laboratory Standards Institute; CN: Culture negative; CN: Gentamicin; CP: Ciprofloxacin; CR: Ceftriaxone; ER: Erythromycin; GNO: Gram negative organism; GPB: Gram positive bacilli; HA-MRSA: Healthcare-associated methicillin-resistant *Staphylococcus aureus*; HRG: High risk group; IDSA: Infectious Disease Society of America; IE: Infective Endocarditis; IVI: Invasive vascular interventions; MIC: Minimal inhibitory concentration; MoDC: Modified Duke's criteria; MRSA: Methicillin-resistant *Staphylococcus aureus*; MSSA: Methicillin-Sensitive *Staphylococcus aureus*; NCDs: Non-communicable diseases; NVE: Native valve endocarditis; NVG: Native valve group; OX: Oxacillin; PE: Penicillin; PVE: Prosthetic valve disease; RHD: Rheumatic heart disease; TE: Thromboembolic; VA: Vancomycin

Acknowledgements

Ahmed Rahim for sample size calculation and data management.

Authors' contributions

US, EK, HS, were involved in conception and design of the study, US collected clinical and Lab data, HS and BJ contributed by identifying the clinical cases according to modified Dukes Criteria, JF contributed in data analysis and interpretation, EK, US drafted the manuscript, JF, BJ and HS did critical revision, all gave final approval of the version to be published and agreed to be accountable on all aspects of the work in ensuring that questions. All authors read and approved the final manuscript.

Competing interests

The authors declare that they have no competing interests.

Author details

[1]Section of Microbiology, Department of Pathology and Laboratory Medicine, Aga Khan University, Karachi, Pakistan. [2]Section of Cardiothoracic Surgery, Department of Surgery, Aga Khan University, Karachi, Pakistan. [3]Section of Infectious Diseases, Department of Medicine, Aga Khan University, Karachi, Pakistan.

References

1. Baddour LM, Wilson WR, Bayer AS, Fowler VG, Tleyjeh IM, Rybak MJ, et al. Infective endocarditis in adults: diagnosis, antimicrobial therapy, and management of complications. Circulation. 2015;132(15):1435–86.
2. Habib G, Lancellotti P, Antunes MJ, Bongiorni MG, Casalta JP, Del Zotti F, Dulgheru R, El Khoury G, Erba PA, Iung B, Miro JM. 2015 ESC guidelines for the management of infective endocarditis: the task force for the management of infective endocarditis of the European Society of Cardiology (ESC) endorsed by: European Association for Cardio-Thoracic Surgery (EACTS), the European Association of Nuclear Medicine (EANM). Eur Heart J. 2015;36(44):3075-128.
3. Tariq M, Alam M, Munir G, Khan MA, Smego RA Jr. Infective endocarditis: a five-year experience at a tertiary care hospital in Pakistan. Int J Inf Dis : IJID : official publication of the International Society for Infectious Diseases. 2004; 8(3):163–70. Epub 2004/04/28
4. Arshad S, Awan S, Bokhari SS, Tariq M. Clinical predictors of mortality in hospitalized patients with infective endocarditis at a tertiary care center in Pakistan. JPMA The J Pak Med Assoc. 2015;65(1):3–8. Epub 2015/04/04
5. Tariq M, Siddiqui BK, Jadoon A, Alam M, Khan SA, Atiq M, et al. Clinical profile and outcome of infective endocarditis at the Aga Khan University Hospital. International Journal of Collaborative Research on Internal Medicine & Public Health. 2009;1(3):84.
6. Sadiq M, Nazir M, Sheikh SA. Infective endocarditis in children—incidence, pattern, diagnosis and management in a developing country. Int J Cardiol. 2001;78(2):175–82.
7. Faheem M, Iqbal MA, Saeed R, Asghar M, Hafizullah M. Profile of infective endocarditis in a tertiary care hospital. Pak Heart J. 2014;47(1).
8. Naber CK, Erbel R. Infective endocarditis with negative blood cultures. Int J Antimicrob Agents. 2007;30:32–6.
9. Manne MB, Shrestha NK, Lytle BW, Nowicki ER, Blackstone E, Gordon SM, et al. Outcomes after surgical treatment of native and prosthetic valve infective endocarditis. Ann Thorac Surg. 2012;93(2):489–93. Epub 2011/12/31
10. Brennan JM, Edwards FH, Zhao Y, O'Brien S, Booth ME, Dokholyan RS, Douglas PS, Peterson ED. Long-Term Safety and Effectiveness of Mechanical versus Biologic Aortic Valve Prostheses in Older Patients: Results from the Society of Thoracic Surgeons (STS) Adult Cardiac Surgery National Database. Circulation. 2013:CIRCULATIONAHA-113.
11. User Manual for AUTOMATED BLOOD CULTURE BACTEC™ 9240/9120/9050. BD Diagnostics; 2000. legacy.bd.com/ds/technicalCenter/clsi/clsi-9000bc2.pdf.
12. Ahmad A, Iram S, Hussain S, Yusuf NW. Diagnosis of paediatric sepsis by automated blood culture system and conventional blood culture. JPMA The J Pak Med Assoc. 2017;67(2):192–5. Epub 2017/02/01
13. Habib G. Management of infective endocarditis. Heart. 2006;92(1):124–30.
14. Jafar TH, Haaland BA, Rahman A, Razzak JA, Bilger M, Naghavi M, et al. Non-communicable diseases and injuries in Pakistan: strategic priorities. Lancet. 2013;381(9885):2281–90. Epub 2013/05/21
15. Xu H, Cai S, Dai H. Characteristics of infective endocarditis in a tertiary Hospital in East China. PLoS One. 2016;11(11):e0166764. Epub 2016/11/20
16. Garg N, Kandpal B, Tewari S, Kapoor A, Goel P, Sinha N. Characteristics of infective endocarditis in a developing country-clinical profile and outcome in 192 Indian patients, 1992-2001. Int J Cardiol. 2005;98(2):253–60. Epub 2005/02/03
17. Li L, Wang H, Wang L, Pu J, Zhao H. Changing profile of infective endocarditis: a clinicopathologic study of 220 patients in a single medical center from 1998 through 2009. Tex Heart Inst J. 2014;41(5):491–8. Epub 2014/11/27
18. Barrau K, Boulamery A, Imbert G, Casalta JP, Habib G, Messana T, et al. Clin Microbiol Infect : the official publication of the European Society of Clinical Microbiology and Infectious Diseases. 2004;10(4):302–8. Epub 2004/04/03
19. Slipczuk L, Codolosa JN, Davila CD, Romero-Corral A, Yun J, Pressman GS, et al. Infective endocarditis epidemiology over five decades: a systematic review. PLoS One. 2013;8(12):e82665. Epub 2013/12/19
20. Cresti A, Chiavarelli M, Scalese M, Nencioni C, Valentini S, Guerrini F, et al. Epidemiological and mortality trends in infective endocarditis, a 17-year population-based prospective study. Cardiovasc Diagn Ther=. 2017;7(1): 27–35. Epub 2017/02/07
21. Nakatani S, Mitsutake K, Ohara T, Kokubo Y, Yamamoto H, Hanai S, et al. Recent picture of infective endocarditis in Japan. Circ J. 2013;77(6):1558–64.
22. Doern GV, Ferraro MJ, Brueggemann AB, Ruoff KL. Emergence of high rates of antimicrobial resistance among viridans group streptococci in the United States. Antimicrob Agents Chemother. 1996;40(4):891–4. Epub 1996/04/01
23. Simsek-Yavuz S, Sensoy A, Kasikcioglu H, Ceken S, Deniz D, Yavuz A, et al. Infective endocarditis in Turkey: aetiology, clinical features, and analysis of risk factors for mortality in 325 cases. Int J Infect Dis : IJID : official publication of the International Society for Infectious Diseases. 2015;30:106–14. Epub 2014/12/03
24. Chen CJ, Huang YC. New epidemiology of Staphylococcus aureus infection in Asia. Clin Microbiol Infect : the official publication of the European Society of Clinical Microbiology and Infectious Diseases. 2014;20(7):605–23. Epub 2014/06/04
25. Deprele C, Berthelot P, Lemetayer F, Comtet C, Fresard A, Cazorla C, et al. Risk factors for systemic emboli in infective endocarditis. Clin Microbiol Infect : the official publication of the European Society of Clinical Microbiology and Infectious Diseases. 2004;10(1):46–53. Epub 2004/01/07

21

Mitral valve repair, how to make volume not matter; techniques, tendencies, and outcomes, a single center experience

Manuel Giraldo-Grueso[1], Néstor Sandoval-Reyes[2], Jaime Camacho[2], Ivonne Pineda[3] and Juan P. Umaña[4*]

Abstract

Background: Recent evidence has showed us that quality of mitral valve repair is strongly related to volume. However, this study shows how low-volume centers can achieve results in mitral valve repair surgery comparable to those reported by referral centers. It compares outcomes of mitral valve repair using resection versus noresection techniques, tendencies, and rates of repair.

Methods: Between 2004 and 2017, 200 patients underwent mitral valve repair for degenerative mitral valve disease at Fundación Cardioinfantil-Institute of Cardiology. Fifty-eight (29%) patients underwent resection and 142 (71%) noresection.

Results: Follow-up was 94% complete, mean follow-up time was 2.3 years. There was no 30-day mortality. Five patients required mitral valve replacement after an average of 5.3 years (Resection = 2; Noresection = 3). Freedom from severe mitral regurgitation was 98% at 6.6 years of follow-up for the noresection group, and 92.5% at 7 years for the resection group (log rank: 0.888). At last follow-up, two patients died of cardiovascular disease related to mitral valve, 181 patients (86%) showed no or grade I mitral regurgitation. Patients with previous myocardial infarction had increased risk of recurrent mitral regurgitation ($p = 0,030$). Within four years, we inverted the proportion of mitral valve replacement and repair, and in 2016 we achieved a mitral valve repair rate of 96%.

Conclusion: This study suggests that resection and noresection techniques are safe and effective. Recurrence of severe mitral regurgitation and need for mitral valve replacement are rare. We show that low-volume centers can achieve results comparable to those reported worldwide by establishing a mitral valve repair team. We encourage hospitals to follow this model of mitral valve repair program to decrease the proportion of mitral valve replacement, while increasing mitral valve repair.

Keywords: Mitral regurgitation, Mitral valve annulus repair, Prolapsed mitral valve

Background

Mitral valve repair (MVr) is the gold standard for the treatment of mitral regurgitation (MR) secondary to degenerative mitral valve (MV) disease. MVr was initially performed by Alain Carpentier in 1983, who developed a standardized approach to correct MR, dubbed "the French correction". It involved leaflet resection followed by annular plication with or without sliding plasty in order to restore the coaptation surface [1].

Excellent, reproducible results led to this technique becoming the gold standard to treat mitral valve prolapse. In 1998, Tirone David et al. proposed a novel repair technique using extended polytetrafluoroethylene (ePTFE) sutures for chordal replacement, preserving leaflet tissue and improving surface of coaptation [2].

Subsequent studies have shown excellent results for both techniques in terms of mortality, morbidity, and freedom from recurrent MR [3]. Controversy remains as to which technique is superior given lack of long-term follow-up with creation of neochordae and the perception that this technique is more difficutl to standardize, preventing widespread application.

* Correspondence: jpumana@cardioinfantil.org
[4]Director Cardiovascular Medicine, Cardiac Surgery Department, Fundación Cardioinfantil- Instituto de Cardiologia, Bogotá, Colombia
Full list of author information is available at the end of the article

In Latin America, long-term results of MVr remain unknown and the established practice is to replace rather than repair the MV. The present study was carried out to evaluate the short and long-term results of MVr using resection (R) versus noresection (NR) techniques in a low-volume center and resolve if a low-volume center can achieve MVr results comparable to those reported worldwide. We analyzed freedom from reoperation, recurrent MR, and functional status, as well as the change in the tendency of MVr and mitral valve replacement (MVR) at our institution over the study period. The findings of the study seek to improve cardiac surgery.

Methods
Patients
From January of 2004 to June 2017, 200 patients underwent MVr due to degenerative MV disease at Fundación Cardioinfantil- Institute of Cardiology, in Bogotá Colombia. Patients were identified through an institutional cardiac surgery database. Operational definitions, demographic variables, preoperative, intraoperative characteristics, and 30-day outcomes were obtained retrospectively according to the Society of Thoracic Surgeons database guidelines [4].

Fifty-eight patients (29%) were in the R group and 142 (71%) in the NR group (chordal replacement or just ring annuloplasty). Twelve patients (6%) were lost to follow up.

Interventions
Operations were performed through a conventional median sternotomy or minimally invasive techniques (right lateral minithoracotomy or periareolar approach). In the conventional approach, cardiopulmonary bypass was established through standard bicaval and aortic cannulation with moderate hypothermia. Intraoperative transesophageal echocardiography was used routinely in all patients. Access to the MV was performed through a left atriotomy. Next, segmental analysis of the MV was performed as described by Carpentier and colleagues [5]. In all patients, ring annuloplasty was performed with a semi-rigid, complete ring Fig. 1.

When the repair was performed minimally invasively, the femoral vessels were cannulated using modified Seldinger technique under echocardiographic guidance. A Chitwood clamp was used and cardiac arrest achieved using HTK or Del Nido cardioplegia. Video assistance was used routinely.

Chordal replacement was performed with 5.0 ePTFE sutures without pledgets, passed as a figure of eight through the tip of the papillary muscle, followed by a figure of eight through the free edge of the prolapsing segment. A minimum of two neochordae were placed, and sutures were added depending on the size of the prolapsing segment. The height of the neochordae was established by filling the ventricle with a cold cardioplegic solution to test the valve hydrostatically. The number of neochordae ranged from one to seven pairs (mean: 1.88). A single pair of neochordae was used in 29% and multiple in 71%. The decision to perform either a R or NR technique was left to the surgeon's criteria.

Surgical data were obtained by systematic chart review, emphasizing the MVr technique and approach.

Data collection
Preoperative (age, previous cardiac operation, functional class, Euroscore II, left ventricular ejection fraction, previous arrhythmia, and medical history) and postoperative variables (length of stay, cross-clamp and cardiopulmonary bypass time, reoperation for bleeding and 30-day mortality) were described.

Follow up was performed by telephone or in person (clinic visits). Endpoints were recurrent MR, reoperation or death. Echocardiographic evaluations were performed postoperatively before discharge, 30 to 90 days after surgery, then annually thereafter. The severity of MR was classified as none/trivial (0), mild (I), moderate (II) or severe (III). New York Heart Association (NYHA) functional class was assessed in all the patients. Echocardiographic data were used for analysis only if there were at least two echocardiographic reports available.

We described tendencies and number of cases of MVR and MVr for degenerative MV disease from 2004 to 2016. Data were obtained from the institutional cardiac surgery database.

Statistical analysis
Baseline demographics and clinical characteristics were summarized using descriptive statistics. For continuous variables, data were presented as mean or median and standard deviations or interquartile range. Categorical variables were presented as absolute numbers and percentages. The frequency of MR was described. The difference between the groups R and NR were ascertained using chi-square test or Fisher test, and Mann-Whitney U test. The endpoint of interest was recurrent severe MR, MV reoperation or death. Patients that did not reach the endpoint were censored at the end of study time. Survival was analyzed through Kaplan-Meier method; the log-rank test was used to determine differences between groups. Statistical analysis was done with Stata SE 14 (program). A significance level of 0.05 was used throughout the analysis.

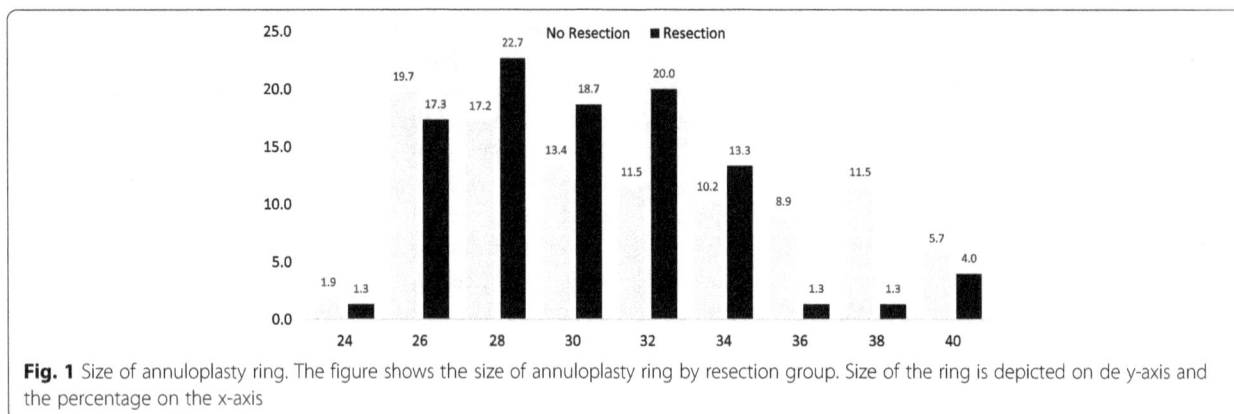

Fig. 1 Size of annuloplasty ring. The figure shows the size of annuloplasty ring by resection group. Size of the ring is depicted on de y-axis and the percentage on the x-axis

Results

Demographic data

Follow-up was 94% complete with a mean time of 2.33 years. Preoperative variables are summarized in Table 1. Of all patients, 122(61%) were male, and the average age at operation was 58 (48–58) years for the NR group and 56 (50–65) years for the R group. Before surgery, NYHA functional class was assessed in all the patients, 21 (10.5%) were in NYHA class I, 135 (67,5%) class II and 33 (16,5%) class III. Three (1.5%) patients had a history of myocardial infarction before surgery, all of them belong to the NR group. We found differences in the left ventricular ejection fraction (LVEF) between groups; 55% (50–60%) and 60% (51–65) for the NR group and R group, respectively ($p = 0.013$).

Euroscore II was calculated in all patients before surgery. 50.4% in the NR group were classified as low risk, compared to 25,9% in the R group (risk < 2%) Fig. 2.

Perioperative outcomes

Perioperative variables are summarized in Table 1. One hundred and seven patients (75%) of the NR group and 48 (84.5%) of the R group underwent isolated MVr. Mean cardiopulmonary bypass time was similar for both groups, 117 min (IQR 95–141) and 117 min (IQR 105–143) for the NR and R groups respectively. Forty-seven (33.1%) patients from NR group and 35 (60%) from R group had a posterior leaflet prolapse ($p = 0,004$). There was a statistically significant difference in the number of minimally invasive procedures performed in each group, with 51 (32.9%) in the NR group and 7 (12.1%) in the R group ($p = 0.001$). Overall 30-day mortality was 0%.

Survival outcomes

NYHA class and incidence of MR at last follow-up in 188 patients are reported in Table 2. Functional class was assessed in all the patients, most of whom showed significant improvement: 156 (83%) had NYHA class I, 25 (13%) class II, 5 (3%) class III and 2 (1%) class IV. Patients in NYHA class IV had concomitant chronic

obstructive pulmonary disease (COPD). Ninety-eight patients (52%) had none/trace MR, mild MR in 70 (37%), and moderate/severe in 20 (10%).

There were only two cardiac-related deaths at last follow-up. Freedom for severe MR was 98% at 6.6 years of follow-up for the NR group, and 92.5% at 7 years of follow-up for the R group. Based on MVr technique, patients in the R group had the same likelihood of developing MR compared to patients in NR group (log rank: 0.881). Five patients required an MV replacement after an average of 5.3 years, 3 belonged to the NR group and 2 to the R group Fig. 3.

Bivariate analysis

In the bivariate analysis, patients with previous myocardial infarction had an increased risk of developing at least moderate recurrent MR ($p = 0,030$). Preoperative variables such as diabetes, dialysis, dyslipidemia, hypertension and previous arrhythmia, were not associated with an increased risk of developing recurrent MR after MVr. Patients that underwent minimally invasive repair, had a lower risk of developing recurrent MR ($p = 0,040$) Table 3.

Mitral valve surgery tendencies and repair rate

Tendencies and number of cases of MVr and MVR for degenerative MV disease are shown in Fig. 4. Within four years, we inverted the tendency and were able to maintain MVr as preferred technique of MV intervention. The MVr rates at our institution are shown in Fig. 5. Over the years there has been a constant increase in MVr rate, achieving a 96% repair rate in 2016.

Discussion

MV regurgitation is frequently caused by degenerative MV disease leading to myxomatous changes with chordal elongation with or without rupture [6–8]. R and NR techniques have shown excellent results, with low incidence of progression to severe MR and need for MVR [7–9]. In our series, five patients required MVR

Table 1 Preoperative, clinical, and perioperative variables of the patients

Variable n (%)	No resection n = 142	Resection n = 58	P value
Preoperative variables			
Male sex	83 (58.4)	39 (67,2)	0,247
Age years, median IQR	58 (48–66)	56 (48–66)	0,969
Diabetes	9 (6,3)	1 (1,7)	0,287
Dyslipidemia	18 (12,7)	11 (18,9)	0,252
Dialysis	2 (1,4)	3 (5,2)	0,147
Hypertension	59 (41,5)	20 (34,5)	0,354
COPD	7 (4,9)	4 (6,9)	0,580
Creatinine	1 (0,9-1,08)	0,95 (0,9–1)	0,821
Previous myocardial infarction	0	3 (5,2)	0,023
Previous cardiac operation	4 (2.8)	1 (1,7)	0,999
NYHA functional class			0,079
I	12 (8,7)	9 (17,3)	
II	99 (72,3)	36 (69,2)	
III	26 (19)	7 (13,5)	
Previous arrhythmia	48 (33,8)	19 (32,8)	0,887
LVEF, median IQR	55 (50–60)	60 (51–65)	0,013
Perioperative variables			
Isolated ring annuloplasty	14 (9,8)	0 (0,0)	< 0,001
Isolated MV repair	107 (75)	49 (84,5)	0,108
Non-Isolated MV repair	35 (25)	9 (15,5)	0,235
ASD closure	7 (4,9)	0 (0,0)	0,086
Tricuspid repair	24 (16,9)	9 (15,5)	0,809
Tricuspid replacement	1 (0,7)	0 (0,0)	0,001
Tricuspid repair+ASD closure	3 (2,1)	0 (0,0)	0,013
Minimally invasive	51 (35,9)	7 (12.1)	< 0,001
ICU stay days	1 (1–4)	1 (1–3)	0,495
Post ICU stay (days)	3 (2–5)	4 (3–5)	0,674
Degenerative MV pathology			
Posterior leaflet prolapse	47 (33,1)	35 (60,3)	0,004
Anterior leaflet prolapse	23 (16,1)	4 (6,8)	0,079
Bileaflet prolapse	17 (11,9)	3 (5,1)	0,144
Elongated/ruptured chord(s)	29 (20,4)	10 (17,2)	0,604
Annular dilation	25 (17,6)	2 (3,4)	0,014
Unknown	1 (0,7)	4 (6,9)	0,011
Postoperative complications			
Reoperation for bleeding	0 (0,0)	2 (3,4)	0,083
Renal impairment	2 (1,4)	0 (0,0)	0,503
Hospital length of stay	8 (5–15)	8 (5–14)	0,906
Mortality 30 days	0 (0,0)	0 (0,0)	

Categorical data are expressed as number (%) and continuous data as median (Interquartile range)

COPD Chronic Obstructive Pulmonary Disease, *ICU* Intensive Care Unit, *IQR* Interquartile Range, *LVEF* Left Ventricular Ejection Fraction, *NYHA* New York Hear Association

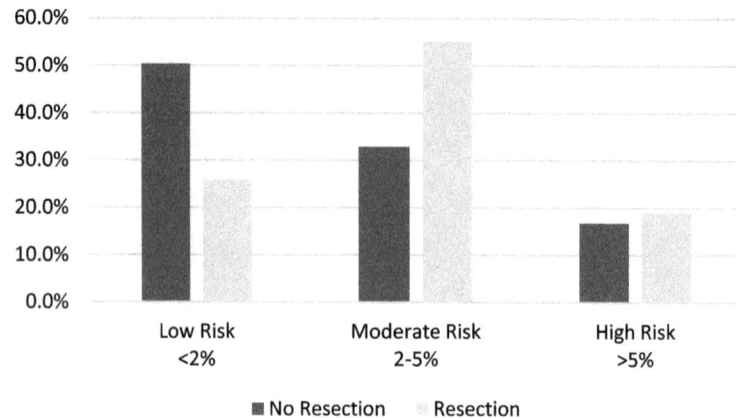

Fig. 2 Preoperative Euroscore II risk assessment. Figure shows Euroscore II risk assessment in NR and R groups

after an average of 5.3 years, three belonged to the NR group and two to the R group, one patient from the NR group had an ePTFE chord rupture. Schwartz et al. [10] described similar results with a freedom from reoperation of 89% at ten years. There was no 30-day mortality in our series; Lange et al. [11] showed comparable results with 30-day mortality of 1%. We were able to achieve MVr results with R and NR techniques similar to those reported by referral institutions, despite being a low-volume center.

NR techniques, like chordal replacement, preserve leaflet mobility increasing coaptation surface and avoiding outflow tract obstruction. How to standardize length of the neochordae and the long-term durability of the reapir remain subjects of debate [11, 12]. In our series survival rates of NR techniques for severe MR were 77% (CI 95% 0.38–0.93) at 6.6 years of follow-up and freedom from reoperation was 98.40%. Salvador et al. [13] reported 608 consecutive MVr with NR techniques, with a freedom from reoperation of 92% after 15 years.

Table 2 Postoperative occurrence of mitral regurgitation and assessment of NYHA class

Variable	No resection n = 136	Resection n = 52	P value
NYHA functional class			0.797
I	115 (84.5)	41 (78.8)	
II	16 (11.7)	9 (17.3)	
III	3 (2.2)	2 (3.8)	
IV	2 (1.5)	0	
Mitral valve regurgitation			0.267
None/Trace	76 (56.0)	22 (42.3)	
Mild	48 (35.3)	22 (42.3)	
Moderate	9 (6.6)	6 (11.5)	
Severe	3 (2.1)	2 (3.8)	

Categorical data are expressed as number (%)
NYHA New York Hear Association

R techniques have exhibited excellent results [1, 11], however, these techniques sometimes sacrifice a large amount of valve tissue, resulting in leaflet restriction, and requires a skilled and experienced surgeon. New techniques, like butterfly resection, have been shown to prevent systolic anterior motion, decreasing the need for annular plication [14, 15]. In our series survival rates of R techniques for severe MR were 92.4% (CI 95% 0.69–0.98) at 8.3 years of follow-up, with a freedom from reoperation of 96%. Sakamoto et al. [16] reported the long-term results of this techniques, with a freedom from reoperation of 92,3% at 10 years.

In the matter of functional class, the results are excellent; the majority of patients showed considerable improvement after surgery. In our series, at last follow-up, 156 (82,9%) were in NYHA class I and 181 patients (86%) showed no or grade I MR, with no difference between groups. Lange et al. [11] described similar results, at last follow-up 94% of their patients showed no or grade I MR. The literature supports that the incidence of severe MR, need for reoperation, and death are equally low with R and NR techniques [11, 17–21]. However, the institutions were these investigations were conducted had high-volumes of MVr. It was uncertain if centers with low-volume could reproduce these results.

In our bivariate analysis, we found that patients that underwent minimally invasive repair had a lower risk of developing recurrent moderate MR. This could be explained by the fact that in our practice, minimally invasive MVr is performed by a single surgeon (JPU), who also has the most experience. Further analysis has also shown, that minimally invasive MVr has resulted in earlier referral of patients by cardiologists, leading to patients being healthier, with less comorbidities. Since the NR group had more minimally invasive repairs, this could explain the difference in euroscore II assessments between groups.

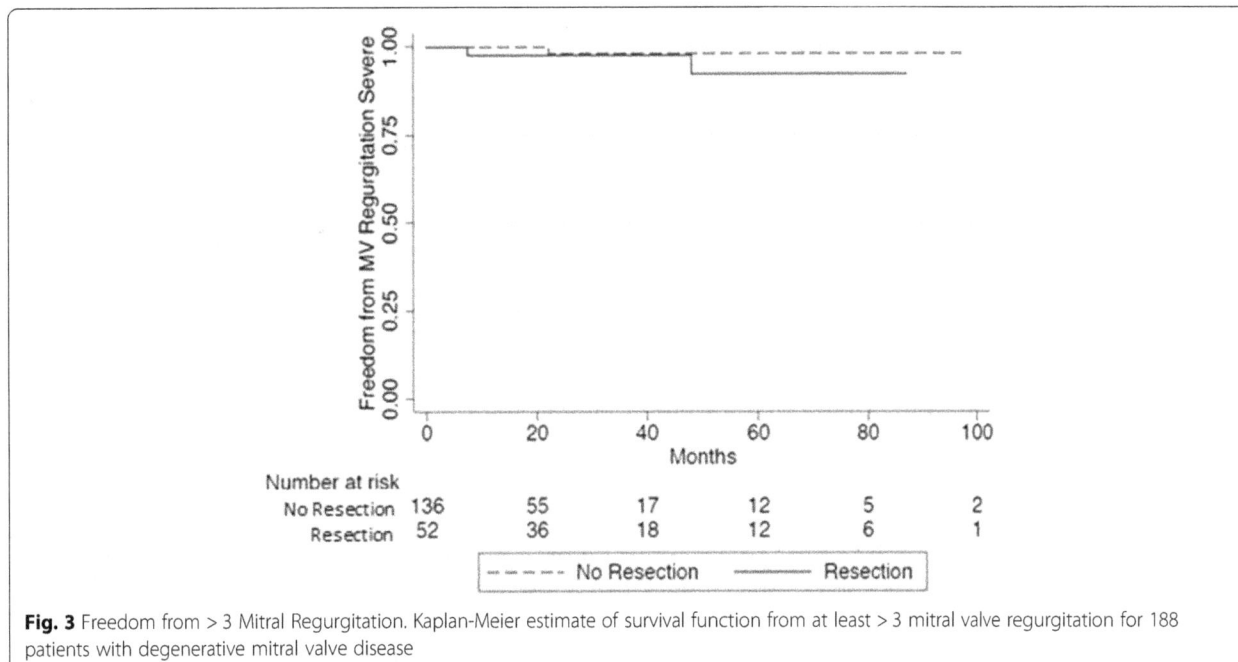

Fig. 3 Freedom from > 3 Mitral Regurgitation. Kaplan-Meier estimate of survival function from at least > 3 mitral valve regurgitation for 188 patients with degenerative mitral valve disease

Our results show that, despite low volumes in the earlier years of our experience, MVr results achieved can be comparable to those reported by referral centers worldwide, leading to an inversion in the tendency of MVR vs MVr in our Institution and an excellent MVr rates. We attribute this change to the creation of a MVr program, with a dedicated team lead by a MV surgeon (JPU) resulting in better patient selection, standardization of processes and procedures, education of referring physicians, earlier patient referral, and better postoperative care and follow-up.

To improve volume and results of the MVr program, we began to encourage targeted referral and guideline-based assessment of MV pathology. Cardiology, imaging, and critical care teams were optimally equipped and physicians were trained so an earlier referral could be achieved. All MV cases were analyzed by the MVr program before the procedure, and the repair was performed by an experienced surgeon. Cardiac anesthesiologists in charge of the cases were fully prepared to perform echocardiograms in the operating room so the quality of the MVr could be assessed before the patient was weaned of CPB. Junior cardiac surgeons were mentored and technically supported. A valvular heart clinic was created so MV patients could be properly followed and controlled.

With target and earlier referral, we improved patient selection and MVr rates. We were able to operate healthier patients, with less comorbidities, better functional class, younger, and with better LVEF. This was a key factor for achieving and maintaining good results, since patients with previous myocardial infarction, dyslipidemia, dialysis, and hypertension have an increased risk of developing at least moderate recurrent MR, as shown before in different studies [20–23]. The literature has suggested a close relationship between preoperative comorbidities and the odds of developing recurrent MR. Fukuda et al. [24] found a close relationship between type 2 diabetes and the progression of MR. We performed an exploratory logistic binary regression, finding that previous myocardial infarction by itself increases the risk up to 18% and can be modified in the presence of variables such as age, gender, and surgical approach.

Different articles [25, 26] have shown that individual surgeon volume is a determinant of MVr rates, freedom from reoperation, and survival. A total of < 25 MVr per year has been associated with poor results and low MVr rates. When no volume-outcome relationships were available, the United Kingdom proposed a volume threshold of 25 MVr/year for surgeon, so better results

Table 3 Bivariate analysis identifying factors related to at least moderate MV regurgitation in 188 patients

Bivariate analysis	OR	CI 95%	P value
Previous myocardial infarction	18,55	1602-214,857	0,030
Diabetes	0,93	0.112–7.747	1000
Dialysis	2,15	0.03–20,314	0,043
Minimally invasive technique	0,22	0,051-1019	0,040
Dyslipidemia	1,65	0.508–5.420	0,489
Hypertension	1,29	0,509-3299	0,585
Arrhythmia	1,01	0,294-3518	1000

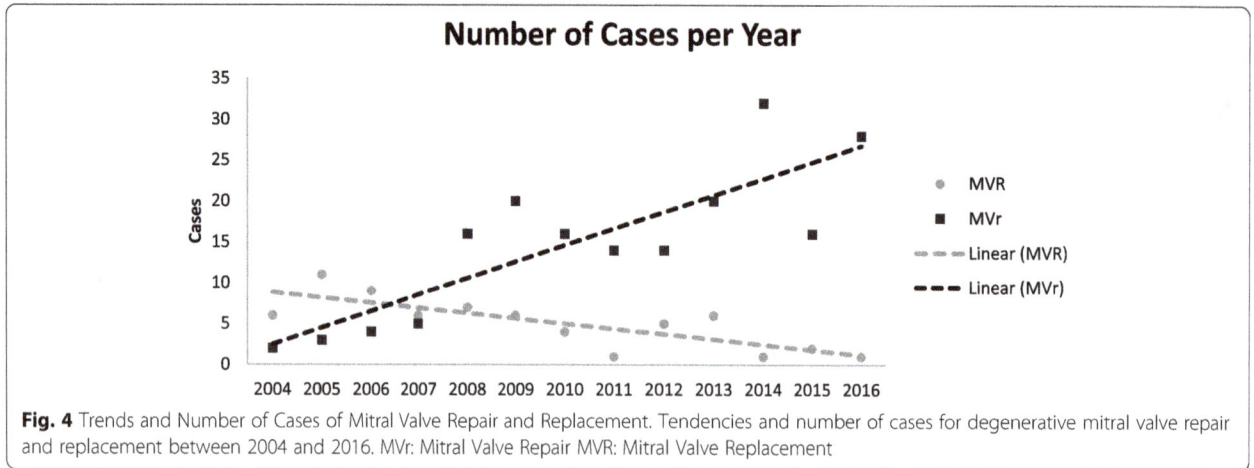

Fig. 4 Trends and Number of Cases of Mitral Valve Repair and Replacement. Tendencies and number of cases for degenerative mitral valve repair and replacement between 2004 and 2016. MVr: Mitral Valve Repair MVR: Mitral Valve Replacement

could be achieved. In the United States, there is no minimum volume standardized for MVr [26]. At our institution, since the creation of the MVr program, patient volume has grown and MVr rate has improved. We have been able to maintain MVr as preferred technique of MV intervention, and satisfactory results have been obtained. With the creation of a well prepared, well equipped and experienced MVr program, that has a guideline-assessment of MV pathology and is lead by an experienced MV surgeon, adequate MVr results can be accomplished in low-volume centers.

Daneshmand et al. [25] conducted a 20-year study, and concluded that MVr patients have better survival and functional outcomes, especially after 10–15 years, compared to MVR. In keeping with this, Gammie et al. [27] presented the trends of MV surgery in the United States, showing progressive adoption of MVr. In Latin America, however, trends of MV surgery remain unknown, with little data showing trends in MVr vs MVR and different studies have suggested the number of MVr should be increased [27].

This paper has some limitations, it was a retrospective study performed over a period of 15 years. Changes in surgical techniques and postoperative management of the patients might have affected the incidence of recurrent MR.

Conclusions

In conclusion, short and long-term results with either the R or the NR techniques are equivalent. Recurrence of severe MR and the need for MVR are rare. Significant symptomatic improvement can be achieved in more than 80% of the patients, and the majority will present with no or grade I MR. Risk factors for MR after surgery should be analyzed. The most reliable and durable repair technique for degenerative MV disease is the one that the surgeon feels more comfortable and has the most experience with. This study shows how low-volume centers can achieve results comparable to those reported worldwide as recently suggested by Bakaeen et al. [28]. We attribute the results presented in this paper to the creation of a MVr team, with a dedicated MVr surgeon as the leader.

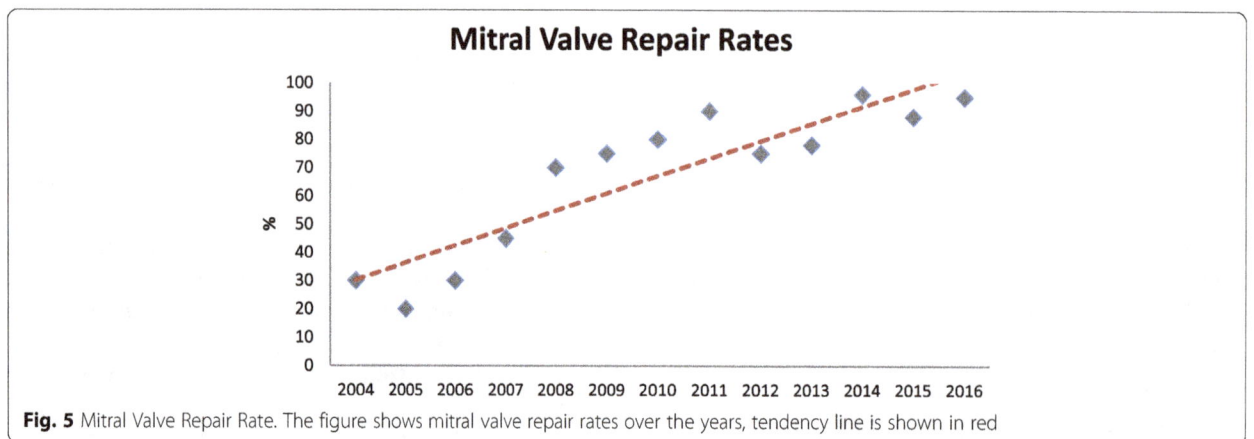

Fig. 5 Mitral Valve Repair Rate. The figure shows mitral valve repair rates over the years, tendency line is shown in red

Abbreviations

ePTFE: Polytetrafluoroethylene; MR: Mitral regurgitation; MV: Mitral valve; MVr: Mitral valve repair; MVR: Mitral valve replacement; NR: No resection; NYHA: New York Heart Association; R: Resection

Acknowledgments

We will like to thank the anesthesia department, the valvular heart disease clinic and the research department for the advisory and corrections for this manuscript.

Authors contributions

JU, JC, NS, were the cardiac surgeons in charge of the patients. MG IP JU structured the article and wrote it. All authors read and approved the final manuscript.

Competing interests

Dr. Juan P. Umana is a consultant for Edwards Lifesciences. Other authors declare that they have no competing interests.

Author details

[1]Vascular Function Research Laboratory, Fundación Cardioinfantil- Instituto de Cardiologia, Bogotá, Colombia. [2]Cardiac Surgery, Fundación Cardioinfantil- Instituto de Cardiologia, Bogotá, Colombia. [3]Cardiac Surgery Department, Fundación Cardioinfantil- Instituto de Cardiologia, Bogotá, Colombia. [4]Director Cardiovascular Medicine, Cardiac Surgery Department, Fundación Cardioinfantil- Instituto de Cardiologia, Bogotá, Colombia.

References

1. Carpentier A. Cardiac valve surgery--the "French correction". J Thorac Cardiovasc Surg. 1983;86(3):323–37.
2. Perier P, Hohenberger W, Lakew F, Batz G, Urbanski P, Zacher M, et al. Toward a new paradigm for the reconstruction of posterior leaflet prolapse: midterm results of the "respect rather than resect" approach. Ann Thorac Surg. 2008;86(3):718 -25-25.
3. Perier P, Hohenberger W, Lakew F, Diegeler A. Prolapse of the posterior leaflet: resect or respect. Ann Cardiothorac Surg. 2015;4(3):273–7.
4. Society of Thoracic Surgeons [Internet] . [cited 2017 Oct 10]. Available from: https://www.sts.org/registries-research-center/sts-national-database/adult-cardiac-surgery-database/data-collection. Accessed 07 Oct 2017.
5. Carpentier AF, Lessana A, Relland JYM, Belli E, Mihaileanu S, Berrebi AJ, et al. The "physio-ring": an advanced concept in mitral valve annuloplasty. Ann Thorac Surg. 1995;60(5):1177–86.
6. Davies MJ, Moore BP, Braimbridge MV. The floppy mitral valve. Study of incidence, pathology, and complications in surgical, necropsy, and forensic material. Br Heart J. 1978;40(5):468–81.
7. Sawazaki M, Tomari S, Zaikokuji K, Imaeda Y. Controversy in mitral valve repair, resection or chordal replacement? Gen Thorac Cardiovasc Surg. 2014;62(10):581–5.
8. Tomita Y, Yasui H, Iwai T, Nishida T, Morita S, Masuda M, et al. Extensive use of polytetrafluoroethylene artificial grafts for prolapse of posterior mitral leaflet. Ann Thorac Surg. 2004;78(3):815–9.
9. Deloche A, Jebara VA, Relland JY, Chauvaud S, Fabiani JN, Perier P, et al. Valve repair with Carpentier techniques. The second decade. J Thorac Cardiovasc Surg. 1990;99(6):990–1001-2.
10. Schwartz CF, Grossi EA, Ribakove GH, Ursomanno P, Mirabella M, Crooke GA, et al. Ten-year results of folding Plasty in mitral valve repair. Ann Thorac Surg. 2010;89(2):485–8.
11. Lange R, Guenther T, Noebauer C, Kiefer B, Eichinger W, Voss B, et al. Chordal replacement versus quadrangular resection for repair of isolated posterior mitral leaflet prolapse. Ann Thorac Surg. 2010;89(4):1163–70.
12. Kobayashi J, Sasako Y, Bando K, Minatoya K, Niwaya K, Kitamura S. Ten-year experience of chordal replacement with expanded polytetrafluoroethylene in mitral valve repair. Circulation. 2000;102(19 Suppl 3):III30–4.
13. Salvador L, Mirone S, Bianchini R, Regesta T, Patelli F, Minniti G, et al. A 20-year experience with mitral valve repair with artificial chordae in 608 patients. J Thorac Cardiovasc Surg. 2008;135(6):1280–7.
14. Jebara VA, Mihaileanu S, Acar C, Brizard C, Grare P, Latremouille C, et al. Left ventricular outflow tract obstruction after mitral valve repair. Results of the sliding leaflet technique. Circulation. 1993;88(5 Pt 2):II30–4.
15. Grossi EA, Galloway AC, Kallenbach K, Miller JS, Esposito R, Schwartz DS, et al. Early results of posterior leaflet folding plasty for mitral valve reconstruction. Ann Thorac Surg. 1998;65(4):1057–9.
16. Sakamoto Y, Hashimoto K, Okuyama H, Ishii S, Kawada N, Inoue T, et al. Mitral valve reconstruction: long-term results of triangular resection for degenerative prolapse. Gen Thorac Cardiovasc Surg. 2008;56(2):63–7.
17. David TE, Omran A, Armstrong S, Sun Z, Ivanov J. Long-term results of mitral valve repair for myxomatous disease with and without chordal replacement with expanded polytetrafluoroethylene sutures. J Thorac Cardiovasc Surg. 1998;115(6):1279–85.
18. Falk V, Seeburger J, Czesla M, Borger MA, Willige J, Kuntze T, et al. How does the use of polytetrafluoroethylene neochordae for posterior mitral valve prolapse (loop technique) compare with leaflet resection? A prospective randomized trial. J Thorac Cardiovasc Surg. 2008;136(5):1205–6.
19. Dogan S, Aybek T, Risteski PS, Detho F, Rapp A, Wimmer-Greinecker G, et al. Minimally invasive port access versus conventional mitral valve surgery: prospective randomized study. Ann Thorac Surg. 2005;79(2):492–8.
20. Sündermann SH, Czerny M, Falk V. Open vs. minimally invasive mitral valve surgery: surgical technique, indications and results. Cardiovasc Eng Technol. 2015;6(2):160–6.
21. Svensson LG, Atik FA, Cosgrove DM, Blackstone EH, Rajeswaran J, Krishnaswamy G, et al. Minimally invasive versus conventional mitral valve surgery: a propensity-matched comparison. J Thorac Cardiovasc Surg. 2010;139(4):926–32.
22. Singh RG, Cappucci R, Kramer-Fox R, Roman MJ, Kligfield P, Borer JS, et al. Severe mitral regurgitation due to mitral valve prolapse: risk factors for development, progression, and need for mitral valve surgery. Am J Cardiol. 2000;85(2):193–8.
23. Wilcken DE, Hickey AJ. Lifetime risk for patients with mitral valve prolapse of developing severe valve regurgitation requiring surgery. Circulation. 1988;78(1):10–4.
24. Fukuda N, Oki T, Iuchi A, Tabata T, Manabe K, Kageji Y, et al. Predisposing factors for severe mitral regurgitation in idiopathic mitral valve prolapse. Am J Cardiol. 1995;76(7):503–7.
25. Daneshmand MA, Milano CA, Rankin JS, Honeycutt EF, Swaminathan M, Shaw LK, et al. Mitral valve repair for degenerative disease: a 20-year experience. Ann Thorac Surg. 2009;88(6):1828–37.
26. Gammie JS, Sheng S, Griffith BP, Peterson ED, Rankin JS, O'Brien SM, et al. Trends in mitral valve surgery in the United States: results from the Society of Thoracic Surgeons adult cardiac surgery database. Ann Thorac Surg. 2009;87(5):1431–7.
27. Chikwe J, Toyoda D, Anyanwu A, et al. Relation of mitral valve surgery volume to repair rate, durability, and survival. JACC. 2017;69:2397–409.
28. Bakaeen FG, Shroyer AL, Zenati MA, Badhwar V, Thourani VH, Gammie JS, et al. Mitral valve surgery in the US veterans administration health system: 10-year outcomes and trends. J Thorac Cardiovasc Surg. 2018;155(1):105–17.

22

Junctional ectopic tachycardia following tetralogy of fallot repair in children under 2 years

Mohamed Fouad Ismail[1,2], Amr A. Arafat[3], Tamer E. Hamouda[1,4], Amira Esmat El Tantawy[5], Azzahra Edrees[1], Abdulbadee Bogis[1], Nashwa Badawy[1,5], Alaa B. Mahmoud[1,3], Ahmed Farid Elmahrouk[1,3*] (iD) and Ahmed A. Jamjoom[1]

Abstract

Background: Junctional ectopic tachycardia is a serious arrhythmia that frequently occurs after tetralogy of Fallot repair. Arrhythmia prophylaxis is not feasible for all pediatric cardiac surgery patients and identification of high risk patients is required. The objectives of this study were to characterize patients with JET, identify its predictors and subsequent complications and the effect of various treatment strategies on the outcomes in selected TOF patients undergoing total repair before 2 years of age.

Methods: From 2003 to 2017, 609 patients had Tetralogy of Fallot repair, 322 were included in our study. We excluded patients above 2 years and patients with preoperative arrhythmia. 29.8% of the patients ($n = 96$) had postoperative JET.

Results: JET patients were younger and had higher preoperative heart rate. Independent predictors of JET were younger age, higher preoperative heart rate, cyanotic spells, non-use of B-blockers and low Mg and Ca ($p = 0.011$, 0.018, 0.024, 0.001, 0.004 and 0.001; respectively). JET didn't affect the duration of mechanical ventilation nor hospital stay ($p = 0.12$ and 0.2 respectively) but prolonged the ICU stay ($p = 0.011$). JET resolved in 39.5% ($n = 38$) of patients responding to conventional measures. Amiodarone was used in 31.25% ($n = 30$) of patients and its use was associated with longer ICU stay ($p = 0.017$). Ventricular pacing was required in 4 patients (5.2%). Median duration of JET was 30.5 h and 5 patients had recurrent JET episode. Timing of JET onset didn't affect ICU ($p = 0.43$) or hospital stay ($p = 0.14$) however, long duration of JET increased ICU and hospital stay ($p = 0.02$ and 0.009; respectively).

Conclusion: JET increases ICU stay after TOF repair. Preoperative B-blockers significantly reduced JET. Patients with preoperative risk factors could benefit from preoperative arrhythmia prophylaxis and aggressive management of postoperative electrolyte disturbance is essential.

Keywords: Congenital heart disease, Arrhythmia, Junctional ectopic tachycardia; tetralogy of Fallot

Background

Postoperative junctional ectopic tachycardia (JET) is a potential life-threatening arrhythmia occurring after congenital cardiac surgery. [1] The incidence of JET following congenital cardiac surgery varies widely in literature which can be attributed to the different diagnostic criteria and the great variability in the patients' characteristics among the published studies. [2] Incidence of JET is higher when the intervention is close to the atrioventricular node and bundle of Hiss as in tetralogy of Fallot (TOF) and complete atrioventricular canal (AVC) repair. [1, 3] Several treatment strategies ranging from pharmacologic agents to atrial cardiac pacing are used sequentially to lower the ventricular rate and re-establish atrioventricular synchrony. [4–6] Recently, the effect of several pharmacologic agents on reducing postoperative JET was evaluated. [7–9]

Generalization of preoperative prophylaxis for arrhythmia in all patients undergoing surgery for congenital heart

* Correspondence: A_marouky@hotmail.com;
Ahmed.elmahrouki1@med.tanta.edu.eg; Ael-Mahrouk@KFSHRC.edu.sa
[1]Cardiothoracic Surgery Department, King Faisal Specialist Hospital and Research Center, MBC J-16, P.O Box: 40047, Jeddah 21499, Saudi Arabia
[3]Cardiothoracic Surgery Department, Tanta University, Tanta, Egypt
Full list of author information is available at the end of the article

defects is non-practical and preoperative identification of high risk patients is essential. Although many studies were concerned with postoperative arrhythmia, little have focused on JET following total TOF repair in infants. [1, 10] The objectives of this study were to characterize patients with JET, identify its predictors and subsequent complications and the effect of various treatment strategies on the outcomes in selected TOF patients undergoing total repair before 2 years of age.

Methods

Study population

This is a retrospective cohort study performed at King Faisal Specialized Hospital and Research Centre in Jeddah, Saudi Arabia. A total of 609 patients underwent surgical TOF repair between January 2003 and December 2017. We excluded patients older than 2 years ($n = 231$) and patients with rhythm disturbances or heart block preoperative ($n = 16$). Moreover; patients with serious postoperative arrhythmia other than JET ($n = 17$) and patients with missing postoperative JET diagnosis criteria from the medical records ($n = 23$) were excluded. A total of 322 patients were included in the study. Approval of the institutional review board was obtained before data collection and the need for patients' consents was waived due to the retrospective nature of the study.

Operative technique

Surgical repair was performed by consultant level cardiac surgeons through median sternotomy. Bicaval cannulation was performed and cardioplegic arrest was done by antegrade cold crystalloid cardioplegia. Median temperature of the perfusate was 32 °C. Right atrial incision was performed in 98% of the patients for resection of the RVOT obstructing bundles and closure of the ventricular septal defect and trans-annular patch (TAP) was used in 64% of the patients. Patients who required TAP were mainly operated upon during the early study period and our current strategy is to avoid TAP and preserve the pulmonary valve when possible. Pulmonary valvotomy was performed in 71 patients (22.5%) and resection of the right ventricular outflow tract (RVOT) obstructing bundles was done in 94.7% ($n = 305$). Concomitant tricuspid valve repair was performed in 55 patients (17.4%).

Data collection

Patients' medical charts were retrospectively reviewed to collect preoperative variables including patients age at the time of surgery, gender, weight (Kg), body surface area (BSA) (m2), preoperative B-blockers administration, associated cardiac anomalies and previous palliative surgical procedures as modified Blalock-Tausig Shunt. Preoperative 12 leads electrocardiogram were reviewed in all patients to identify the preoperative rhythm and PR interval, QRS duration were calculated. Preoperative heart rate was reported from the anesthesia records after sedating the patients. Intraoperative variables include cardiopulmonary bypass (CPB) time (minutes), aortic cross clamp time (minutes), temperature of the perfusate, use of transannular patch (TAP) and resection of right RVOT obstructing muscle bundle and the use of right atrial or right ventricular approach.

Postoperative data

We included all patients who had JET whatever its duration and the onset of JET whether intraoperatively or postoperatively in the intensive care unit (ICU) was determined. The criteria used for JET diagnosis were i) Heart rate > 175 Bpm ii) Absent P wave from lead II of EKG iii) Narrow QRS complexes iv) Ventricular rate faster than atrial rate with AV dissociation.

Protocol of JET management included discontinuation of unnecessary inotropes, infusion of IV fluids boluses for hypovolemic patients with low central venous pressure, cooling (reducing temperature to 36–36.5 °C), and sedation. At the same time postoperative electrolyte imbalance was aggressively corrected with K, Ca, and magnesium. Our Intensive care protocol is to maintain serum K > 4.1 mmol/L, ionized Ca > 1.1 mmol/L and serum Mg > 1.1 mg/dL. During early study period, digoxin was administered at 5 μcg /kg/dose IV once to control the ventricular rate. Amiodarone was administered as a bolus with 5 mg / kg IV over one hour and if JET persisted, further infusion at 5 μcg /kg/min was given till sinus rhythm was established or the heart rate slowed to an acceptable rate with stable hemodynamic. Our policy for possible postoperative pacing is to insert ventricular pacing wire unless the patient showed heart block immediately on recovery from CPB, in this case we insert both atrial and ventricular pacing wires. Dopamine, dobutamine, milrinone, epinephrine administration was reported, and we calculated the inotropic score at the time of onset of arrhythmia using the following formula: {(dopamine + dobutamine) × 1} + (milrinone X 20) + {(epinephrine + norepinephrine) × 100}.

Study endpoints

Preoperative, operative and postoperative variables were used to predict the occurrence of JET. The impact of JET on duration of mechanical ventilation (hours), ICU stay (days) and total duration of hospital stay (days) were analyzed.

Statistical analysis

Data presentation

Continuous variables were presented as mean ± Standard deviation and categorical variables as number and percent.

Data analysis

Mann-Whitney test was used to compare continuous variables and for categorical variables Chi2 was used or Fisher Exact test if the frequency is less than 5. Multiple imputation was used to handle the missing variables. Multivariable logistic regression models were used to identify the predictors of postoperative JET. Three models were constructed from the preoperative, operative and postoperative variables respectively and the variables in each model didn't exceed 9 variables to power the multivariable analysis. Odds ratio, p-value and 95% confidence interval were reported. The effect of JET on the postoperative outcomes was assessed using propensity score analysis. The probability of having JET was calculated using multivariable logistic regression model after adjustment of the measured preoperative confounders. Propensity score was used in the adjusted model to predict the effect of JET on the postoperative outcomes. To fulfil the linearity assumptions of the model, non-normally distributed continuous variables were rescaled by, inverse squared and inverse transformations. P-value lesser than 0.05 was considered significant. All statistical analyses were performed using STATA 14 software (Statacorp, Texas- USA).

Results

A total of 322 patients had tetralogy of Fallot repair during the study period and met the inclusion criteria. Patients' age at time of operation ranged from 2 to 23 months and male to female ratio was 1.6: 1. JET occurred in 96 patients (29.9%) and patients were classified into JET and non-JET groups.

Patients' characteristics

Patients who had postoperative JET were significantly younger ($p = 0.01$) and had higher preoperative heart rate ($p = 0.03$). Associated lesions were Atrial Septal Defect ($n = 6$), complete AVC ($n = 3$), persistent Left Superior Vena Cava ($n = 1$), Patent Ductus Arteriosus ($n = 7$), Multiple Aorto- Pulmonary Collateral Arteries ($n = 2$), peripheral pulmonary artery stenosis ($n = 3$), pulmonary atresia ($n = 5$) and 12 patients had prior modified Blalock Taussig shunt. There was no statistically significant difference in associated lesion between patients with and without postoperative JET ($p = 0.8$). Fifteen patients in JET group had preoperative B-blockers (19.5%) versus 62 patients (80.5%) in Non-JET group ($p = 0.015$). (Table 1).

Operative variables are comparable between both groups with no statistically significant difference in the measured variables. Table 1 shows the comparison of the preoperative and operative variables. Postoperative inotropes administered before the onset of JET were compared between groups and showed no significant

Table 1 Comparison of the preoperative and operative data between JET and non-JET patients

Variable	JET group ($n = 96$)	Non-JET ($n = 226$)	P
Male (n)	56 (58.3%)	144 (63.7%)	0.36
Age (months)	7.5 ± 3	8.35 ± 2.99	0.01
Weight (Kg)	6.95 ± 1.8	7.37 ± 2.1	0.11
BSA (m2)	0.36 ± 0.07	0.37 ± 0.6	0.42
Oxygen saturation (%)	82.4 ± 7.7	82.8 ± 8	0.14
Cyanotic spells (n)	20 (21.7%)	42 (19%)	0.58
EKG			
Heart Rate (b/m)	103.7 ± 13.5	99.97 ± 12.97	0.03
P duration	0.06 ± 0.01	0.06 ± 0.01	0.7
P-R interval	0.13 ± 0.02	0.13 ± 0.03	0.7
QRS	0.06 ± 0.02	0.06 ± 0.01	0.5
Pulmonary annulus (mm)	6.36 ± 2	6.47 ± 2.1	0.57
RVOT gradient (mmHg)	70.8 ± 14.6	71.5 ± 15.1	0.61
Cross-Clamp time (min)	74.4 ± 2.6.5	75.3 ± 27.1	0.77
Cardiopulmonary bypass (min)	102.1 ± 31.1	101.3 ± 32	0.7
Temperature (Celsius)	32 ± 1.5	31.7 ± 1.5	0.12
Tricuspid valve repair (n)	13 (13.5%)	42 (19%)	0.24
Pulmonary valvotomy (n)	25 (26.6%)	47 (20.7%)	0.25
RA approach (n)	93 (96.9%)	223 (98.7%)	0.28
RVOT resection (n)	91 (94.8%)	214 (94.7%)	0.97
Trans-annular patch (n)	66 (68.75%)	141 (62.39%)	0.27

Continuous variables are presented as mean ± SD and categorical variables as number (%)
RA right atrial, *RVOT* right ventricular outflow tract

difference in patients who received dopamine, dobutamine, epinephrine and milrinone between JET and non-JET patients. Levels of serum potassium, calcium and magnesium before the onset of JET were compared and showed significantly lower magnesium level in patients who developed JET ($p = 0.001$). (Table 2).

Factors associated with JET

By multivariable analysis of the measured preoperative variables, younger age, cyanotic spells, non-use of B-blockers and higher preoperative heart rate predicted the postoperative JET ($p = 0.011, 0.024, 0.001$ and 0.018; respectively). By constructing a separate model for the operative variables, none of the measured operative variables predicted the postoperative JET. In the postoperative variables model; low magnesium and calcium independently predicted the occurrence of JET ($p = 0.004$ and 0.001; respectively). (Table 3).

Effect of JET

Ventilation time didn't differ significantly between JET patients ($23.4 ± 24.7$ h) vs non-JET patients ($19.5 ±

Table 2 Comparison of the inotropes and serum electrolytes in JET and non-JET groups

Variable	JET group ($n = 96$)	Non-JET ($n = 226$)	P
Inotropes			
Dopamine (n)	22 (23.4%)	65 (29.28%)	0.28
Dobutamine (n)	47 (49.5%)	91 (41%)	0.16
Epinephrine (n)	34 (36.6%)	85 (37.8%)	0.84
Milrinone (n)	47 (50%)	127 (58.3%)	0.18
Inotrope score	12.3 ± 14	9.2 ± 6	0.17
Electrolytes			
PH	7.36 ± 0.066	7.37 ± 0.06	0.16
Potassium (mmol/L)	3.98 ± 0.45	4.07 ± 0.56	0.17
Magnesium (mEq/L)	1.01 ± 0.39	1.14 ± 0.43	0.001
Calcium (mmol/L)	2.32 ± 0.32	2.24 ± 0.35	0.08

Continuous variables are presented as mean ± SD and categorical variables as number (%)

11.6 h, $p = 0.11$). Patients with JET had longer ICU stay (6.1 ± 5.8 vs 5 ± 1.9 days, $p = 0.01$) and longer hospital stay (15.1 ± 11.2 vs 13.4 ± 6.5 days, $p = 0.04$). Propensity score matching was used to estimate the effect of JET on the duration of ventilation, ICU and hospital stay after adjustment of the measured preoperative variables. JET didn't affect the duration of mechanical ventilation nor hospital stay ($p = 0.12$ and 0.2 respectively) but significantly prolonged ICU stay ($p = 0.011$). (Table 4) Hospital mortality occurred in 10 patients (3.11%), 4 patients with JET (4.1%) versus 6 patients without JET (2.65%) ($p = 0.49$). (Table 4).

Course of JET

JET was diagnosed post cardiopulmonary bypass and inside the operation room in 30 patients (30.25%) and in the ICU in 66 patients (68.75%). Subgroup analysis was done to identify the difference between patients who had JET intraoperatively and those who had JET in the ICU. No difference between both groups as regard age ($p =$

Table 3 Predictors of postoperative JET

Variable	OR	P	95% CI
Pre-operative			
Age	0.86	0.011	0.76–0.97
Cyanotic spells	2.9	0.024	1.15–7.41
B-blockers	0.2	0.001	0.08–0.51
Preoperative HR	1.02	0.018	1.004–1.04
Post-operative			
Mg	0.37	0.004	0.19–0.7
Ca	0.4	0.001	0.23–0.7

OR odds ratio, CI confidence interval

Table 4 Effect of JET on duration of mechanical ventilation, ICU and hospital stay

Variable	Coefficient	P	95% CI
Ventilation time[a]	−1.5	0.123	−0.036–0.004
ICU stay[b]	−0.3	0.011	−0.057–−0.007
Hospital stay[a]	− 0.009	0.2	−.025–.007

[a]inverse squared
[b]inverse

0.17), gender ($p = 0.82$), body surface area ($p = 0.89$), preoperative heart rate ($p = 0.86$), preoperative oxygen saturation ($p = 0.37$), cyanotic spells ($p = 0.86$), B blockers ($p = 0.65$), CPB time ($p = 0.11$) and ischemic time ($p = 0.24$). After adjustment of the preoperative variables, no difference was found in duration of JET ($p = 0.91$), ICU stay ($p = 0.43$), ventilation time ($p = 0.52$) and hospital stay (0.14) between both groups.

JET resolved in 39.5% ($n = 38$) of patients responding to conventional measures. At the same time, postoperative electrolyte imbalance was aggressively corrected with K, Ca, and Mg. Fifty-nine patients (61.5%) received digoxin and digoxin administration was not significantly associated with the duration of mechanical ventilation ($p = 0.77$), ICU stay ($p = 0.43$) nor hospital stay ($p = 0.98$) in patients with JET. Amiodarone was used in 31.25% ($n = 30$) of patients and no relation was found between the use of amiodarone and the duration of mechanical ventilation ($p = 0.07$) nor hospital stay ($p = 0.35$). However, amiodarone use was significantly associated with longer ICU stay ($p = 0.017$). Betablockers were used in 58 patients (64.2%) with no significant association with the duration of mechanical ventilation ($p = 0.8$), ICU ($p = 0.37$) or hospital stay ($p = 0.07$). Ventricular pacing was required in 4 patients (4.16%) because of progression into heart block. Five patients (5.2%) had a second episode of JET, 3 of them were males. Their median age was 7 months (ranged from 6 to 15 months) and median oxygen saturation was 80% (ranged from 79 to 85%). None of these patients had preoperative B-blockers, 3 of them had TAP and JET occurred intraoperatively in 3 patients. Full recovery occurred in 4 patients and 1 patients progressed to complete heart block and required permanent pace maker.

The median duration of JET was 30.5 h and ranged from 3 to 96 h. Longer duration of postoperative JET "i.e. above the median value" was significantly associated with lower preoperative oxygen saturation ($p = 0.01$). After adjustment of the pre- JET variables, longer duration of JET was significantly associated with prolonged ICU ($p = 0.02$) and hospital stay ($p = 0.009$) but had no significant association with the duration of mechanical ventilation ($p = 0.21$) compared with patients with short JET duration.

Discussion

Prophylaxis of arrhythmia after pediatric cardiac surgery became the focus of many trials recently. [7, 8, 11, 12] Generalization of prophylaxis in all patients undergoing surgery for congenital heart disease is difficult and may increase the hazard of surgery. In literature, various factors were found associated with the genesis of JET after surgical repair of congenital heart disease. Most of these studies [1, 10, 13–15] were performed in a wide variety of congenital heart defects. Including all types of congenital heart defects in risk models to predict postoperative JET underpowers the results as the incidence of JET varies widely in different congenital heart diseases and procedures. Based on several reports, JET is commonly associated with TOF [1, 10] therefore we included in our series TOF patients who underwent corrective surgery before 2 years of age. In our series the incidence of JET was 29.8% and this high incidence of JET can be explained by our strict selection criteria of those high-risk patients. The incidence of JET following TOF repair varied in the published series and ranged from 4 to 37%. [8, 16–18] The great variability in JET incidence could be attributed to the diagnostic criteria used and the wide variability in patients' characteristics especially age. [2] Another explanation for this variability is the low patients number, it is remarkable that lower incidence of JET post TOF repair was documented with less number of TOF patients included in the study. Moreover, we included all patients who expressed JET whether were hemodynamically stable or not. In our study; younger age was significantly associated with increased risk of postoperative JET and this finding is consistent with other studies [14]. Younger patients are generally sicker and smaller hearts are more prone to damage by surgical technique and retraction. Increased preoperative heart rate predicted postoperative JET. Normal range of heart rate depends on patients' age and the definition of tachycardia is not consistent. In order to have a standardized condition for all patients, we reported the operation room heart rate after the patients were properly sedated. This also could explain the insignificant findings of the preoperative ECG measurements as usually they are not taken under standardized conditions and patients conditions during ECG recording significantly affected these ECG intervals.

Preoperative B-blockers were associated with significant reduction of postoperative JET in our patients which is consistent with a previous report. [19] Further randomized studies are required to evaluate Bblockers as a preoperative prophylaxis against JET in those high-risk patients.

Trans-atrial approach is our standardized approach for closure of ventricular septal defect and relief of RVOT obstruction and 98% of our patients were operated through RA. Although RA approach in a study of 343 patients independently predicted postoperative JET in the total patient series, no correlation was made with their 114 subsets of TOF patients. [20] Our surgical strategies have been shifted from the use of TAP to preservation of the pulmonary valve if possible as it has a proved efficacy in reducing the incidence of postoperative pulmonary regurgitation. [21] Nevertheless, TAP was not associated with JET in our series. Some authors documented a significant association between JET and prolonged ischemic and cardiopulmonary bypass time and higher bypass temperature [17, 22–24]. In our study, none of the operative variables predicted the postoperative JET. Cardiopulmonary bypass time affected JET in studies which included all congenital heart disease patients. In those patients, CPB time differed significantly between different lesions due to the different surgical procedure specific to each lesion Inotropes didn't predict JET in our patients. In contrary to this, dopamine or inotropic score were risk factors for JET in other series. [14, 17] Revision of electrolyte profiles in the sample just prior to JET occurrence proved that JET group had statistically significant lower serum magnesium and Calcium. Serum magnesium carries a lot of debate among authors, some documented its significance as a risk factor or as prophylactic therapy for JET, [25–27] others documented that magnesium and calcium levels were not significantly different between the two groups. [22]

Our experience in management of JET is to imply conventional strategies as correction of reduced intravascular volume, reduce body temperature, titrate inotropes to off if not affecting hemodynamic status of patients and aggressively correct electrolyte imbalance. In the early period of our study we used digoxin before the administration of amiodarone. Some authors [14] didn't recommend the use of digoxin in JET because its direct action of increasing excitability of all forms of myocardium, however, it was used to delay atrioventricular node bundle conduction maintaining a reasonable ventricular rate and to counteract the negative inotropic effect of Class III antiarrhythmic (sotalol and amiodarone). Recently amiodarone has gained popularity in JET treatment or prophylaxis. [5, 8] Many authors stated that class III antiarrhythmic drugs (sotalol and amiodarone) when given orally or intravenous, were shown to be almost devoid of negative inotropic effects [14, 18], however amiodarone use was associated with prolonged ICU stay in our JET patients.

In our series the median duration of JET was 30.5 h and many cases resolved smoothly without any hemodynamic instability with recurrence of a second episode of JET in 5.2% of the patients. Complications in the form of heart block requiring pacemaker insertion was encountered in 4 patients of the JET group.

Junctional ectopic tachycardia significantly increased ICU stay but not the duration of the mechanical ventilation of hospital stay. This is explained by the benign course of our JET patients and the additional treatment required lead to increased ICU stay while there was no effect on total hospital stay. No difference in patients' characteristics or the outcome of JET in patients who had JET onset intraoperatively versus those who had JET onset in the ICU. This can be explained by the overlap of the time frame between both groups and it is recommended for future to classify JET into early and late onset based on time of onset rather than the place of onset. Moreover, the duration of JET had an impact on the patients' outcome since longer JET episodes lead to prolonged ICU and hospital stay which is expected due to the increase in time required for treating those patients compared with shorter JET episodes.

In summary, JET post tetralogy of Fallot repair can be predicted based on the preoperative variables. Preoperative cyanotic spells were associated with postoperative JET and preoperative B-blockers significantly reduced postoperative JET. Postoperative electrolytes imbalance played a role in JET pathogenesis. JET had a benign course and didn't increase hospital mortality but it prolonged ICU stay. The outcome of JET was affected by the duration of JET episode but not the time of onset.

Study strength and limitations

The major limitation of the study is the retrospective design with its inherited biases. However, this is an acceptable design for rare outcomes. Many of the limitations of previously published reports were managed in our study including limiting selection to a specific age and pathology in contrast to other studies which included all types of congenital heart disease and wide range of age. The relatively large number in our series and the high incidence of JET in this subset of patients properly powered the multivariable analysis. Missing of some variables is another limitation however missing values didn't exceed 8% (1–7.1%) in the variables used in the analysis and multiple imputation is a suitable method to handle these missing variables. Recent studies [7, 9] showed that Dexmedetomidine has a role as a prophylactic and therapeutic agent for postoperative JET, however we didn't use it in our patients which could be another limitation of the study.

Conclusion

Junctional ectopic tachycardia is a frequent complication after Tetralogy of Fallot repair. It has a benign course; however, it prolongs ICU stay after TOF repair. Preoperative B-blockers reduced postoperative JET and

patients with preoperative risk factors could benefit from preoperative arrhythmia prophylaxis. JET can be prevented by aggressive management of postoperative electrolyte disturbance. The outcome of JET was not affected by time of JET onset however, prolonged duration of JET had a negative impact of ICU and hospital stay.

Abbreviations

BSA: Body surface area; CPB: Cardiopulmonary bypass; ICU: Intensive care unit; JET: Junctional Ectopic Tachycardia; RVOT: Right ventricular outflow tract; TAP: Trans-annular patch; TOF: Tetralogy of Fallot

Funding

This research received no specific grant from any funding agency in the public, commercial, or not-for-profit sectors.

Authors' contributions

IM Conducted the literature search analysis and interpretation of data, AA, Conducted the statistical analysis and interpretation of data, HT: Conducted the literature search, EAE: Designed the study, IA, Data Collection, BA, Data Collection, NB, conducted the literature search, MAB, Analysis and interpretation of data, EA, Involved in the study design, and drafted the manuscript "corresponding author", JA, Supervised the study and conducted the review of data. All authors read and approved the final manuscript.

Competing interests

The authors declare that they have no competing interests.

Author details

[1]Cardiothoracic Surgery Department, King Faisal Specialist Hospital and Research Center, MBC J-16, P.O Box: 40047, Jeddah 21499, Saudi Arabia. [2]Cardio-thoracic Surgery Department, Mansoura University, Mansoura, Egypt. [3]Cardiothoracic Surgery Department, Tanta University, Tanta, Egypt. [4]Cardio-thoracic Surgery Department, Benha University, Benha, Egypt. [5]The Department of Pediatrics, Faculty of Medicine Cairo University, Cairo, Egypt.

References

1. Sahu MK, Das A, Siddharth B, Talwar S, Singh SP, Abraham A, et al. Arrhythmias in children in early postoperative period after cardiac surgery. World J Pediat Congenit Heart Surg. 2018;9(1):38–46.
2. Entenmann A, Michel M, Egender F, Hessling V, Kramer HH. Impact of different diagnostic criteria on the reported prevalence of junctional ectopic tachycardia after pediatric cardiac surgery. Pediatric Crit Care Med. 2016; 17(9):845–51.
3. Ozyilmaz I, Ergul Y, Ozyilmaz S, Guzeltas A. Junctional ectopic tachycardia in late period after early postoperative complete atrioventricular block: messenger of return to normal sinus rhythm? : Explanation with four case series. J Electrocardiol. 2017;50(3):378–82.
4. Imamura T, Tanaka Y, Ninomiya Y, Yoshinaga M. Combination of flecainide and propranolol for congenital junctional ectopic tachycardia. Pediat Int. 2015;57(4):716–8.

5. Kovacikova L, Hakacova N, Dobos D, Skrak P, Zahorec M. Amiodarone as a first-line therapy for postoperative junctional ectopic tachycardia. Ann Thorac Surg. 2009;88(2):616–22.

6. Saiki H, Nakagawa R, Ishido H, Masutani S, Senzaki H. Landiolol hydrochloride infusion for treatment of junctional ectopic tachycardia in post-operative paediatric patients with congenital heart defect. Europace. 2013;15(9):1298–303.

7. El Amrousy DM, Elshmaa NS, El-Kashlan M, Hassan S, Elsanosy M, Hablas N, et al. Efficacy of prophylactic Dexmedetomidine in preventing postoperative junctional ectopic tachycardia after pediatric cardiac surgery. J Am Heart Assoc. 2017;6:e004780. https://doi.org/10.1161/JAHA.116.004780.

8. Imamura M, Dossey AM, Garcia X, Shinkawa T, Jaquiss RD. Prophylactic amiodarone reduces junctional ectopic tachycardia after tetralogy of Fallot repair. J Thorac Cardiovasc Surg. 2012;143(1):152–6.

9. Kadam SV, Tailor KB, Kulkarni S, Mohanty SR, Joshi PV, Rao SG. Effect of dexmeditomidine on postoperative junctional ectopic tachycardia after complete surgical repair of tetralogy of Fallot: a prospective randomized controlled study. Ann Card Anaesth. 2015;18(3):323–8.

10. Cools E, Missant C. Junctional ectopic tachycardia after congenital heart surgery. Acta Anaesthesiol Belg. 2014;65(1):1–8.

11. El-Shmaa NS, El Amrousy D, El Feky W. The efficacy of pre-emptive dexmedetomidine versus amiodarone in preventing postoperative junctional ectopic tachycardia in pediatric cardiac surgery. Ann Card Anaesth. 2016;19(4):614–20.

12. Rajput RS, Das S, Makhija N, Airan B. Efficacy of dexmedetomidine for the control of junctional ectopic tachycardia after repair of tetralogy of Fallot. Ann Pediat Cardiol. 2014;7(3):167–72.

13. Andreasen JB, Johnsen SP, Ravn HB. Junctional ectopic tachycardia after surgery for congenital heart disease in children. Intensive Care Med. 2008;34(5):895–902.

14. Batra AS, Chun DS, Johnson TR, Maldonado EM, Kashyap BA, Maiers J, et al. A prospective analysis of the incidence and risk factors associated with junctional ectopic tachycardia following surgery for congenital heart disease. Pediatr Cardiol. 2006;27(1):51–5.

15. Talwar S, Patel K, Juneja R, Choudhary SK, Airan B. Early postoperative arrhythmias after pediatric cardiac surgery. Asian Cardiovasc Thorac Ann. 2015;23(7):795–801.

16. Dodge-Khatami A, Miller OI, Anderson RH, Gil-Jaurena JM, Goldman AP, de Leval MR. Impact of junctional ectopic tachycardia on postoperative morbidity following repair of congenital heart defects. Eur J Cardiothorac Surg. 2002;21(2):255–9.

17. Hoffman TM, Bush DM, Wernovsky G, Cohen MI, Wieand TS, Gaynor JW, et al. Postoperative junctional ectopic tachycardia in children: incidence, risk factors, and treatment. Ann Thorac Surg. 2002;74(5):1607–11.

18. Pfammatter JP, Bachmann DC, Wagner BP, Pavlovic M, Berdat P, Carrel T, et al. Early postoperative arrhythmias after open-heart procedures in children with congenital heart disease. Pediatr Crit Care Med. 2001;2(3):217–22.

19. Mahmoud AB, Tantawy AE, Kouatli AA, Baslaim GM. Propranolol: a new indication for an old drug in preventing postoperative junctional ectopic tachycardia after surgical repair of tetralogy of Fallot. Interact Cardiovasc Thorac Surg. 2008;7(2):184–7.

20. Dodge-Khatami A, Miller OI, Anderson RH, Goldman AP, Gil-Jaurena JM, Elliott MJ, et al. Surgical substrates of postoperative junctional ectopic tachycardia in congenital heart defects. J Thorac Cardiovasc Surg. 2002; 123(4):624–30.

21. Arafat AA, Elatafy EE, Elshedoudy S, Zalat M, Abdallah N, Elmahrouk A. Surgical strategies protecting against right ventricular dilatation following tetralogy of Fallot repair. J Cardiothorac Surg. 2018;13(1):14.

22. Delaney JW, Moltedo JM, Dziura JD, Kopf GS, Snyder CS. Early postoperative arrhythmias after pediatric cardiac surgery. J Thorac Cardiovasc Surg. 2006; 131(6):1296–300.

23. Valsangiacomo E, Schmid ER, Schupbach RW, Schmidlin D, Molinari L, Waldvogel K, et al. Early postoperative arrhythmias after cardiac operation in children. Ann Thorac Surg. 2002;74(3):792–6.

24. Abdelaziz O, Deraz S. Anticipation and management of junctional ectopic tachycardia in postoperative cardiac surgery: single center experience with high incidence. Ann Pediat Cardiol. 2014;7(1):19–24.

25. Dorman BH, Sade RM, Burnette JS, Wiles HB, Pinosky ML, Reeves ST, et al. Magnesium supplementation in the prevention of arrhythmias in pediatric patients undergoing surgery for congenital heart defects. Am Heart J. 2000; 139(3):522–8.

26. He D, Sznycer-Taub N, Cheng Y, McCarter R, Jonas RA, Hanumanthaiah S, et al. Magnesium lowers the incidence of postoperative junctional ectopic tachycardia in congenital heart surgical patients: is there a relationship to surgical procedure complexity? Pediatr Cardiol. 2015;36(6):1179–85.

27. Manrique AM, Arroyo M, Lin Y, El Khoudary SR, Colvin E, Lichtenstein S, et al. Magnesium supplementation during cardiopulmonary bypass to prevent junctional ectopic tachycardia after pediatric cardiac surgery: a randomized controlled study. J Thorac Cardiovasc Surg. 2010;139(1):162–9.e2.

23

Safety, efficacy, and cost-effectiveness of intraoperative blood salvage in OPCABG with different amount of bleeding: a single-center, retrospective study

Huan Wang, Weijian Zheng, Weiping Fang, Gaige Meng, Lei Zhang, Yannan Zhou, Erwei Gu and Xuesheng Liu[*]

Abstract

Background: We sought to evaluate the safety, efficacy, and cost-effectiveness of intraoperative blood salvage (IBS) in off-pump coronary artery bypass grafting (OPCABG) surgery with different amount of bleeding.

Methods: We retrospectively reviewed the medical records of 321 patients who underwent OPCABG between December 2012 and December 2016 at our hospital. Patients treated with IBS or allogeneic blood (AB) transfusions were divided into three groups depending on the amount of bleeding respectively: IBS1 or AB1 group (400–600 ml); IBS2 or AB2 group (600–1000 ml); IBS3 or AB3 group (1000–1500 ml). The intraoperative and postoperative conditions, blood transfusion volume, clinical and hematological outcomes, and total blood transfusion cost were examined.

Results: The amount of allogeneic red blood cell (RBC) transfusion in the IBSs groups were significantly lower than that in the ABs groups ($P < 0.01$). Furthermore, drainage volume 24 h post-surgery ($P < 0.05$) and white blood cell count (WBC) 2 day post-surgery ($P < 0.01$) in IBS3 group were significantly higher compared with the AB3 group. Additionally, when IBS cost was 230 USD per set, the total blood transfusion cost in the IBSs groups was significantly higher than that in the ABs groups ($P < 0.01$); however, when 199 or 184 USD, only the IBS1 group, rather than IBS2 or IBS3, showed significantly higher cost of the total blood transfusion compared with the AB1 group ($P < 0.05$).

Conclusions: When the amount of bleeding was 600–1000 ml, IBS can significantly reduce the demand for allogeneic blood, and has no direct adverse effects on coagulation function and recuperation, and is cost-effective in OPCABG.

Keywords: OPCABG, Autologous blood transfusion, Cost-effectiveness

Background

Increased intraoperative blood loss has been shown in off-pump coronary artery bypass grafting (OPCABG) due to the fact that patients with a high risk of bleeding try to receive surgery [1–3]. Despite the progress in the safety of allogeneic blood (AB) transfusions, there are still some potential risks such as immunological reactions, transfusion-transmitted infection, and bacteria contamination [4, 5]. Intraoperative blood salvage (IBS), also known as autologous blood transfusion or cell salvage, is a medical procedure of collecting, filtering and washing blood gathered from the surgical field to produce autologous blood for transfusion back to the patient [1]. In order to reduce the incidence of adverse events resulting from AB transfusion and to cope with increasing blood shortage and medical costs, IBS has been recently applied in the field of cardiac surgery.

With the progress in surgical technique and the application of advanced equipment, on one hand, the amount of intraoperative bleeding was obviously reduced due to the development of minimally invasive surgery [6]; and

* Correspondence: liuxuesheng@ahmu.edu.cn
Department of Anesthesiology, the First Affiliated Hospital of Anhui Medical University, No. 218 Jixi Road, Hefei, Anhui 230022, People's Republic of China

on the other hand, the amount of intraoperative blood loss is still fluctuating as many patients with high bleeding risk also began to undergo surgical treatment. The cost-effectiveness of IBS differs with the amount of bleeding. Until now, few data evaluating IBS in high-bleeding-risk cardiac surgery has published [7].

Thus, the aim of this study was to evaluate the safety, efficacy, and cost-effectiveness of IBS in OPCABG surgery with different amount of bleeding. To address this, we retrospectively analyzed the medical records of 321 patients who underwent OPCABG at our hospital. Patients treated with IBS or AB transfusions were divided into three groups depending on the amount of bleeding respectively. The intraoperative and postoperative conditions, blood transfusion volume, clinical and hematological outcomes, and total blood transfusion cost were examined.

Methods

Subjects

We retrospectively reviewed the medical records of 321 patients undergoing elective OPCABG surgery under general anesthesia from December 2012 to December 2016 in the First Affiliated Hospital of Anhui Medical University. Of all, there were 206 males and 115 females, with age of 50–75 years, body mass index (BMI) of 16–34, and the American Society of Anesthesiologists' (ASA) physical status of II-IV level. A previous study has indicated that the application of IBS is more meaningful in patients with more than 1000 ml blood loss during surgery [1]. Nevertheless, at present, the intraoperative blood loss is usually less than 1000 ml, and Advanced Trauma Life Support System (ATLS) [8] believe that human conditions are stable only when the blood loss was less than 15% (about 600 ml when calculating with a systemic blood volume of 4000 ml). In clinical applications, we found that when the bleeding volume was less than 600 ml, Cell Saver, in most cases, washed out autologous red blood cells with lower hematocrit, and the application efficiency was poor; when the bleeding volume was less than 400 ml, blood transfusion was usually not needed. Therefore, for patients who underwent IBS, they were divided into IBS1 group (bleeding volume 400–600 ml), IBS2 group (600–1000 ml), IBS3 group (1000–1500 ml) depending on the amount of intraoperative blood loss. Patients with allogeneic blood transfusions blood were divided into AB1 group (bleeding volume 400–600 ml), AB2 group (600–1000 ml), AB3 group (1000–1500 ml).

The exclusion criteria were as follows: (1) cases of abandoning treatment and self-discharge due to the personal wishes of patients and their families; (2) cases of secondary surgery; (3) cases of severe data loss; (4) cases in which the amount of intraoperative blood loss failed to meet the criteria.

The study was approved by the Ethics Committee of the First Affiliated Hospital of Anhui Medical University. Written informed consent was obtained from each patient. The CONSORT diagram of the flow of patients was summarized in Fig. 1.

Surgery and blood transfusion

All patients received intratracheal intubation and combined intravenous with inhalation general anesthesia in each case, the red blood cell salvage was performed using a Cell Saver 5 System (Haemonetics; Braintree, MA). Normal saline (500 ml) containing 15,000 µl heparin was used as the anticoagulant solution. The blood reservoir and tubing are pre-impregnated with 150 ml anticoagulant solution before the start of blood recovery. The drip rate was 1 to 2 per second depending on the speed of blood flow during machine operation. After filtrated, centrifugated, washed, the recovered blood became autologous blood (autologous RBC) with a hematocrit of 50% to 60% [9, 10], and was then transfused back to the patients immediately. All autologous RBC was transfused back before the end of surgery. Blood transfusions were administrated if hemoglobin (HGB) level < 9 g per deciliter. HBG level was maintained at ≥10 g per deciliter [11]. In order to prevent coagulation dysfunction, fresh frozen plasma and platelets were transfused according to thromboelastogram data and the clinician experience when necessary.

Charges

The costs in the ABs group are the sum of the costs of all infusion of allogeneic blood products, including allogeneic red blood cells, fresh frozen plasma and other costs. Each unit of allogeneic red blood cells was 34 USD; fresh frozen plasma per 100 ml was 6 USD; Each dose of therapeutic platelets was 218 USD; Each unit of cold precipitation was 15 USD.

The costs in the IBSs group include cell saver consumables usage fees and allogeneic blood products costs. Each set of consumables includes a collection reservoir, a combination line, a centrifuge cup, a reinfusion bag, and a waste bag. Due to the reduction of costs, the cost of cell saver consumables has been declined year by year. Here, the cost of cell saver was divided into three grades, 230, 199 and 184 USD, which were due to the different prices of cell saver consumables in different periods. Patients in the IBSs group were treated with a recovery autologous blood transfusion technique, which only charged the consumables usage fee, and did not charge the technical and labor costs of the IBS. If a patient in the IBS group receives an allogeneic blood product, it is also charged according to the cost of the allogeneic blood products.

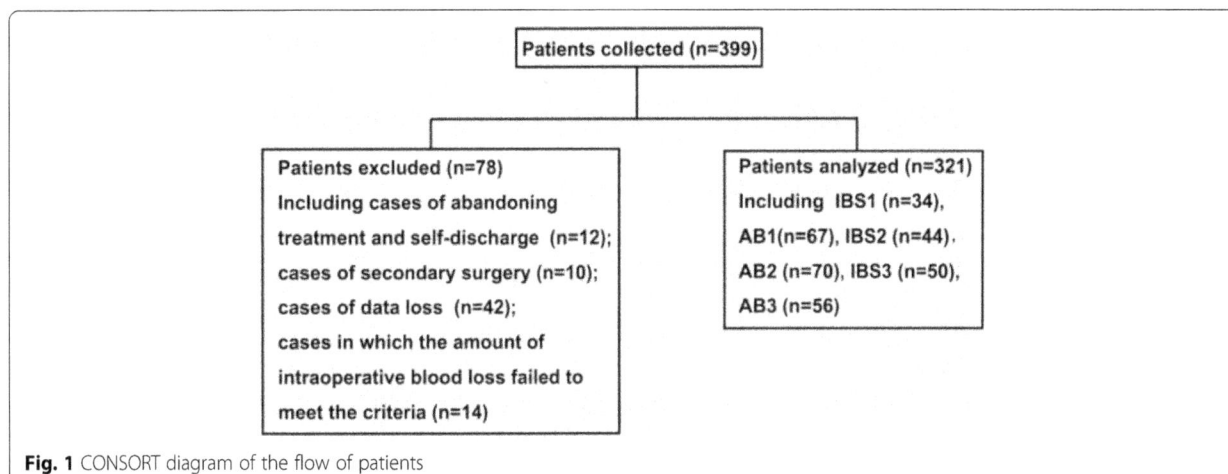

Fig. 1 CONSORT diagram of the flow of patients

Data collection

The main indicators included intraoperative blood loss, hemoglobin (HGB), white blood cell count (WBC), RBC, platelet (PLT) values before and 1, 2, and 7 days after surgery, infusion of allogeneic RBC, PLT, and plasma, and total transfusion costs. The minor indicators included mechanical ventilation duration, intensive care unit (ICU) stay, hospital stay, etc. The intraoperative blood loss is estimated by calculating the sum of the blood in the vacuum aspirator, the blood in the auto-blood reservoir, the gauze, and the blood in the cotton pad.

Statistical analysis

All statistical analyses were performed using SPSS statistical software package standard version 17.0 (SPSS, Inc., Chicago, IL, USA). Normally distributed data are expressed as the mean ± standard deviation (SD). Two independent sample t-tests were used for comparison between groups. χ^2-tests were used for comparison of counting data. $P < 0.05$ was considered to indicate a statistically significant difference.

Results

General conditions of all subjects

As shown in Table 1, there was no significant difference in gender, age, ASA status, cardiac function, and

complications including hypertension and diabetes of all the 321 participants.

Comparison of intraoperative and postoperative conditions as well as blood transfusions

As shown in Tables 2 and 3, there were no significant differences between the ABs and IBSs groups in terms of intraoperative and postoperative conditions in patients, including the number of intra-aortic balloon pump counterpulsation (IABP), number of bridges, operation duration, hospital stay, ICU stay, mechanical ventilation duration, Intraoperative blood loss, total platelet transfusion at therapeutic dose, and total plasma transfusion. As indicated in Table 3, the drainage volume 24 h post-surgery in the IBS3 group was significantly higher than that in the AB3 group ($P < 0.05$). Furthermore, the total infusion of allogeneic red blood cells in the IBSs groups was significantly lower than that in the corresponding ABs groups ($P < 0.01$).

Comparison of hematological outcomes

Next, we compared hematological outcomes of all the patients. Data revealed that the white blood cell count (WBC) 2 day post-surgery in the IBS3 group was significantly higher compared with the AB3 group (Table 4, $P < 0.01$).

Table 1 Comparison of general data

Group	N	Male/Female (N)	Age	BMI (kg/m^2)	ASA II/III/IV	Cardiac function II/III/IV	Hypertension (%)	Diabetes (%)
IBS1	34	21/13	64.82 ± 6.25	23.31 ± 3.36	13/20/1	14/19/1	18 (53)	8 (24)
AB1	67	34/33	62.73 ± 7.04	23.76 ± 3.45	22/43/2	24/41/2	25 (40)	14 (22)
IBS2	44	24/20	62.82 ± 9.45	23.79 ± 3.75	12/32/0	18/26/0	24 (55)	9 (21)
AB2	70	45/25	63.97 ± 6.48	22.96 ± 3.37	17/52/1	25/44/1	42 (60)	13 (19)
IBS3	50	33/17	65.22 ± 8.91	24.32 ± 3.67	10/37/3	16/31/3	30 (60)	11 (22)
AB3	56	39/17	63.41 ± 7.96	23.12 ± 3.39	11/43/2	18/36/2	27 (48)	14 (25)

BMI body mass index, *ASA* the American Society of Anesthesiologists' physical status

Table 2 Comparison of intraoperative and postoperative conditions in patients

Group	N	IABP (%)	Number of bridges	Operation duration (min)	Hospital stay (day)	ICU stay (h)	Mechanical ventilation duration (h)
IBS1	34	9 (27)	3.44 ± 1.23	225.41 ± 47.45	26.88 ± 9.17	55.35 ± 62.97	13.09 ± 4.94
AB1	67	28 (44)	3.25 ± 0.84	239.87 ± 32.46	28.35 ± 9.03	62.97 ± 30.24	13.71 ± 5.07
IBS2	44	15 (34)	3.66 ± 0.88	272.55 ± 47.71	28.45 ± 7.89	70.20 ± 35.08	14.75 ± 5.28
AB2	70	22 (31)	3.47 ± 1.05	259.50 ± 47.70	27.00 ± 8.14	70.00 ± 38.29	13.91 ± 5.94
IBS3	50	23 (46)	3.74 ± 0.77	283.00 ± 50.02	27.54 ± 8.10	73.66 ± 34.30	15.98 ± 4.51
AB3	56	20 (36)	3.63 ± 1.03	284.52 ± 38.15	27.34 ± 8.56	67.34 ± 38.87	15.32 ± 8.00

IABP intra-aortic balloon pump counterpulsation, *ICU* intensive care unit

Comparison of total blood transfusion cost

As reflected in Table 5, the total blood transfusion cost in the IBSs groups was significantly higher than that in the ABs groups when the IBS cost was 230 USD per set ($P < 0.05$). However, when 199 or 184 USD per set, only the IBS1, rather than IBS2 or IBS3 group, showed significantly higher cost of the total blood transfusion compared with the AB1 group ($P < 0.05$).

Discussion

Previous studies have shown that infusion of allogeneic blood has adverse effects on the long-term prognosis of patients [12, 13], especially for patients with existing cardiac problems, which can increase the mortality within 5 years after surgery [14]. At the same time, autologous blood transfusion has been recently used in the field of cardiac surgery due to the tight blood supply. However, the blind application of IBS technology will not only fail to exert its advantages, but also increase hospitalization costs and increase the burden on patients. Accordingly, in this study, a single OPCABG surgery was conducted, and bleeding was divided into three different hemorrhage layers to evaluate the impact of IBS on outcomes following OPCABG surgery.

The results showed that when the blood loss ranged from 600 to 1000 ml, the application of IBS led to a significant reduction in the transfusion volume of allogeneic blood. Meanwhile, IBS maintained the HGB and RBC values similar to that of the ABs groups. Moreover, IBS did not increase the number of postoperative leukocytes and drainage volume 24 h post-surgery. Additionally, IBS

did not affect the mechanical ventilation duration, ICU stay, hospital stay, and total transfusion cost, showing the best cost-effectiveness.

Our results also revealed that, when the amount of blood loss ranged from 400 to 600 ml, IBS could reduce the total allogeneic RBC infusion to a certain degree. We also found that IBS significantly increased the total transfusion cost compared with the transfusion of allogeneic blood only. In addition, the current standards for blood transfusion for cardiac patients differs depending on the specific conditions, and the comparison of restrictive and loose blood transfusion standards are still to be studied [15]. Therefore, whether or not a patient with less than 600 ml blood loss applies IBS can depend on the condition of the patient and the experience of clinicians.

When the blood loss ranged from 1000 to 1500 ml, the IBS3 group showed higher 24 h post-surgery drainage volume compared with the AB3 group but there was no significant difference in the number of postoperative platelets counts between the two groups. This may be attributed to less infusion of fresh frozen plasma and thus lack of coagulation factors. The results also showed that the IBSs groups had lower plasma transfusion volume than in the ABs groups, indicating that the application of the IBS technique requires a reasonable amount of infusion of blood products such as fresh frozen plasma rich in coagulation factors when the amount of intraoperative blood loss is large, otherwise it may affect the coagulation function of patients. This is consistent with the results of Shen et al. [16]. The cause of this

Table 3 Comparison of bleeding and blood transfusion in patients

Group	N	Intraoperative blood loss (ml)	Drainage volume 24 h post-surgery (ml)	Allogeneic red blood cell transfusion (U)	Total platelet transfusion (therapeutic dose)	Total plasma transfusion (ml)
IBS1	34	476.94 ± 96.75	470.15 ± 154.01	1.97 ± 1.98[b]	0.00 ± 0.00	426.47 ± 260.31
AB1	67	447.49 ± 110.86	469.08 ± 174.37	4.7 ± 1.73	0.02 ± 0.13	518.36 ± 291.45
IBS2	44	796.05 ± 99.58	474.95 ± 129.14	1.86 ± 2.73[b]	0.02 ± 0.15	479.55 ± 383.72
AB2	70	789.77 ± 100.22	511.57 ± 170.90	5.19 ± 2.76	0.06 ± 0.23	596.43 ± 404.35
IBS3	50	1393.26 ± 270.87	626.16 ± 189.38[a]	3.78 ± 4.60[b]	0.08 ± 0.27	738.00 ± 688.87
AB3	56	1331.80 ± 276.39	543.32 ± 185.71	6.52 ± 4.11	0.07 ± 0.26	882.14 ± 465.87

[a]$P < 0.05$, [b]$P < 0.01$ vs. AB group

Table 4 Comparison of hematological outcomes

Indexes	Group	N	Pre-surgery	1 d post-surgery	2 d post-surgery	7 d post-surgery
HGB(g/L)	IBS1	34	126.41 ± 12.03	123.41 ± 15.51	119.24 ± 16.86	124.65 ± 19.05
	AB1	67	127.57 ± 11.38	124.90 ± 12.48	119.24 ± 12.30	127.81 ± 73.53
	IBS2	44	131.43 ± 11.78	123.86 ± 13.98	118.55 ± 17.12	125.30 ± 17.25
	AB2	70	129.97 ± 13.09	124.57 ± 13.21	120.11 ± 14.66	130.17 ± 16.72
	IBS3	50	134.54 ± 13.16	115.62 ± 19.41	113.22 ± 14.18	126.18 ± 14.13
	AB3	56	137.14 ± 13.07	118.71 ± 13.02	116.91 ± 15.12	129.32 ± 16.03
WBC(10^9/L)	IBS1	34	6.39 ± 1.43	14.43 ± 4.00	13.99 ± 4.54	8.99 ± 2.42
	AB1	67	6.18 ± 1.64	13.98 ± 3.67	12.98 ± 4.29	9.62 ± 2.62
	IBS2	44	6.59 ± 1.49	15.52 ± 4.43	14.54 ± 3.70	9.45 ± 2.83
	AB2	70	6.73 ± 1.57	14.52 ± 3.59	13.17 ± 4.66	9.97 ± 2.82
	IBS3	50	6.62 ± 1.76	14.06 ± 3.92	15.08 ± 5.07[b]	10.63 ± 4.45
	AB3	56	6.83 ± 1.78	13.53 ± 3.55	12.53 ± 3.53	9.79 ± 2.77
RBC(10^{12}/L)	IBS1	34	4.17 ± 0.53	4.06 ± 0.44	3.91 ± 0.50	4.11 ± 0.55
	AB1	67	4.23 ± 0.38	4.16 ± 0.41	3.94 ± 0.43	4.20 ± 0.53
	IBS2	44	4.29 ± 0.48	4.07 ± 0.48	3.87 ± 0.56	4.19 ± 0.64
	AB2	70	4.30 ± 0.45	4.08 ± 0.39	3.92 ± 0.47	4.21 ± 0.53
	IBS3	50	4.36 ± 0.45	3.80 ± 0.39	3.56 ± 0.39	4.10 ± 0.41
	AB3	56	4.51 ± 0.41	3.97 ± 0.43	3.65 ± 0.51	4.18 ± 0.60
PLT(10^9/L)	IBS1	34	200.15 ± 65.35	191.68 ± 72.16	152.76 ± 58.65	209.12 ± 65.99
	AB1	67	213.25 ± 65.21	167.84 ± 55.63	135.76 ± 73.53	203.24 ± 73.53
	IBS2	44	212.45 ± 57.45	184.39 ± 61.64	156.68 ± 69.92	212.30 ± 97.22
	AB2	70	219.91 ± 71.88	184.43 ± 55.13	150.47 ± 54.44	220.09 ± 80.20
	IBS3	50	212.26 ± 50.83	172.58 ± 57.43	142.82 ± 52.47	236.44 ± 97.12
	AB3	56	208.68 ± 61.78	156.20 ± 38.59	137.63 ± 47.12	213.23 ± 91.22

HGB hemoglobin, *WBC* white blood cell count, *RBC* red blood cell count, *PLT* platelet
[b]*P* < 0.01 vs. AB group

phenomenon may also include an increase in autologous blood transfusion, which dilutes blood coagulation factors and platelets, increases the heparin content that enters the body [17], thereby promoting damage to the coagulation system. Furthermore, the number of white blood cells in the IBS3 group was higher than that in the AB3 group on the second postoperative day. In addition, we found the WBC value 2 day post-surgery was in the

Table 5 Comparison of the total blood transfusion cost

Group	N	Total blood transfusion cost (USD)		
		230	199	184
IBS1	34	327.5 ± 96.9 [a]	297.0 ± 96.9 [a]	281.7 ± 96.9 [a]
AB1	67	233.7 ± 107.9	233.7 ± 107.9	233.7 ± 107.9
IBS2	44	333.8 ± 145.1 [a]	303.2 ± 145.1	287.9 ± 145.1
AB2	70	260.9 ± 157.5	260.9 ± 157.5	260.9 ± 157.5
IBS3	50	439.2 ± 276.2 [a]	408.6 ± 276.2	393.3 ± 276.2
AB3	56	332.3 ± 219.8	332.3 ± 219.8	332.3 ± 219.8

[a]*P* < 0.05 vs. AB group

IBS3 group was significantly higher compared with the AB3 group which is different from the findings of Cui et al. [18]. The different results may be attributed to several factors, including less blood loss (700 ± 50 ml), and reduced blood transfusion volume, and the different type of surgery in the study by Cui et al. Currently used autologous blood transfusion apparatus can destroy cell components during blood recovery and centrifugation, activate platelets and leukocytes. Conventional washing fails to completely remove activated leukocytes, so reinfusion into patients can promote the release of inflammatory mediators and further aggravated the systemic inflammatory response. Clinically, WBC is widely used for the auxiliary diagnosis of infection, and the degree of WBC elevation is directly related to the degree of trauma [19]. IBS may retain more white blood cells and inflammatory mediators compared with allogeneic blood products with leukocyte-depleted red blood cells. Therefore, the addition of a leukocyte filter would be more beneficial to patients when using IBS in high-bleeding-risk cardiac surgery [20].

Moreover, we also observed that the total blood transfusion cost in the IBSs groups was significantly higher than that in the ABs groups when the IBS cost was 230 USD per set. However, when 199 or 184 USD per set, the IBS1 group showed significantly higher cost of the total blood transfusion compared with the AB1 group. With the reduction of IBS charges and the increase of the blood loss amount, the cost-effectiveness of IBS has gradually emerged. Xie et al. [21] demonstrated that the use of IBS in OPCABG surgery reduced the chances of patients exposure to allogeneic blood, decreased the incidence of transfusion-related diseases and transfusion reactions, but it increased the total transfusion costs. Attaran et al. [22] also stated that the routine use of IBS is not cost-effective. Malhotra *et al.* [1] proposed that the application of IBS is more meaningful in patients with more than 1000 ml blood loss during surgery. Wang et al. [23] reported that a cell saver may be beneficial only when it is used for shed blood and/or residual blood or during the entire operative period. Processing cardiotomy suction blood with a cell saver only during cardiopulmonary bypass has no significant effect on blood conservation and increases fresh frozen plasma transfusion. These abovementioned findings are s not exactly the same as our findings. This may be attributed to the large difference in charges for IBS and allogenic blood products between at home and abroad, as well as the higher charge of IBS and the low cost of allogeneic blood products at home. In addition, the decrease in intraoperative blood loss or inappropriate use of blood transfusion apparatus results in less autologous blood recovery and even failure to wash autologous blood, which may also affect the cost. Moreover, the limited sample size in this study should also be noted. We propose that the results of cost-benefit analysis may differ when the bleeding amount is higher or the IBS charge is lower.

This study was a retrospective analysis, in which patients in the IBS group were started to use autologous blood transfusions immediately after surgery. Due to the inability to predict intraoperative blood loss, we used the commonly used loose blood transfusion standard. That is, when the patient's HGB value was < 9 g/L, blood transfusion can be started. In addition, it is necessary to refer to the preoperative and intraoperative HGB values and the specific operation situation. According to the restrictive blood transfusion standard, patients who may have less than 600 ml of blood loss do not need blood transfusions, and thus do not need to apply IBS. This is the reason why this paper analyzes the cost-effectiveness of stratified blood loss analysis.

Conclusions

In conclusion, IBS has different efficacy in different bleeding situations. Particularly, when the amount of bleeding ranges from 600 to 1000 ml, IBS can significantly reduce the demand for allogeneic blood, and has no direct adverse effects on coagulation function and postoperative recovery of patients, and is cost-effective in OPCABG under the current charge standard. The role and cost-effectiveness of using IBS in patients with old age and high-bleeding risks need to be further analyzed. Furthermore, how to accurately screen high-bleeding-risk patients is still a question worthy of study. In addition, a prospective, multi-center, randomized, controlled study is also needed to clarify the best application guidelines for IBS technology so that the technology could be applied more accurately.

Abbreviations
AB: allogeneic blood; ATLS: Advanced Trauma Life Support System; HGB: hemoglobin; IBS: intraoperative blood salvage; ICU: intensive care unit; OPCABG: off-pump coronary artery bypass grafting; PLT: platelet; RBC: red blood cell; WBC: white blood cell count

Authors' contributions
HW designed the study, HW, WZ, WF, XL collected the data, GM, LZ, YZ, EG analyzed the data, XL wrote the paper. All authors read and approved the final manuscript.

Competing interests
The authors declare that they have no competing interests.

References
1. Malhotra A, Garg P, Bishnoi AK, Sharma P, Wadhawa V, Shah K, et al. Dialyzer-based cell salvage system: a superior alternative to conventional cell salvage in off-pump coronary artery bypass grafting. Interact Cardiovasc Thorac Surg. 2017;24(4):489–97.
2. Mehr-Aein A, Sadeghi M, Madani-civi M. Does tranexamic acid reduce blood loss in off-pump coronary artery bypass? Asian Cardiovasc ThoracAnn. 2007; 15(4):285–9.
3. Dai Z, Chu H, Wang S, Liang Y. The effect of tranexamic acid to reduce blood loss and transfusion on off-pump coronary artery bypass surgery: a systematic review and cumulative meta-analysis. J Clin Anesth. 2018; 44:23–31.
4. Shafiee A, Nazari S, Mogharreban M, Koupaei MT. Evaluating medical interns' knowledge of common blood transfusion complications. Transfus Apher Sci. 2013;48(2):253–6.
5. Hassall O, Maitland K, Pole L, Mwarumba S, Denje D, Wambua K, et al. Bacterial contamination of pediatric whole blood transfusions in a Kenyan hospital. Transfusion. 2009;49(12):2594–8.
6. Sulu B, Aytac E, Stocchi L, Vogel JD, Kiran RP. The minimally invasive approach is associated with reduced perioperative thromboembolic and bleeding complications for patients receiving preoperative chronic oral anticoagulant therapy who undergo colorectal surgery. Surg Endosc. 2013; 27(4):1339–45.
7. Weltert L, Nardella S, Rondinelli MB, Pierelli L, De Paulis R. Reduction of allogeneic red blood cell usage during cardiac surgery by an integrated intra- and postoperative blood salvage strategy: results of a randomized comparison. Transfusion. 2013;53(4):790–7.
8. ATLS Subcommittee, American College of Surgeons' Committee on Trauma, International ATLS working group. Advanced trauma life support (ATLS(R)): the ninth edition. J Trauma Acute Care Surg. 2013;74(5):1363–6.
9. Vonk AB, Meesters MI, Garnier RP, Romijn JW, van Barneveld LJ, Heymans MW, et al. Intraoperative cell salvage is associated with reduced postoperative

blood loss and transfusion requirements in cardiac surgery: a cohort study. Transfusion. 2013;53(11):2782–9.

10. Djaiani G, Fedorko L, Borger MA, Green R, Carroll J, Marcon M, et al. Continuous-flow cell saver reduces cognitive decline in elderly patients after coronary bypass surgery. Circulation. 2007;116(17):1888–95.

11. Mutneja HR, Arora S, Vij A. Liberal or restrictive transfusion after cardiac surgery. N Engl J Med. 2015;373(2):190.

12. Karkouti K, Stukel TA, Beattie WS, Elsaadany S, Li P, Berger R, et al. Relationship of erythrocyte transfusion with short- and long-term mortality in a population-based surgical cohort. Anesthesiology. 2012;117(6):1175–83.

13. Feng S, Machina M, Beattie WS. Influence of anaemia and red blood cell transfusion on mortality in high cardiac risk patients undergoing major non-cardiac surgery: a retrospective cohort study. Br J Anaesth. 2017; 118(6):843–51.

14. Schwann TA, Habib JR, Khalifeh JM, Nauffal V, Bonnell M, Clancy C, et al. Effects of blood transfusion on cause-specific late mortality after coronary artery bypass grafting-less is more. Ann Thorac Surg. 2016;102(2):465–73.

15. Mazer CD, Whitlock RP, Fergusson DA, Hall J, Belley-Cote E, Connolly K, et al. Restrictive or Liberal red-cell transfusion for cardiac surgery. N Engl J Med. 2017;377(22):2133–44.

16. Shen S, Zhang J, Wang W, Zheng J, Xie Y. Impact of intra-operative cell salvage on blood coagulation in high-bleeding-risk patients undergoing cardiac surgery with cardiopulmonary bypass: a prospective randomized and controlled trial. J Transl Med. 2016;14(1):228.

17. Buys WF, Buys M, Levin AI. Reinfusate heparin concentrations produced by two autotransfusion systems. J Cardiothorac Vasc Anesth. 2016;31(1):90–98.

18. Cui B, Zhao P, Wang C. The different influence of inflammatory response after transfusion with autologous blood and stored blood. J Clin Anesthesiol. 2015;31(3):247–9.

19. Paladino L, Subramanian RA, Bonilla E, Sinert RH. Leukocytosis as prognostic indicator of major injury. West J Emerg Med. 2010;11(5):450–5.

20. Gu YJ, de Vries AJ, Boonstra PW, van Oeveren W. Leukocyte depletion results in improved lung function and reduced inflammatory response after cardiac surgery. J Thorac Cardiovasc Surg. 1996;112(2):494–500.

21. Xie Y, Shen S, Zhang J, Wang W, Zheng J. The efficacy, safety and cost-effectiveness of intra-operative cell salvage in high-bleeding-risk cardiac surgery with cardiopulmonary bypass: a prospective randomized and controlled trial. Int J Med Sci. 2015;12(4):322–8.

22. Attaran S, McIlroy D, Fabri BM, Pullan MD. The use of cell salvage in routine cardiac surgery is ineffective and not cost-effective and should be reserved for selected cases. Interact Cardiovasc Thorac Surg. 2011;12(5):824–6.

23. Wang G, Bainbridge D, Martin J, Cheng D. The efficacy of an intraoperative cell saver during cardiac surgery: a meta-analysis of randomized trials. Anesth Analg. 2009;109(2):320–30.

24

Differences of patients' characteristics in acute type A aortic dissection – surgical data from Belgian and Japanese centers

Motohiko Goda[1,3*], Tomoyuki Minami[2], Kiyotaka Imoto[2], Keiji Uchida[2], Munetaka Masuda[3] and Bart Meuris[1]

Abstract

Background: It is well known that there are major differences between the Japanese and Western population regarding the incidence of ischemic heart disease and stroke. The purpose of this study was to evaluate differences of patients' characteristics between Belgian and Japanese cohort with acute type A aortic dissection.

Methods: In 487 patients (297 male patients, mean age 61.9 ± 12.2 yrs) who underwent surgery for acute type A aortic dissection, baseline preoperative and intraoperative data were collected. Belgian patients ($n = 237$) were compared to Japanese patients ($n = 250$). Clinical data included patient demographics, history, status at presentation, imaging study results and intraoperative findings.

Results: The Japanese cohort had significantly more women (48.8% vs. 28.7%, $p < 0.0001$), lower BMI (24.2 vs. 26.4, $p < 0.0001$) and lower prevalence of hypertension (49.2% vs. 65.8%, $p = 0.0002$). More DeBakey type I dissections and less type III dissections with retrograde extension were reported in Belgium than in Japan (77.2% vs. 48.4%, $p < 0.0001$, 3.4% vs. 38.7%, $p < 0.0001$, respectively). More entries were found in the ascending aorta (78.5% vs. 58.5%, $p < 0.0001$) and aortic arch (24.9% vs. 13.7%, $p = 0.0018$) in Belgian patients than in Japanese patients, who had more entries in the descending aorta or undetected entries.

Conclusions: In acute type A aortic dissection, Belgian patients reveal striking differences from Japanese patients regarding gender distribution, entry tear location and type of dissection. Japanese women are more likely to develop acute type A aortic dissection than Belgian women. (234 words).

Keywords: Acute aortic dissection, Epidemiology, Gender differences

Background

It is well known that the prevalence of ischemic heart disease and its mortality are significantly lower in Japan compared to the United States or to other Western populations [1–4]. On the contrary, Japanese people suffer significantly more from stroke, mainly the hemorrhagic type of stroke [1–4]. Within these two major cardiovascular disease types, there is a clear East/West divide [1]. Next to obvious and important differences in dietary habits (lower saturated fat and higher salt intake for the Japanese with subsequently much lower serum cholesterol levels), there might be genetic differences between Japanese and Western people that underlie the observed differences in cardiovascular diseases [1–4]. But the actual causes for these differences in cardiovascular risk profile remain unknown and any explanation remains speculative. There is a higher prevalence of arterial hypertension within the general Japanese population, but this is insufficient to explain all phenomena. And although the Japanese dietary pattern has westernized these days, the trends in cardiovascular risk still last [4].

Acute type A aortic dissection (TA-AAD) is a life-threatening cardiovascular catastrophe which often requires emergency surgery to prevent death [5]. Within the International Registry of Acute Aortic Dissection (IRAD), geographic differences in clinical presentation, treatment and outcome in type A dissection have been studied, comparing European patients to North Americans. This study

---

* Correspondence: gogomotto@gmail.com
[1]Department of Cardiac Surgery, University Hospitals Leuven, Leuven, Belgium
[3]Department of Cardiovascular Surgery, Yokohama City University Hospital, Yokohama, Japan
Full list of author information is available at the end of the article

was able to reveal small differences in presentation and methods used for diagnosis, but overall these two Western patient cohorts were quite comparable [6]. Despite the known and described differences in ischemic heart disease and stroke between Asian and Western people, a comparison within patients with type A dissection has not been performed yet. The purpose of the present study is to evaluate differences in baseline patient characteristics and TA-AAD profile between Belgian and Japanese patient cohort.

Methods

Study population

We collected data from 487 patients (297 male; mean age 61.9 ± 12.2 y; range 14–88 y) with TA-AAD who underwent emergency surgery at a Belgian center (University Hospital Leuven, Leuven, Belgium) or at a Japanese center (Yokohama City University Medical Center, Yokohama, Japan). Surgical interventions were performed in a time frame between January 1986 to September 2011 in the Belgian center and from January 2003 to December 2010 in the Japanese center. Diagnosis was made by imaging studies including computed tomography, magnetic resonance imaging and/or echocardiography. TA-AAD was defined as any dissection that involved the ascending aorta with presentation within 14 days of its onset. Approval by the local ethics committee was granted to collect and analyze patient data.

Data collection

Baseline clinical data on enrolled patients, including patient demographics, medical history, clinical findings at presentation, imaging study results, preoperative complications and intraoperative findings were collected and stored by retrospective chart review. Body mass index (BMI) was calculated (weight(kg)/height(m)^2).

Literature and cardiac surgical society data

In order to cross-check the baseline characteristics from our study cohort with current literature, a Pubmed search was performed for recent reports on TA-AAD within either Western centers (Europe, USA) or Eastern centers (Japan, Korea). Also, recent data on TA-AAD incidence from both the Belgian [6] and Japanese [7] cardiac surgical societies were used to estimate nationwide absolute incidence values.

Statistical analysis

All statistical analyses were performed using StatView J-5.0 (SAS Institute Inc., Cary, NC). Continuous variables were expressed as mean ± standard deviation and were compared using the student's t test. Categorical variables are expressed as absolute numbers or percentages and were compared using chi-square testing. The level of statistical significance was set at $p < 0.05$.

Results

Demographics and patient history

Of the 487 patients enrolled in this study, 237 were from Belgium, and 250 were from Japan. All studied variables are listed in Tables 1 and 2. The proportion of women was significantly higher in Japan than in Belgium (48.8% vs. 28.7%, $p < 0.0001$). Belgian women were younger than Japanese women at the time of operation (61.2 vs. 67.6y, $p = 0.0006$). Belgian patients had a higher BMI (26.4 vs. 24.2, $p < 0.0001$), they were taller (men; 1.76 cm vs. 1.68 cm, $p < 0.0001$, women; 1.64 cm vs. 1.54 cm, $p < 0.0001$), and heavier (men; 82.5 kg vs. 72.2 kg, $p < 0.0001$, women; 70.2 kg vs. 54.5 kg, $p < 0.0001$) than Japanese patients.

Belgian patients had more preoperatively documented arterial hypertension (65.8% vs. 49.2%, $p = 0.0002$), while in Japanese previously documented aortic aneurysms were more prevalent (59.6% vs. 21.5%). Belgian patients had more previous cardiac operations (6.3% vs. 1.6%, 0.0071) than Japanese patients and there were more iatrogenic dissections (1.7% vs. 0%, $p = 0.0391$). There were no significant differences with regard to history of bicuspid aortic valve, Marfan syndrome, pregnancy, drug abuse or trauma.

Table 1 Demographics and patient history for Belgian and Japanese patients

Variables	Belgium (n = 237)	Japan (n = 250)	p Value
Gender (Men/Women)	169/68	128/122	< 0.0001
Age (yrs)	59.3 ± 12.7	63.3 ± 11.3	< 0.0001
Age < 40 yrs	13 (5.5%)	5 (2%)	0.0416
Age ≥ 80 yrs	10 (4.2%)	19 (7.6%)	0.1151
Body Mass Index	26.4 ± 4.1	24.2 ± 3.7	< 0.0001
Hypertension	156 (65.8%)	123 (49.2%)	0.0002
Known aortic aneurysm (≥ 4 cm)	51 (21.5%)	149 (59.6%)	< 0.0001
Bicuspid aortic valve	5 (2.1%)	1 (0.4%)	0.1008
Marfan syndrome	7 (3%)	7 (2.8%)	0.9192
Other connective tissue disease	2 (0.8%)	0 (0%)	0.1455
Pregnant	2 (0.8%)	0 (0%)	0.1455
Drug	2 (0.8%)	0 (0%)	0.1455
Trauma	1 (0.4%)	0 (0%)	0.3039
Iatrogenic	4 (1.7%)	0 (0%)	0.0391
Previous cardiac operation	15 (6.3%)	4 (1.6%)	0.0071
Post cardiac operation within hospital stay	3 (1.3%)	0 (0%)	0.0744
Post cardiac operation within 2 years	13 (5.5%)	1 (0.4%)	0.0008

Table 2 Demographics by gender

Variables	Belgium	Japan	p Value
Men	n = 169	n = 128	
Age (yrs)	58.6 ± 11.8	61.1 ± 11.1	0.0607
Age < 40 yrs	8 (4.7%)	3 (2.3%)	0.2801
Age ≥ 80 yrs	6 (3.6%)	5 (3.9%)	0.8722
Length (m)	1.75 ± 0.07	1.68 ± 0.06	< 0.0001
Weight (kg)	82.5 ± 14.1	72.2 ± 11	< 0.0001
Body Mass Index	26.5 ± 3.9	25.5 ± 3.4	0.0166
Hypertension	107 (63.3%)	62 (48.4%)	0.0104
Women	n = 68	n = 122	
Age (yrs)	61.2 ± 14.5	67.6 ± 10.5	0.0006
Age < 40 yrs	5 (7.4%)	2 (1.6%)	0.0045
Age ≥ 80 yrs	4 (5.9%)	14 (11.5%)	0.2059
Length (m)	1.64 ± 0.08	1.54 ± 0.07	< 0.0001
Weight (kg)	70.2 ± 13.6	54.5 ± 10.5	< 0.0001
Body Mass Index	26.5 ± 3.9	25.5 ± 3.4	< 0.0001
Hypertension	49 (72.1%)	61 (50%)	0.0082

Table 3 Type of aortic dissection and complications for Belgium and Japanese patients

Variables	Belgium (n = 237)	Japan (n = 250)	p Value
DeBakey I	183 (77.2%)	121 (48.4%)	< 0.0001
DeBakey II	43 (18.1%)	31 (12.4%)	0.084
Stanford type B with retrograde extension	8 (3.4%)	96 (38.4%)	< 0.0001
Entry			
Ascending aorta	186 (78.5%)	145 (58%)	< 0.0001
Aortic arch	59 (24.9%)	34 (13.6%)	0.0018
Descending aorta	8 (3.4%)	25 (10%)	0.0084
Not found	0 (0%)	44 (17.6%)	< 0.0001
Shock	67 (28.3%)	47 (18.8%)	0.0136
Cardiac tamponade	41 (17.3%)	74 (29.6%)	0.0014
Cardiopulmonary resuscitation	6 (2.5%)	14 (5.6%)	0.0881
Stroke	16 (6.8%)	16 (6.4%)	0.8758
Paraparesis/paraplegia	9 (3.8%)	2 (0.8%)	0.0261
Lower limb ischemia	27 (11.4%)	30 (12%)	0.8349
Renal ischemia	13 (5.5%)	3 (1.2%)	0.008
Mesenteric ischemia	4 (1.7%)	9 (3.6%)	0.1907
Myocardial ischemia	15 (6.3%)	13 (5.2%)	0.5926

Type of aortic dissection and preoperative complications

Table 3 shows that DeBakey type I dissections were more frequent in Belgium (77.2% vs. 48.4%, $p < 0.0001$) while Type III dissections with retrograde extension were less frequent in Belgium than in Japan (3.4% vs. 38.7%, $p < 0.0001$). More entries were found in the ascending aorta (78.5% vs. 58.5%, $p < 0.0001$) and aortic arch (24.9% vs. 13.7%, $p = 0.0018$) in Belgian patients than in Japanese patients.

Shock was more frequent in Belgian patients than in Japanese patients (28.3% vs. 18.8%, $p = 0.0136$), however, cardiac tamponade was more frequent in Japan than in Belgium (29.6% vs. 17.3%, $p = 0.0014$). As to complications associated with impaired arterial blood flow, the prevalence of renal ischemia (5.5% vs. 1.2%. $p = 0.008$) and paraparesis/paraplegia (3.8% vs. 0.8%, $p = 0.0261$) were more frequent in Belgium than in Japan. There were no significant differences with regard to development of stroke, myocardial ischemia, mesenteric ischemia, and limb ischemia.

Discussion

The occurrence of cardiovascular diseases is certainly associated with genetic factors, life style, dietary factors, environmental conditions and coexisting diseases. Therefore, it is reasonable that there are regional differences in incidence and mortality of different cardiovascular pathologies. The fact that Japan has less ischemic heart disease and more hemorrhagic stroke has been epidemiologically studied and is well recognized these days [1–4, 8, 9]. In the present study we highlight that also acute type A dissection is a disease with regional differences in patient characteristics when Belgian and Japanese patient cohort are compared.

The larger proportion of women in Japanese TA-AAD patients is a remarkable demographic finding in this study. Based on reports from predominantly Western centers, the gender distribution in TA-AAD has always been described as a 2:1 male:female ratio [10–12]. This 2:1 male/female ratio is frequently reported by IRAD and can be found in many textbooks of cardiac surgery [13, 14]. But does this ratio hold true for the Eastern population? The Japanese series in this study showed 48.8% female patients (who were also significantly older). Other reports from Japanese centers (with at least 80 surgical TA-AAD cases) also reported as many as 39.1 to 58.8% of female patients [15–20]. Similarly, recent reports from Korea [21–24] described proportions of female patients up to 42.4 to 52.7%, very similar to the reports from Japan. Therefore, it seems that within the East-Asian population, the gender distribution male:female in TA-AAD patients is more a 1:1 ratio, or Asian women are more likely to develop TA-AAD compared to Western women. According to the organization for economic co-operation and development (OECD) [25], the number of annual deaths from circulatory system diseases in Japanese women was 380 per 1,000,000 persons per year, which is much less than the 940 deaths per million per year in Belgian women. With a significantly lower overall death from cardiovascular diseases, it is paradoxical that Japanese women are more likely to develop TA-AAD, but the etiology behind it might be similar to that causing the higher numbers of hemorrhagic stroke in Japanese women [4]. One can hypothesize that Japanese woman have a more pronounced vessel wall fragility.

The detected differences in the incidence of arterial hypertension are paradoxical, because Japanese have a higher nationwide prevalence of hypertension [25]. Also the fact that more Japanese had previously documented aneurysms is enigmatic. The remaining observed differences in number of redo cases, iatrogenic cases, occurrence of malperfusion and tamponade should be interpreted with caution, given the relatively low number of observations.

It is impossible to investigate the absolute incidence or prevalence of acute aortic dissection. Reported incidences may underestimate the 'real' population value, because TA-AAD also causes sudden death before any diagnostic investigation has been performed. Textbooks teach us an 'estimated worldwide incidence' of 5 to 29.5 per 1,000,000 per year [26]. But also figures between 29 to 52 per 1,000,000 per year have been reported [27–30]. It is important to know that some of these values originate from observations of relatively small patient cohorts and are then extrapolated to the general population of a country. Current data from two Western cardiac surgical societies and registries teach us the following incidences per 1,000,000 persons per year: Belgium 8.1 [7]. The IRAD registry reports an annual incidence of 4.1 per million and data from the USA show an estimated incidence of 2 to 8 per million per year [26]. Surprisingly, Japan reports 27.2 operated TA-AAD cases per million persons in 1 year [31], which is 4 to 7 times higher compared to the current Western data. It seems that the worldwide incidence of acute aortic dissections is indeed - like the textbooks show - within a range 5 to 30 per million per year, but that the incidence in Western people is more on the lower side of this spectrum while Japanese people are on the higher side.

Within TA-AAD patients, type I dissections are the predominant form (in Western series), and in up to 60–68% of cases, the location of the entry tear is within the ascending aorta [13, 14, 26]. Our observation confirmed this pattern and the main entry tear location. But the Japanese data show a different pattern: fewer entries were found in the ascending aorta and more retrograde dissections extending from the descending aorta were observed. Also in a high proportion of patients, no entry tear was found at all, suggesting a tear in the lower descending aorta. The retrograde extension of aortic dissection leads patients with type B dissection to type A. This may partly explain the higher number of TA-AAD cases in Japan compared to other western countries.

Both more prevalent of documented aortic aneurysm and the retrograde extension of aortic dissection are possibly attributed to a vessel fragility of Japanese people. The reason why there would be higher vessel fragility in Japanese remains unknown. Hypotheses have been provided linking low serum cholesterol levels to altered mechanical properties of endothelium and vessel wall quality. Further investigation with comparison of biomechanical characteristics of tissue within both populations is needed to elaborate our findings further.

Conclusion

Belgian patients with TA-AAD differ from Japanese patients with respect to gender, entry tear location and type of dissection. The absolute incidence of TA-AAD in Japan is higher. Especially Japanese women are more likely to develop TA-AAD than Belgian women.

Study limitations

This study included single center data from each country and the numbers of the subjects are relatively small. Only patient data with TA-AAD were evaluated in this study, medically treated cases, chronic dissections or type B dissection data was not included. Pre- and intraoperative factors alone were gathered and studied, without outcome data. The study periods were different between the two centers. No pathological or biomechanical investigations were performed.

Abbreviations

BMI: Body mass index; IRAD: The International Registry of Acute Aortic Dissection; OECD: the organization for economic co-operation and development; TA-AAD: Acute type A aortic dissection

Authors' contributions

Concept/design: MG, BM, Data collection: MG, TM, KU, BM, Data analysis/interpretation: MG, Drafting article: MG, Critical revision of the article: MG, KU, MM, Approval of the article: BM. All authors read and approved the final manuscript.

Competing interests

The authors declare that they have no competing interests.

Author details

[1]Department of Cardiac Surgery, University Hospitals Leuven, Leuven, Belgium. [2]Cardiovascular Center, Yokohama City University Medical Center, Yokohama, Japan. [3]Department of Cardiovascular Surgery, Yokohama City University Hospital, Yokohama, Japan.

References

1. Kita T. Coronary heart disease risk in Japan - an east/west divide? Eur Heart J Suppl. 2004;6:A8–A11.

2. Ueshima H. Explanation for Japanese paradox: prevention of increase in coronary heart disease and reduction in stroke. J Atheroscler Thromb. 2007; 14:278–86.

3. Ueshima H, Sekikawa A, Miura K, Turin TC, Takashima N, Kita Y, Watanabe M, Kadota A, Okuda N, Kadowaki T, Nakamura Y, Okamura T. Cardiovascular disease and risk factors in Asia: a selected review. Circulation. 2008;118: 2702–9.

4. Shinohara Y. Regional differences in incidence and management of stroke-is there any difference between western and Japanese guidelines and antiplatelet therapy? Cerecrovasc Dis. 2006;21:17–24.

5. Goda M, Imoto K, Suzuki S, Uchida K, Yanagi H, Yasuda S, Masuda M. Risk analysis for hospital mortality in patients with acute type a aortic dissection. Ann Thorac Surg. 2010;90:1246–50.

6. Raghupathy A, Nienaber CA, Harris KM, Myrmel T, Fattori R, Sechtem U, Oh J, Trimarchi S, Cooper JV, Booher A, Eagle K, Isselbacher E, Bossone E. Geographic differences in clinical presentation, treatment, and outcome in acute type a aortic dissection (from the international registry of acute aortic dissection). Am J Cardiol. 2008;102:1562–6.

7. Report on the demographics, management and outcome of the surgical treatment for acute type A aortic dissection. A prospective study in Belgian cardiac surgical centers over a one-year period (2008–2009) with a one-year follow-up. Available at http://www.bacts.org/documents/PDF/Database/typeAreport.pdf. Accessed 31 Aug 2018.

8. Ueshima H, Okayama A, Saitoh S, Nakagawa H, Rodrigues B, Sakata K, Okuda N, Choudhury SR, Curb JD, for the INTERLIPID Resaech group. Differences in cardiovascular disease risk factors between Japanese in Japan and Japanese-Americans in Hawaii: the INTERLIPID study. J Hum Hypertens. 2003;17:631–9.

9. Nakamura H, Arakawa K, Itakura H, Kitabatake A, Goto Y, Toyota T, Nakaya N, Nishimoto S, Muranaka M, Yamamoto A, Muzuno K, Ohashi Y, for the MEGA Study Group. Primary prevention of cardiovascular disease with pravastatin in Japan (MEGA study): a prospective randomised controlled trial. Lancet. 2006;368:1155–63.

10. Nienaber CA, Fattori R, Mehta RH, Richartz BM, Evangelista A, Petzsch M, Cooper JV, Januzzi JL, Ince H, Sechtem U, Bossone E, Jianming F, Smith DE, Isselbacher EM, Pape LA, Eagle KA. Gender-related differences in acute aortic dissection. Circulation. 2004;109:3014–21.

11. LeMaire SA, Russell L. Epidemiology of thoracic aortic dissection. Nat Rev Cardiol. 2011;8:103–13.

12. Tsai TT, Trimarchi S, Nienaber CA. Acute aortic dissection: perspectives from the international Registry of acute aortic dissection (IRAD). Eur J Vasc Endovasc Surg. 2009;37:149–59.

13. Reece TB, Green GR, Kron IL. Aortic dissection. In: Cohn LH, editor. Cardiac surgery in the adult. 3rd ed. New York: McGraw-Hill; 2003. p. 53–84.

14. Eang DS, Kake MD. Endovacular therapy for aortic Disection. In Rousseau H, Verhoye JP, Heautor JF. Thoracic aortic diseases. New York: Springer Berlin Heidelberg; 2006. p. 189–97.

15. Uchida N, Shibamura H, Katayama A, Shimada N, Sutoh M, Ishihara H. Operative strategy for acute type a aortic dissection: ascending aortic or hemiarch versus total arch replacement with frozen elephant trunk. Ann Thorac Surg. 2009;87:773–7.

16. Tanaka M, Kimura N, Yamaguchi A, Adachi H. In-hospital and long term results of surgery for acute type a aortic dissection: 243 consecutive patients. Ann Thorac Cardiovasc Surg. 2012;18:18–23.

17. Yamanaka K, Hori Y, Ikarashi J, Kusuhara T, Nakastuka D, Hirose K, Nishina F, Fujita M. Durability of aortic valve prevervartion with root reconstruction for acute type a aortic dissection. Eur J Cardiothorac Surg. 2012;41(4):e32–36.

18. Hata M, Suzuki M, Sezai A, Niino T, Yoshitake I, Unosawa S, Shimamura K, Minami K. Outcome of less invasive proximal arch replacement with moderate hypothermic circulatory arrest followed by aggressive rapid re-warming in emergency surgery for acute type a aortic dissection. Circ J. 2009;73:69–72.

19. Minatoya K, Ogino H, Matsuda H, Sasaki K. Rapid and safe establishment of cardiopulmonary bypass in repair of acute aortic dissection: improved results with double cannulation. Interact Cardiovasc Thorac Surg. 2008;7: 951–3.

20. Kazui T, Yamashita K, Washiyama N, Terada H, Bashar AH, SuzukiT OK. Impact of an aggressive surgical approach on surgical outcome in type a aortic dissection. Ann Thorac Surg. 2002;74:S1844–7.

21. Song JK, Yim JH, Ahn JM, Kim DH, Kang JW, Lee YT, Song JM, Choo SK, Kang DH, Chung CH, Lee JW, Lim TH. Outcome of patients with acute type a aortic intramural hematoma. Circulation. 2009;120:2046–52.

22. Ryu HM, Lee JH, Kwon SY, Park SH, Lee SH, Bae MH, Lee JH, Yang DH, Park HS, Cho Y, Chae SC, Jun JE, Park WH. Examing the relationship between triggering activities and the circadian distribution of acute aortic dissection. Korean Circ J. 2010;40:565–72.

23. Kim JB, Chung CH, Moon DH, Ha GJ, Lee TY, Jung SH, Choo SJ, Lee JW. Total arch repair versus hemiarch repair in the management of acute DeBakey type I aortic dissection. Eur J Cardiothorac Surg. 2011;40:881–7.

24. Kim EK, Choi ER, Ko SM, Jang SY, Choi SH, Ki CS, Choe YH, Kim WS, Sung K, Oh JK, Kim DK. Comparison of aortic dissection in Korean patients with versus without the marfan syndrome. Am J Cardiol. 2012;109:423–7.

25. OECD. Society at a Glance 2011 - OECD Social Indicators. 2011. Available at: https://www.oecd-ilibrary.org/social-issues-migration-health/society-at-a-glance-16. Accessed 31 Aug 2018.

26. Coady MA, Rizzo JA, Goldstein LJ, Elefterades JA. Natural history, pathogenesis, and etiology of thoracic aortic aneurysm and dissections. Cardiol Clin. 1999;17:615–35.

27. Meszaros I, Morocz J, Szlavi J, Schmidt J, Tornoci L, Nagy L, Szep L. Epidemiology and clinicopathology of aortic dissection: a population-based longitudinal study over 27 years. Chest. 2000;117:1271–8.

28. Clouse WD, Hallett JW Jr, Schaff HV, Spittel PC, Rowland CM, Ilstrup DM, Melton LJ 3rd. Acute aortic dissection: population-based incidence compared with degenerative aortic aneurysm rupture. Mayo Clin Proc. 2004; 79:176–80.

29. Guidelines for Diagnosis and Treatment of Aortic Aneurysm and Aortic Dissection (JCS 2006). J Cardiol. 2007;50:547–77.

30. Yu HY, Chen YS, Huang SC, Wang SS, Lin FY. Late outcome of patients with aortic dissection: study of a national database. Eur J Cardiothoracic Surg. 2004;25:683–90.

31. Sakata R, Fujii Y, Kuwano H. Thoacic and cardiovascular surgery in Japan during 2009. Gen Thorac Cardiovasc Surg. 2011;59:636–67.

25

Early-BYRD: alternative early pacing and defibrillation lead replacement avoiding venous puncture

Andreas Keyser[1]*, Simon Schopka[1], Carsten Jungbauer[2], Maik Foltan[1] and Christof Schmid[1]

Abstract

Background: In cases of lead failure after implantation of pacemakers (PM) or implantable cardioverter defibrillators (ICD) early lead replacement may be challenging. Puncture of the subclavian vein bears possible complications such as pneumothorax, hematothorax, and damage of leads to be left in place. To avoid venous puncture PM or ICD leads were replaced using a flexible polypropylene sheath (Byrd-sheath).

Method: From January 2010 through December 2017, 55 patients underwent early lead exchange avoiding venous puncture. Early lead exchange for this study was defined as a reintervention within 14 days after the initial lead implantation. The connector of the malfunctioning lead was cut off, and stabilized by a stiff stylet. After having cut off the plastic knob of the stylet, the lead was passed through the polypropylene sheath and the latter advanced into the subclavian vein with gentle rotational movements to gain access to the subclavian vein. After lead removal the polypropylene sheath was replaced by a peel away sheath a new lead inserted.

Results: Overall, 23 defibrillation leads and 34 pacing leads (16 right atrial leads, 17 right ventricular leads, and 1 left ventricular lead) were successfully explanted. Access to the subclavian vein was uneventful, and blood loss minimal. Radiation exposure and fluoroscopy time were also negligible.

Conclusion: The Byrd-sheath technique proved to be safe and successful in providing vein access within 2 weeks after initial lead implantation using the previously implanted lead and thus avoiding puncture of the subclavian vein.

Keywords: Pacemaker, Implantable cardioverter defibrillator, Lead exchange, Polypropylene sheath, Venous puncture

Background

Malfunction or dislodgement of pacemaker (PM) or implantable defibrillator/cardioverter (ICD) leads should be corrected as they may result in significant morbidity. However, lead replacement procedures may pose certain risks after implantation of PMs or ICDs. Access to the subclavian vein may cause bleeding at the puncture site, as well as a hematothorax or pneumothorax especially in patients with chronic obstructive pulmonary disease, frailty, or cachexia [1–4]. Furthermore, the leads remaining can be damaged. Anticoagulants or platelet inhibitors increase the risk of bleeding complications with accidental puncture of the adjacent subclavian artery [4].

The manuscript presents results using a modified previously described method of exchanging pacemaker or defibrillator/cardioverter leads maintaining the venous access, and eliminating the need of venous puncture (Byrd-sheath technique) [5, 6].

Method

From January 2010 to December 2017, 55 patients underwent early lead exchange avoiding venous puncture. Early lead exchange for this study was defined as reintervention up to 14 days after the initial lead implantation. All data had been prospectively collected in the institutional database.

Patient data

Demographic data included age, gender, underlying diseases, and anticoagulation as well as the necessary

---

* Correspondence: andreas.keyser@ukr.de
[1]Department of Cardiothoracic Surgery, University Medical Center Regensburg, Franz-Josef-Strauss-Allee 11, 93053 Regensburg, Germany
Full list of author information is available at the end of the article

information with regard to the initial implantation procedure. Procedural data contained time of procedure, time to gain access to the attempted vein, sheaths used, and fluoroscopy time. The procedural success and blood loss during the procedure were documented as well as postoperative pocket hematoma and infection.

Surgical procedure

After having opened the generator pocket any sutures were removed from the lead to be replaced. Any other sutures (e.g. ligature of the cephalic vein) compromising the lead were also removed. Active fixations of leads were loosened. The connector of the lead was cut off and the suture sleeve removed. The lead was stabilized by a standard stiff stylet which was usually provided along with the new lead. The stiff stylet provided enough stiffness to allow advancement of a sheath over the lead. After the plastic knob of the stylet had been cut off, the insulation of the lead was fixed with a suture long enough to pass a flexible polypropylene sheath (Fig. 1). A polypropylene sheath of the size just to slide over the lead was chosen (Byrd Dilator Sheath Polypropylene, Cook Medical, Cook Inc., Bloomington, IN, USA). The sheath was gently advanced towards the subclavian vein with rotational movements using fluoroscopic control and assuring a gentle longitudinal movement without dislodging or distorting of the lead (Fig. 2). As soon as access to the vein was gained, the lead was removed. Access to the vein was indicated by dripping of blood from the polypropylene sheath (Fig. 3). Attention was drawn not to advance the sheath any further. A j-tipped guide wire was placed through the polypropylene sheath and a hemostatic peel-away introducer carefully advanced into the vein (SafeSheath®, Pressure Products Medical

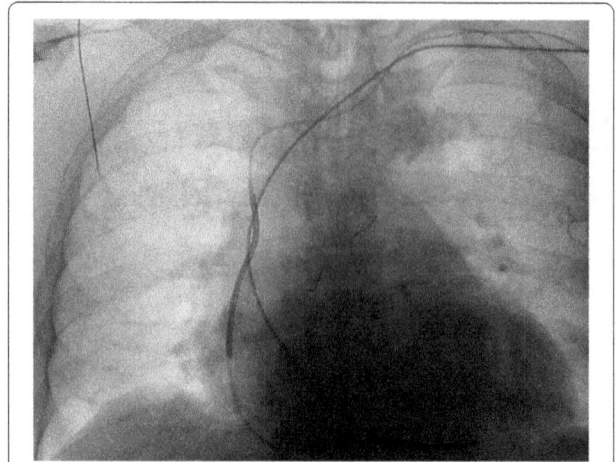

Fig. 2 Radiofluoroscopy. Radioflouroscopic image of Byrd-sheath having been advanced over the lead (note the artrial lead had been loosened from active fixation for removal purose, the ICD lead remaining in place)

Supplies, Inc., Santa Barbara, USA or Prelude SNAP splittable sheath introducer, Merit Medical Systems Inc., Malvern, PA, USA).

Statistical analysis

Statistical analysis was performed with Stata 10.1 SE for Windows (StataCorp., College Station, TX, USA). Continuous data were first tested for normality with the Shapiro–Wilk test. If normally distributed, these data are presented as means ± SD. Dichotomous data are expressed as numbers and percentages. The Mann–Whitney Rank sum test was used for non-normally distributed data. The tests were performed two-sided, and a p-value of < 0.05 was considered to be statistically significant.

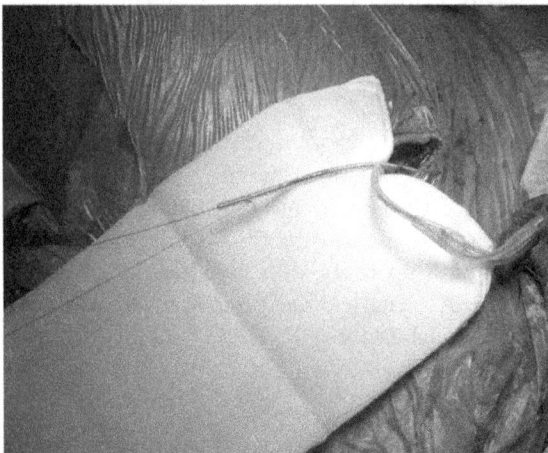

Fig. 1 Preparation of the lead to be exchanged. Stiff stylet in lead to be exchanged, lead insulation fixed with suture (note ICD-lead being left in place)

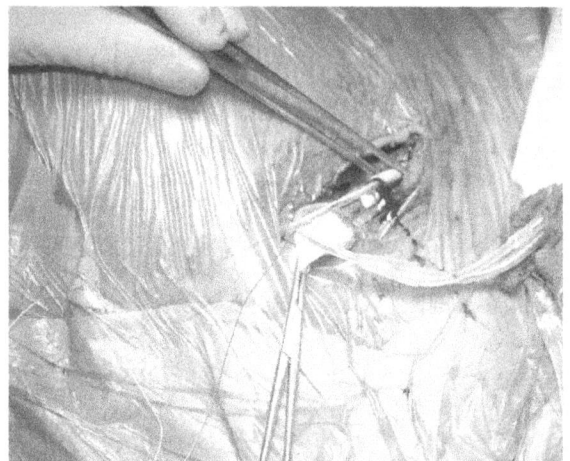

Fig. 3 Access to vein. Byrd-sheath in subclavian vein (note blood dripping from sheath)

Results

Over a period of 8 years, 1946 patients with cardiac implantation of electrical devices were treated, thereof 525 revision procedures including all lead replacements. We detected 55 patients (35 male, 18 female) with early lead malfunction. Mean patient age was 67 ± 11 years (range 36 through 94 years). Twenty-four patients had a Phenprocumon or duel / triple platelet inhibition medication therapy.

Overall, 57 leads had to be replaced. Lead replacement was performed in 25 pacemaker systems (5 VVI, 20 DDD), and 30 ICD systems (14 VVI ICD, 10 DDD ICD, 6 CRT-D). Fifteen patients were referred to our institution for early lead exchange from other hospitals (27%). The indications for replacement were dislocation ($n = 21$), insufficient threshold ($n = 22$), and over-/undersensing ($n = 14$). Accordingly, 23 defibrillation leads, 16 right atrial leads, 17 right ventricular pace-sense leads, and 1 left ventricular lead had to be replaced. The mean dwell time of the leads after implantation was 3.6 ± 3.4 days (range 0 through 12 days). During the procedures, 40 leads in 34 patients remained in place. In 45 patients, the pacemaker or ICD was on the left side (82%), whereas 10 patients had a right-sided implantation (18%). A primary access via the cephalic vein was present in 15 patients (27%).

All procedures were successful. Mean time to gain access to the venous system was 2 ± 1 min. Blood loss was negligible in all cases. X-ray burden of the entire reintervention varied from 75.7 cGy*cm^2 through 6740.7 cGy*cm^2 (mean 1021.2 ± 1095.65 cGy*cm^2) with time of fluoroscopy ranging from 0.24 min to 15.4 min (mean 3.28 ± 3.02 min). No postoperative pocket hematoma or infection developed. There were neither major nor minor complications.

We could not find a significant difference between patients with pacemaker or implantable cardioverter-defibrillator concerning the body mass index or age ($p = 0.165$; $p = 0.479$ respectively). Mean of ejection fraction was better in pacemaker patients compared to ICD patients ($p = < 0.001$). However, there was no difference when comparing pacemaker and ICD patients with respect to access time ($p = 0.392$), procedural time ($p = 0.375$), X-ray time ($p = 0.819$) and X-ray burden ($p = 0.642$).

Significant differences were also not found when comparing male with female patients with respect to ejection fraction ($p = 0.189$), as well as access and procedure time ($p = 0.757$; $p = 0.785$ respectively). Female patients though had a significant higher X-ray time ($p = 0.026$), but the X-ray burden appeared to be comparable and lacked statistical significance ($p = 0.111$).

An immediate lead exchange during the initial implant procedure occurred in 11 of the 55 patients. The procedure time was significantly higher in these patients ($p = < 0.001$). Likewise, the X-ray time and X-ray burden were significantly higher ($p = < 0.001$; $p = 0.003$ respectively).

Discussion

Since Furman and Chardack introduced the first implantable pacemakers in the 1960s [7], the venous access has been improved by King [8] and Belott [9]. With increasing numbers of pacemakers and implantable cardioverter/defibrillators the quantity of lead malfunction steadily rises, and lead replacement remains a necessity and a challenge.

Puncture of the subclavian vein is common to gain access to the venous system in order replace malfunctioning leads. Complications associated with venous puncture are well described. Pneumothorax and hematothorax as major complications are rather infrequent, the incidence is described in 0.1–1.3% [1, 4]. Bleeding at the puncture pocket site as minor complication occurs in up to 2% [10, 11]. Most of the pocket hematomas are related to pocket formation rather than back from the venous system. Further, collateral lead damage is possible to other leads. This is exceedingly rare, though.

Major complications such as perforation of central veins and cardiac cavities have been described in causal connection with lead extraction or replacement [12]. Minor complications, such as pericardial effusion not requiring pericardiocentisis or surgical intervention, and hematothorax not requiring a chest tube, are linked to lead extraction [12]. Arm swelling or thrombosis of implant veins resulting in medical intervention, hematoma at the surgical site requiring reoperation for drainage, vascular repair near the implant site or venous entry site, blood transfusion related to blood loss during surgery, and pulmonary embolism not requiring surgical intervention are further adverse events classified as minor complications [12].

Using polypropylene sheaths to gain access to the venous system also bears the risk of bleeding, too, as the outer diameter is significantly larger than the lead body itself. Thorough surgery may well prevent bleeding back from the venous system even if a polypropylene sheath with is used. Sliding a properly sized peel-away introducer over the lead after it has been stabilized with a stiff stylet does not achieve the same results. The stiff stylet and the proximal end of the lead will have to be brought forward through the introducer cap in a retrograde manner. Especially when gaining the access to the subclavian vein, the rather soft tip of the peel-away introducer tends to be damaged by surrounding tissue. The damaged tip of the peel-away introducer may inhibit further advancement or even serious injury to the wall of the subclavian vein.

According to the analysis of Sant'Anna et al. we assume the proposed procedure safer, as we observed no bleeding complication with respect to our patients, as half of them were treated with oral anticoagulation or dual / triple platelet inhibition [13]. Neither bleeding from the puncture site nor bleeding as result of puncture of the axillary artery occurs when lead exchange is performed avoiding puncture techniques.

Air embolism is a rare but possible complication when using the polypropylene sheath technique. This complication did not occur and is avoided by keeping the patient in a slight Trendelenburg position during the procedure.

For primary venous access a retained guide wire technique is described by Byrd [14]. It may be helpful as a back-up method to avoid a second venous puncture in cases when the lead planted first has to be exchanged [15]. The guide wire is left in place in the sheath after the dilator is withdrawn, thus allowing the introduction of a second sheath to pass through a new pacing lead. However, this technique requires a larger intruding sheath and can be utilized only during the same implantation procedure when the first implanted lead is problematic. The guide wire itself may interfere with the lead placement. Having placed two guide wires with one introducer and using separate introducers for lead placement does not solve the interference and friction of multiple leads. In any case, these techniques may only be considered for primary implantation procedures.

A wire under the insulation technique to maintain venous access for the purpose of lead exchange has been previously described by Steinberg [16]. This technique may be employed in redo procedures. Yet, lead-on-lead interaction may render this approach challenging having two leads in place. Lead-on-lead interaction especially applies to silicone insulation layers. Even if the lead can be easily moved from the endocardium to the superior vena cava using direct traction, dislocation of the wire is possible with advancement of the lead. As the Byrd-technique indicates venous access as soon as blood is dripping out of the sheath, no further advancement of the sheath is required, thus simplifying he process. After the j-tipped guide-wire has been advanced, the access is secured. Once the access is assured, the situation will equal a normal lead implantation.

Leads with efficient passive fixation leads may be difficult to remove 4–6 months after implantation [14]. Fibrotic attachments develop between chronically implanted leads and venous, valvular and cardiac structures may pose obstacles to successful lead extraction [15]. The same applies to active fixation, as the fixation mechanism, the screw, may not be readily loosened. The reported technique is a modification of the described methods of Byrd and Bongiorni which allows overcoming these obstacles and may easily be used *during* or *early after* lead implantation, sacrificing the original lead(s) [5, 17].

This method may be employed within 1 year whenever lead malfunction occurs [14]. We focussed on early lead exchange ranging from intraoperatively to a maximum of 14 days since the initial implantation to eliminate adhesions possibly occurring within the first year of implant. The indication to sacrifice a lead with early malfunction is seen in bits of myocardium and/or small thrombi compromising the fixation mechanism. This applies to both active and passive fixation mechanisms of leads. Both fixation mechanisms may be impaired and unsatisfactory for proper and safe repositioning of a lead.

We could exchange all leads intended to be replaced leaving additional leads in place. Virtually any leads could be replaced, and any lead could be left in place without dislocation. It seems obvious, that obligate intraoperative lead exchanges proof to have the highest X-ray doses due to the difficulties in achieving a sufficient threshold and/or sensing during lead placement. As only a few seconds of additional time of fluoroscopy are required to gain access to the vein the additional X-ray burden remains negligible, especially when considering the entire procedural X-ray doses of lead exchanges [18]. None of the patients experienced complications due to the redo procedure.

As the implanted pacemaker devices are located in a layer under the pectoral fascia, the procedure of pacemaker lead replacement is well performed in local anaesthesia. We generally implant ICD devices in a sub muscular layer and accordingly approached defibrillator lead replacement in general anaesthesia, which is not mandatory. In any case, the technique of using a sheath for lead replacement itself does not oblige to a certain form of anaesthesia.

Limitation

Our study has several limitations. It was designed as a retrospective study and conducted at one single medical centre. The number of reinterventions and referred patients for early lead exchange appears to be rather high. We interpret the referral of complex patients as a part of the duties of a department of cardiothoracic surgery. The study does not compare venous puncture with the described approach; there may be a selection bias. Experience in lead extraction may be of advantage.

Conclusion

The technique of lead replacement using a flexible polypropylene sheath (Byrd-sheath) proved to be safe and successful in providing venous access using the previously implanted lead and thus avoiding puncture of a vein. The technique is simple and can be performed with standard operating room instruments. When clinically indicated, we advocate our method of replacing pacemaker or defibrillator/cardioverter leads in order to facilitate the procedure and minimize intraoperative complications.

Abbreviations
CRT-D: cardiac resynchronization therapy defibrillator cardioverter; DDD
ICD: duel chamber implantable cardioverter defibrillator; DDD: duel chamber

pacemaker; ICD: implantable defibrillator cardioverter; PM: Pacemaker; VVI ICD: single chamber implantable cardioverter defibrillator; VVI: single chamber pacemaker

Authors' contributions

AK and SS designed the study and are responsible for finalizing the protocol, analysis, and completion of the final manuscript. AK and MF developed the search strategy in consultation with CS. AK conceived the project, developed the protocol, wrote and revised the manuscript. CJ and CS contributed to writing the manuscript. All authors provided critical revision of the protocol and final manuscript. All authors read and approved the final manuscript,

Competing interests

The authors declare that they have no competing interests.

Author details

[1]Department of Cardiothoracic Surgery, University Medical Center Regensburg, Franz-Josef-Strauss-Allee 11, 93053 Regensburg, Germany. [2]Department of Internal Medicine II/Cardiology, University Medical Center, Regensburg, Germany.

References

1. Eerola R, Kaukinen L, Kaukinen S. Analysis of 13800 subclavian vein cathetherisations. Acta Anaesthesiol Scand. 1985;29:193–7.
2. Byrd CL. Safe introducer technique for pacemaker lead implantation. Pace. 1992;15:262–9.
3. Haapaniemi L, Slatis P. Supraclavivular cathetherisation of the superior vena cava. Acta Anaesthesiol Scand. 1974;18:12–22.
4. Ruesch S, Walder B, Tramer MR. Complications of central venous catheters: internal jugular versus subclavian access — a systematic review. Crit Care Med. 2002;30:454–60.
5. Fearnot NE, Smith HJ, Goode LB, Byrd CL, Wilkoff BL, Sellers TD. Intravsascular lead extraction using locking sylets, sheaths, and other techniques. PACE. 1990;13:1871–5.
6. Love CJ. Current concepts in extraction of transvenous pacing and ICD leads. Cardiol Clin. 2000;18:193–217.
7. Furman S, Schwedel JB. An intracardiac pacemaker for stokes-Adams seizures. N Engl J Med. 1959;261:943–8 Pacing Clin Electrophysiol. 2006 May; 29(5):453–8.
8. King SM, Arrington JO, Dalton ML. Permanent transvenous cardiac pacing via the left cephalic vein. Ann Thorac Surg. 1968;5:469–73.
9. Belott PH. A variation to introducer technique for unlimited access to the subclavian vein. Pacing Clin Electrophysiol. 1981;1:43–8.
10. Koh Y, Bingham NE, Law N, Le D, Mariani JA. Cardiac implantable electronic device hematomas: risk factors and effect of prophylactic pressure bandaging. Pacing Clin Electrophysiol. 2017;40:857–67.
11. Masiero S, Connolly SJ, Birnie D, Neuzner J, Hohnloser SH, Vinolas X, Kautzner J, O'Hara G, VanErven L, Gadler F, Wang J, Mabo P, Glikson M, Kutyifa V, Wright DJ, Essebag V, Healey JS. Wound hematoma following defibrillator implantation: incidence and predictors in the Shockless implant evaluation (SIMPLE) trial. Europace. 2017;19:1002–6.
12. Maytin M, Epstein LM. The challenges of tranvenous lead extraction. Heart. 2011;97:425–34.
13. Sant'Anna RT, Leiria TL, Nascimento T, Sant'Anna JOM, Kalil RAK, Lima GG, Verma A, Healey JS, Birnie DH, Essebag V. Meta-analysis of continuous Oral anticoagulants versus heparin bridging in patients undergoing CIED surgery: reappraisal after the BRUISE study. Pace. 2015;38:417–23.
14. Byrd CL. Managing device-related complications and transvenous lead extraction. In: Ellenbogen, et al., editors. Clinical cardiac pacing, defibrillation and resynchronization therapy. 3rd ed. Philadelphia: Saunders Elsevier; 2007. p. 855–930.
15. Wilkoff BL, Byrd CL, Love CJ, Hayes DL, Sellers TD, Schaerf R, Parsonnet V, Epstein LM, Sorrentino RA, Reiser C. Pacemaker Lead extraction with the laser sheath: results of the pacing Lead extraction with the Excimer sheath (PLEXES) trial. J Am Coll Cardiol. 1999;33:1671–6.
16. Steinberg SD, Mayer DA, Tsapogas MJ, Wallack MK. Pacemaker leads: a simple atraumatic method for replacing pacemaker electrodes. Ann Thorac Surg. 2000;70:1426–8.
17. Bongiorni MG. Personal technique and experience: The Pisa approach. In: Bongiorni MG, editor. Tranvenous lead extraction. Milan: Springer-Verlag Italia; 2011. p. 85–7.
18. Perisinakis K, Theocharopoulos N, Damilakis J, Manios E, Vardas P, Gourtsoyiannis N. Fluoroscopically guided implantation of modern cardiac resynchronization devices. Radiation Burden to the Patient and Associated Risks. J Am Coll Cardiol. 2005;46:2335–9.

26

The role of deep hypothermic circulatory arrest in surgery for renal or adrenal tumor with vena cava thrombus: a single-institution experience

Peng Zhu[1], Songlin Du[1], Shijun Chen[2], Shaobin Zheng[2], Yu Hu[1], Li Liu[1] and Shaoyi Zheng[1]* (ID)

Abstract

Background: The aim of this study was to review our experience in managing renal or adrenal tumors with level III or IV inferior vena cava thrombus by using deep hypothermic circulatory arrest (DHCA), and to evaluate survival outcomes.

Methods: Between September 2004 and March 2016, we treated 33 patients with renal or adrenal malignancy tumor and thrombus extending into the inferior vena cava. Patients were identified according to radiographic records and operative findings. Clinicopathological and operative characteristics were recorded, and comparisons of clinical and operative characteristics through DHCA were performed. A Cox regression model was used to determine predictors of perioperative mortality.

Results: Twenty-one out of 33 patients with level III ($n = 15$), level IV ($n = 5$), or level II ($n = 1$) renal or adrenal tumors were treated surgically through cardiopulmonary bypass (CPB) with DHCA, and 12 patients with level II or III tumors were treated surgically through normothermic CPB. Three complications were observed, and one death occurred perioperatively, owing to multiple organ failure. The overall perioperative mortality was 4.7%. There were significant differences in the clinicopathological characteristics, operative duration, estimated blood loss, transfusions and hospital stay depending on use of DHCA. Multivariate analysis indicated that the operative duration (OR, 3.78; $P < 0.001$), estimated blood loss (OR, 1.08; $P = 0.02$), and transfusion (OR, 2.13; $P = 0.038$) during/after surgery were positively associated with higher mortality and morbidity. DHCA failed to reach statistical significance ($P = 0.378$).

Conclusions: Use of CPB and DHCA to treat renal or adrenal tumors allows for complete tumor resection, especially at the T4 stage. Although it can cause physical damage, this technique does not increase operative risk and is a relatively safe approach.

Keywords: Hypothermic arrest, Renal tumor, Thrombectomy, Cardiopulmonary bypass

Background

Tumor thrombus in the inferior vena cava (IVC) occurs in 4–10% of patients with renal cell carcinoma (RCC) and poses a challenge for surgical teams [1]. Because there is no systemic therapy available to significantly decrease tumor burden, surgical intervention is the standard treatment [2]. However, the surgical approach

is associated with substantial morbidity and mortality. To minimize operative complications, ensuring adequate exposure and a virtually bloodless surgical field in the upper abdomen and retroperitoneum is essential.

The IVC must be opened when it is associated with tumors. Surgeons therefore must preoperatively determine the precise extent of the tumor and thrombus, to plan their approach accordingly [3]. The use of cardiopulmonary bypass (CPB) with accompanying deep hypothermic circulatory arrest (DHCA) is a recommended and established adjunct technique for surgical management of patients with renal or adrenal

---

* Correspondence: shaoyizheng@yahoo.com
[1]Department of Cardiovascular Surgery, NanFang hospital, Southern Medical University, 1838 North Guangzhou Avenue, Guangzhou 510515, People's Republic of China
Full list of author information is available at the end of the article

tumors and large IVC tumor thrombi [4]. This approach requires close collaboration between urologic and cardiac surgical teams. In our center, the technique of CPB with DHCA is selected by patients undergoing removal of non-metastatic RCC with intrahepatic or subhepatic IVC thrombus. Furthermore, this approach has been used for selected patients with other types of retroperitoneal malignancy with a large IVC thrombus.

Here, we describe our experience with CPB and DHCA in the management of 33 patients with retroperitoneal tumors and large caval thrombi. The aim of this retrospective study was to elucidate the roles of extracorporeal circulation and deep hypothermic total circulatory arrest in surgical treatment for tumor thrombi extending into the retrohepatic caval vein or right atrium. The investigation was performed with special reference to surgical complications, primary mortality and long-term survival.

Methods

From September 2004 to March 2016, 33 patients with large vena caval tumor thrombi from renal or adrenal malignancy underwent surgical resection and removal of thrombi in our center. Among those, 21 patients were treated with the CPB and DHCA techniques. After institutional review board approval was obtained, the demographics, operative data, and postoperative outcomes of these patients were collected retrospectively from our computerized patient database. All surgical procedures were performed by the urologic surgery team in conjunction with the cardiovascular surgery team. Tumor staging was identified on the basis of radiographic records and/or operative findings, and IVC tumor thrombi were classified according to the Mayo Classification of macroscopic venous invasion in RCC (Fig. 1) [5]. Patient and pathological characteristics including age, sex, T classification (T2, T3, or T4), Eastern Cooperative Oncology Group Performance Status (ECOG PS; 0.1, > 1), tumor size, metastatic status (M0 or M1) estimated blood loss (EBL), intraoperative blood transfusions, and perioperative mortality were recorded. The use of DHCA and the length of stay in the intensive care unit were recorded. Patient demographics and perioperative courses are shown in Tables 1 and 2, respectively.

The preoperative evaluation included abdominal magnetic resonance imaging (MRI) and/or computed tomography (CT) scan, and renal arteriography and/or inferior vena cavography (Fig. 2). Evaluation of the proximal extent of the thrombus is essential for planning appropriate surgical strategies. Right heart catheterization with injection of the superior aspect of the IVC was performed if there was IVC occlusion or if MRI did not

clearly demonstrate the distal extent of the thrombus. In current standard practice, when MRI or CT findings are not definitive, transesophageal echocardiography also has reasonable accuracy in assessing the presence and extent of tumor thrombi. X-ray, brain and lung CTs, as well as Positron Emission Tomography-Computed Tomography (PET-CT), were used to evaluated metastases. Renal arterial embolization was performed 48–72 h before surgery in three patients with evidence of a hypervascular IVC tumor thrombus in renal arteriography.

Seven patients with renal or adrenal tumors and large IVC tumor thrombi showed evidence of distant metastatic disease before surgery. A patient with renal clear cell carcinoma was known to have direct tumor extension into the liver.

The hospital charts of all patients were reviewed, and follow-up information was obtained through direct contact with either the patients or local physicians. Complete follow-up data were available for all patients. The follow-up interval ranged from 6 to 60 months, with a mean of 22 months.

Surgical technique

Radical nephrectomy: Urologists usually choose ventral midline incision, after entering the posterior peritoneal cavity, carefully separating the posterior peritoneal and conglutinated kidney. The IVC showed marked dilation, and tumor thrombi in renal veins or IVC like cords were palpable at that time. Through use of the renal vein as a guide, the renal artery can be accessed and ligated. Separation and perfect traction are important in free renal veins, to allow for ureteral ligation. After opening the sheath of the IVC and the abdominal aorta from the renal hilum, the IVC and renal vein were totally dissociated.

DHCA and removal of tumor thrombi: The anesthetic considerations for CPB with DHCA have been described in detail elsewhere. The surgical technique was performed according to previously described methods [6]. Briefly, a lateral subcostal abdominal incision was made, and the retroperitoneal tumor mass was mobilized. The entire kidney was mobilized and left attached by only the main renal vein to the tumor thrombus. After maximum mobilization of the tumor, a median sternotomy was performed (Fig. 3). The patient was systemically heparinized. The ascending aorta and the right atrium were cannulated. CPB was performed with systemic cooling, using a topical cold solution in the abdomen and chest. After a core temperature of 18 to 20 °C had been achieved, CPB was terminated, and the blood volume was drained into a pump. Before the onset of circulatory arrest, methylprednisolone (1 g) was administered to protect the brain and vital organs during arrest. The ascending aorta was immediately cross-clamped before circulatory arrest.

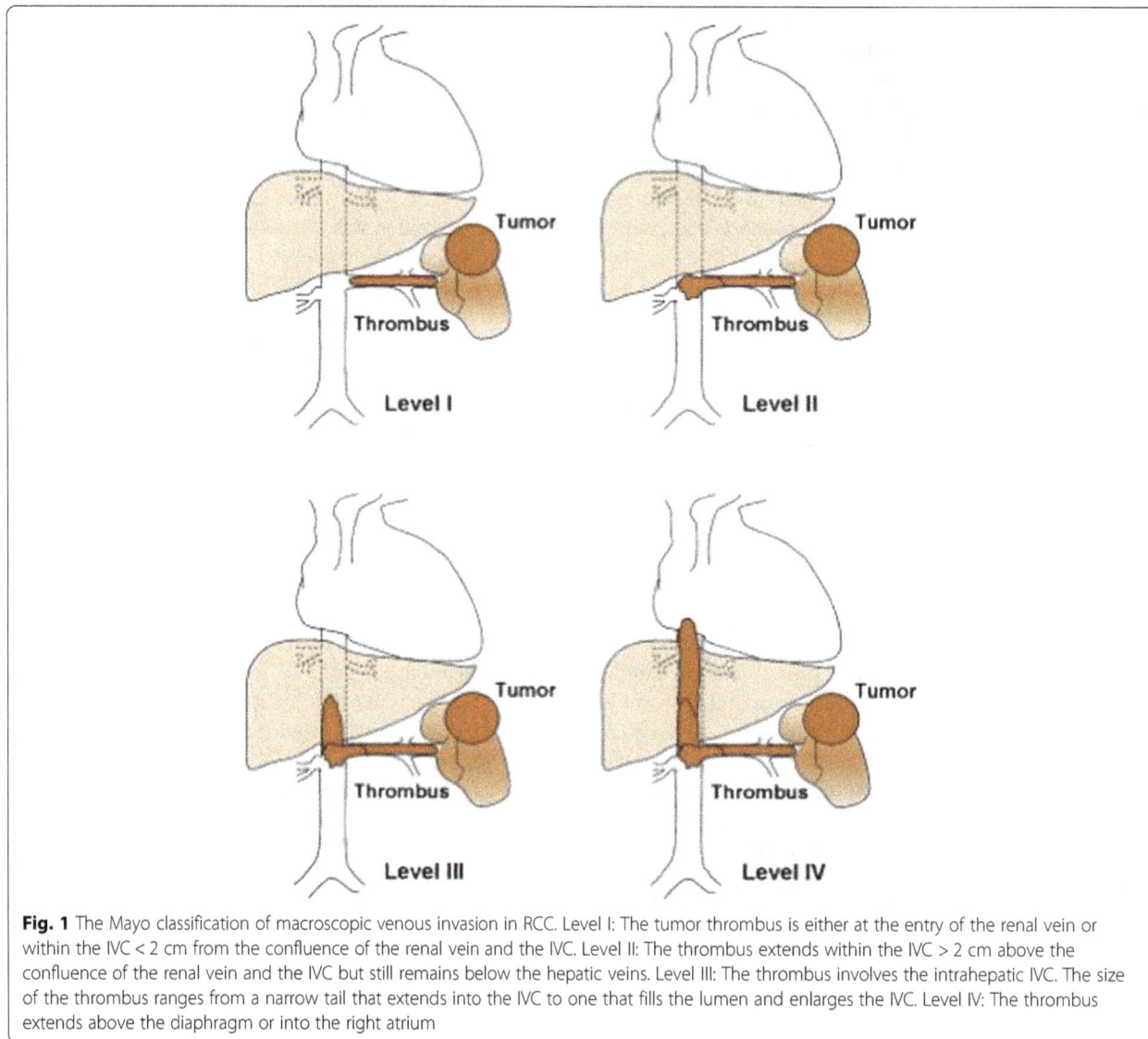

Fig. 1 The Mayo classification of macroscopic venous invasion in RCC. Level I: The tumor thrombus is either at the entry of the renal vein or within the IVC < 2 cm from the confluence of the renal vein and the IVC. Level II: The thrombus extends within the IVC > 2 cm above the confluence of the renal vein and the IVC but still remains below the hepatic veins. Level III: The thrombus involves the intrahepatic IVC. The size of the thrombus ranges from a narrow tail that extends into the IVC to one that fills the lumen and enlarges the IVC. Level IV: The thrombus extends above the diaphragm or into the right atrium

The IVC was mobilized as close to the diaphragm as possible, the RA was opened near the orifice of the IVC, and attention was then directed to the IVC, which was entered near the orifice of the renal vein. The vena caval tumor thrombus was then removed in a bloodless operative field (Fig. 4). After extraction of the thrombus and repair of the caval wall, a two-stage venous cannula was reinserted into the RA, and the right atrium was closed. The CPB was reinstituted, and the patient was rewarmed to a core temperature of 37 °C. During the rewarming procedure, radical nephrectomy was also performed. CPB was then terminated, and heparin was reversed. In all cases, the primary malignancy and IVC tumor thrombus were completely removed (Fig. 5). Atriotomy was performed in five patients with tumor thrombi extending into the right atrium and in selected other patients with friable or adherent thrombi.

Two patients underwent vena caval reconstruction with pericardial grafts. Additional procedures done at the time of CPB with DHCA included coronary artery bypass grafting in one patient with renal clear cell carcinoma, pulmonary resection of metastases in one patient with RCC and hepatic lobectomy in the patient with invasive adrenocortical carcinoma.

Comparisons of patient demographics and operative characteristics were performed between bypass techniques. For the risk analysis, a multiple logistic regression model was developed by using a forward stepwise variable selection method. Fisher's exact test or chi-square test was used for categorical variables, and Student's t-test was used for continuous covariates. P values < 0.05 were considered statistically significant. Analyses were performed in SPSS version 20.0 (IBM Corporation, Somers, NY, USA).

Table 1 The patients clinical, pathological and operative characteristics

	DHCA		P
	No	Yes	
Number of patients	12	21	
Mean(SD)age,years	54.41(15.43)	47.05(13.86)	0.62
Sex M/F,n(%)	6(50%)/6(50%)	14(67%)/7(33%)	0.73
Mean (SD) BMI(kg/m^2)	22.7(4.4)	22.5(4.8)	0.87
T stage,n(%)			0.00
T2	9(75%)	1(5%)	
T3	3(25%)	15(71%)	
T4	0	5(24%)	
Mean(SD)tumour size,mm	8.9(3.4)	9.5(4.2)	0.72
Metastases,n(%)			0.35
No	9(75%)	17(81%)	
Yes	3(25%)	4(19%)	
Fuhrman grade,n(%)			0.63
2	1(8%)	3(14%)	
3	8(67%)	13(61%)	
4	3(25%)	5(24%)	
ECOG PS,n(%)			0.21
0	5(42%)	14(67%)	
1	6(50%)	5(24%)	
>1	1(8%)	2(10%)	
Mean (SD) Serum creatinine,umol/l	76.37(15.26)	77.12(12.54)	0.62

M male, *F* female

Table 2 The operative characteristics of patients compared by use of DHCA

Variable	DHCA		P
	No	Yes	
Operative duration,min			0.00
n	12	21	
Mean(median)	267.9(96.7)	521.9(120.6)	
EBL,ml			0.01
n	12	21	
Mean(median)	854.3(863.8)	5933.7(8040)	
Transfusions,n			
n	5	21	
Mean(median)	4.8(3.1)	17.22(11.67)	
ICU stay,days			
n	1	21	
Mean(median)	6	6.4(1.3)	
Hospital stay,days			0.00
n	12	33	
Mean(median)	13.8(4.4)	28.5(14.3)	
Perioperative mortality,n			0.58
n	12	21	
N(%)deaths	0	1(4.7)	
Tumor pathology			
renal clear cell carcinoma	5(41.7)	8(38.1)	
renal cell carcinoma	3(0.25)	5(23.8)	
adrenocortical	2(16.7)	4(19.0)	
Whilms tumor	2(16.7)	3(14.3)	
renal pelvic transitional carcinoma	0	1(4.7)	

Results

Between September 2004 and March 2016, 33 consecutive patients (20 males, 13 females) undergoing surgery were identified. The clinicopathological characteristics of all patients are summarized in Table 1. At the time of surgery, the median age was 50 years (IQR: 18 to 72 years). The tumor was located on the left in six (18.2%) patients and on the right in 27 (81.8%) patients.

The renal tumors had a median size of 9.3 (IQR: 6–15 cm). The median total operation time was 521 min, with median CPB and DHCA durations of 191 min and 40.5 min, respectively, and the median total operation time was 267 min without CPB.

In the CPB with DHCA group, the median estimated blood loss was 5933 ml (IQR: 1000 to 26,000), and all patients required blood transfusions, with a median estimated RBC transfusion volume of 17.22 U (IQR: 7–45).At the beginning of the study, three patients had uncontrollable hemorrhage during surgical removal of the tumor,and an extracorporeal circulation with DHCA techniques were urgently established to complete the surgery. The blood loss and transfusion volume in the three patients caused statistical fluctuations.The decision to administer blood was based on preoperative hemoglobin levels and the degree of blood loss. The overall perioperative mortality was 4.7%.

Only one operative death occurred, in a 51-year-old woman with severe congestive cardiac failure. This patient experienced intraoperative heart failure and could not be weaned from CPB. Three complications were observed in this patient cohort: re-operation because of bleeding ($n = 1$), acute renal failure (n = 1) and severe post-operative subcutaneous hydrops. All of the remaining complications were resolved with appropriate treatment. There were no other ischemic or neurologic complications. There were no cases of perioperative tumor embolization. The average hospital stay of surviving patients was 20 days (range: 8–56 days), and 6.4 days in the intensive care unit (range: 4 to 8 days). Pathologic examination of the tumors revealed that 13 (39.3%) patients had renal clear cell carcinoma, eight (24.2%) patients had RCC, six (18.1%) patients had

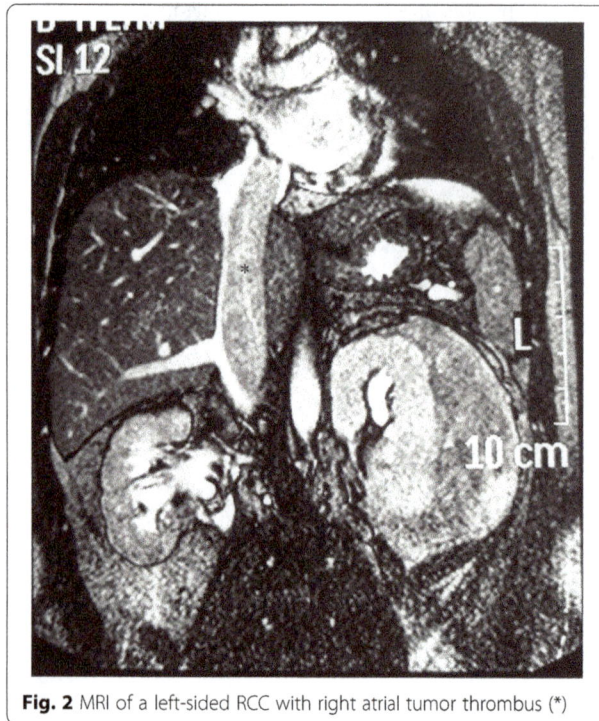

Fig. 2 MRI of a left-sided RCC with right atrial tumor thrombus (*)

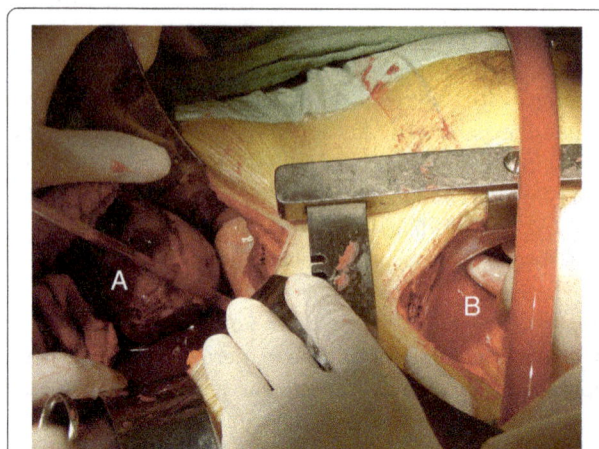

Fig. 4 Without blood, the thrombus (arrow) of the hepatic segment was excised and plastic IVC was performed. The right-sided RCC(*)

adrenocortical carcinoma, five (15.1%) patients had Wilms' tumor, and one (3%) patient had renal pelvic transitional carcinoma.

Comparisons of patient characteristics based on the bypass technique are shown in Table 2. There were no differences in patient perioperative mortality between patients undergoing either bypass technique. The pathological (T stage), operative duration, EBL, transfusion, and hospital stay differed depending on bypass techniques, and tumor pathology were listed in Table 2.

Risk factors potentially contributing to perioperative mortality were assessed. Multivariate analysis indicated that operative duration (OR, 3.78; $P < 0.001$), estimated blood loss (OR, 1.08; $P = 0.02$), and transfusion (OR, 2.13; $P = 0.038$) during/after surgery were each positively associated with increased mortality and morbidity. DHCA failed to reach statistical significance ($P = 0.378$).

The median follow-up time for the patients was 24 months (range: 6–60 months) after surgery. The mean overall survival period of the cohort was 34.5 ± 6.7 months, and the disease-free survival period was 26.6 ± 17.4 months. After surgery, liver metastases were found in five patients, and lung metastases were found in four patients. Abdominal metastases were found in

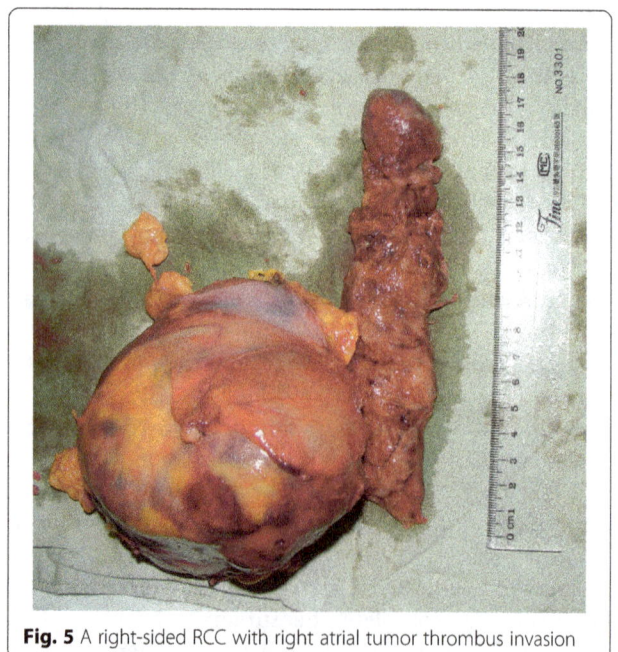

Fig. 3 Incisions used for a right-sided tumor. **a** An abdominal rectus incision was made to expose the right renal and IVC. **b** CPB and DHCA were performed through a chest median incision

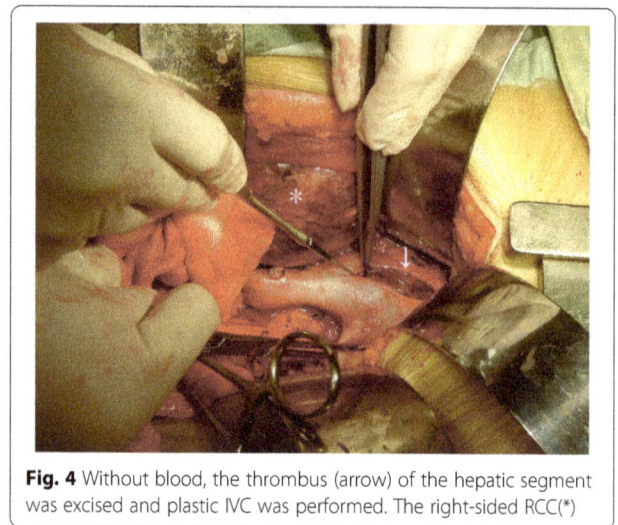

Fig. 5 A right-sided RCC with right atrial tumor thrombus invasion

two patients at 3 months after surgery: one had been alive for 22 months, and the other had been alive for 7 months. The opposite renal metastases were found in two patients at 4 and 36 months after surgery, who had been alive for 6 months and 48 months. Seven patients with metastases refused further treatment, and follow-up was lost; the other patients with metastases were administered chemotherapy and/or targeted therapy. The mean overall survival of patients without metastases was 38.3 ± 22.4 months.

Discussion

Among retroperitoneal tumors, including renal and retroperitoneal sarcoma, renal pelvic transitional cell carcinoma, Wilms' tumor pheochromocytoma, adrenocortical carcinoma and some lymphomas, RCC is most often found to invade the IVC, even in the absence of distant metastases [7]. RCC has a biological propensity toward intravascular invasion of the renal vein and extension into the IVC. Neoplastic invasion of the IVC occurs in 5–15% of patients with renal cancer, and the tumor embolus extends to the right atrium in 14–39% of patients [8]. Renal or adrenal tumor with IVC tumor thrombus often implies an unfavorable prognosis that is unsuitable for surgery. Radical nephrectomy together with thrombectomy is the most effective therapeutic method after medical therapies have proven ineffective [9]. However, surgical management for patients with RCC with a tumor thrombus extending into the IVC, or even the right atrium, poses a major surgical challenge. Although renal tumors often extend into the IVC before clinical diagnosis, unlike other tumors, their prognosis is fairly good if the tumor is surgically resected and metastatic disease is absent [10].

Several surgical techniques for the treatment of these tumors have been proposed, but they are limited by small patient numbers and limited follow-up [1–3]. Additionally, several reports have combined patients with different bypass techniques and different levels of thrombi. Moreover, substantial controversy regarding the best operative management method still persists regarding treatment of RCC patients with level III or IV thrombi. Some surgeons have reported the use of CPB without circulatory arrest and vascular occlusion without CPB to facilitate the removal of tumor thrombi. Level IV thrombi can be managed with veno-venous bypass and/ or caval-atrial shunt [11, 12]. Although high-level thrombi can be removed successfully without CPB and DHCA, kidney health and liver function may be affected postoperatively, even when the procedures are performed by experienced surgeons. In our institution, our experience suggests that use of CPB and DHCA decreases the risk of life-threatening intra-operative hemorrhage and incomplete thrombus removal. As

performed by a urological surgery team in conjunction with a cardiovascular surgery team, CPB and DHCA have been safely used to treat RCC with high-level IVC thrombi.

The use of DHCA has been questioned in surgical resection, because there is concern regarding the risk of hemorrhage with heparinization and neurological sequelae with low-flow cerebral perfusion. CPB with hypothermia may be associated with platelet dysfunction. However, when CPB is combined with systemic use of heparin, coagulopathy and bleeding from the retroperitoneum are risks. The present study and our data demonstrated CPB with DHCA to be safe in cases of level III or IV tumor thrombus. The deep hypothermia in conjunction with circulatory arrest, thought to limit renal and liver ischemia in thrombus removal, may protect the contralateral kidney and decrease postoperative dialysis. Hence, CPB with DHCA may potentially decrease perioperative mortality. Hatcher et al. [13] have reported that patients who underwent extraction of a mobile tumor thrombus from the vena cava had a 69% 5-year survival (median, 9.9 years), whereas patients with tumor thrombi directly invading the vena cava had a 26% 5-year survival (median, 1.2 years), which improved to 57% (median 5.3 years) when the involved vena caval side wall was resected successfully. In such cases, curative resection might be feasible with reasonable long-term survival.

Surgical techniques have been developed to remove tumor thrombi extending into the retrohepatic caval vein and the right atrium [14] These procedures are accompanied by risks of unexpected and life-threatening hemorrhage with hypotension, disruption, and embolization of the tumor into the pulmonary arteries, myocardial infarction, stroke, renal failure, and hepatic dysfunction [15]. In contrast, the use of DHCA can decrease the risks of warm hepatic and renal ischemia and of incomplete tumor extirpation. This technique allows adequate hemodynamics to be maintained during long surgical interventions in several serous cavities. Moreover, it allows for removal of thrombi and tumorous cells from cardiac cavities, and prevention of hematogenous debrimetatases from intravascular tumors. The necessity for DHCA is debatable if the IVC can be completed within 10 min in every case [16]. However, longer times are occasionally needed for meticulous curetting or complicated reconstruction. In addition, because the situation cannot be predicted in advance, we use deep hypothermia to minimize neurologic complications.

Akchurin et al. [17] have demonstrated that CPB and the cell-saver technique in combination with oncologic and cardiovascular surgery does not increase the risk of hematogenous dissemination. They studied eight patients who underwent oncologic surgery and open heart surgery or procedures on major blood vessels. In three patients, the intravascular portion of the tumor was extracted as much as possible through a right atrium approach (in three cases the tumor invaded the IVC). All of the patients had uneventful postoperative periods and were alive 1 year after the procedures. During cytological investigation after each operation, tumor cells were found only on the internal surfaces of the heart-lung machine arterial filters with 20 μm holes. That study suggests that special cardiovascular devices such as the heart-lung machine and cell saver might be used in borderline situations in oncology without increasing the risk of hematogenous tumor dissemination. In our hospital, we suspended blood reclamation when the whole tumor embolus was exposed. After the tumor thrombus was carefully dissected from the IVC wall and removed en bloc, we rinsed the abdominal cavity with saline repeatedly, then resumed blood reclamation. This procedure enables surgeons to re-infuse lost blood and avoid transfusion with donated blood to overcome immune and post transfusion complications. Furthermore, the current approach decreased the risk of hematogenous dissemination resulting from aspiration of the tumor cells from the surgical wound.

Limitations

Our study has several limitations. A limited number of patients were enrolled, and the follow-up time was relatively short. We used CPB with DHCA alone in surgical resection without other techniques. A randomized controlled trial should be conducted in the future to compare this technique with other surgical techniques for the management of RCC with level III or IV tumor thrombus. Finally, we were unable to perform adjustment for surgical-team or surgeon-specific characteristics that might have made the analysis more robust.

Conclusions

Renal carcinoma with tumor extension into the IVC presents a major surgical challenge. Surgery for RCC and high-level tumor thrombus by using CPB with DHCA, a preferred surgical technique, provides better visibility of the vascular anatomy, thus allowing for complete extraction of the thrombus, regardless of its invasiveness and potential for adverse effects. In addition, this technique significantly decreases both the rate of severe intraoperative complications and the perioperative mortality. These results suggest that long-term survival is possible if radical nephrectomy and complete extirpation of the tumor thrombus are performed, and the use of CPB with DHCA and retrograde cerebral perfusion results in favorable outcomes. Further prospective studies are needed to evaluate the possible benefits of DHCA and other surgical techniques to decrease the potential risk of cavoatrial tumor extension.

Abbreviations

CPB: Cardiopulmonary bypass; DHCA: Deep hypothermic circulatory arrest; EBL: Estimated blood loss; IBS: Intraoperative blood salvage; IVC: Inferior vena cava; MRI: Magnetic resonance imaging; OR: Odds Ratic; PET-CT: Positron emission tomography-computed tomography; RCC: Renal cell carcinoma; VVBP: Venovenous bypass

Funding

This work was supported by the President Foundation of NanFang hospital,Southern Medical University (Grant No.2017B022).

Authors' contributions

PZ designed the study, collected the clinical data and performed the statistical analysis, participated in the operation and drafted the manuscript. SLD,SJC, SBZ,YH and LL participated in the operation and revised the paper. ZKW and SYZ designed and supervised the study. All authors read and approved the final manuscript.

Competing interests

The authors declare that they have no competing interests.

Author details

[1]Department of Cardiovascular Surgery, NanFang hospital, Southern Medical University, 1838 North Guangzhou Avenue, Guangzhou 510515, People's Republic of China. [2]Department of Urinary Surgery, NanFang hospital, Southern Medical University, GuangZhou, People's Republic of China.

References

1. Chiappini B, Savini C, Marinelli G, Suarez SM, Di Eusanio M, Fiorani V, Pierangeli A. Cavoatrial tumor thrombus: single-stage surgical approach with profound hypothermia and circulatory arrest, including a review of the literature. J Thorac Cardiovasc Surg. 2002;124:684–8.
2. Blute ML, Leibovich BC, Lohse CM, Cheville JC, Zincke H. The Mayo Clinic experience with surgical management, complications and outcome for patients with renal cell carcinoma and venous tumour thrombus. BJU Int. 2004;94:33–41.
3. Lawindy SM, Kurian T, Kim T, Mangar D, Armstrong PA, Alsina AE, Sheffield C, Sexton WJ, Spiess PE. Important surgical considerations in the management of renal cell carcinoma (RCC) with inferior vena cava (IVC) tumour thrombus. BJU Int. 2012;110:926–39.
4. Pouliot F, Shuch B, Larochelle JC, Pantuck A, Belldegrun AS. Contemporary management of renal tumors with venous tumor thrombus. J Urol. 2010; 184:833–41. quiz 1235
5. Neves RJ, Zincke H. Surgical treatment of renal cancer with vena cava extension. Br J Urol. 1987;59:390–5.
6. Marshall FF, Reitz BA, Diamond DA. A new technique for management of renal cell carcinoma involving the right atrium: hypothermia and cardiac arrest. J Urol. 1984;131:103–7.
7. Siegel RL, Miller KD, Jemal A. Cancer statistics, 2015. CA Cancer J Clin. 2015;65:5–29.
8. Langenburg SE, Blackbourne LH, Sperling JW, Buchanan SA, Mauney MC, Kron IL, Tribble CG. Management of renal tumors involving the inferior vena cava. J Vasc Surg. 1994;20:385–8.
9. Subramanian VS, Stephenson AJ, Goldfarb DA, Fergany AF, Novick AC, Krishnamurthi V. Utility of preoperative renal artery embolization for management of renal tumors with inferior vena caval thrombi. Urology. 2009;74:154–9.
10. Shuch B, Crispen PL, Leibovich BC, LaRochelle JC, Pouliot F, Pantuck AJ, Liu W, Crepel M, Schuckman A, Rigaud J, et al. Cardiopulmonary bypass and renal cell carcinoma with level IV tumour thrombus: can deep hypothermic

circulatory arrest limit perioperative mortality? BJU Int. 2011;107:724–8.

11. Foster RS, Mahomed Y, Bihrle R, Strup S. Use of a caval-atrial shunt for resection of a caval tumor thrombus in renal cell carcinoma. J Urol. 1988; 140:1370–1.

12. Ciancio G, Soloway MS. Renal cell carcinoma with tumor thrombus extending above diaphragm: avoiding cardiopulmonary bypass. Urology. 2005;66:266–70.

13. Marshall FF, Dietrick DD, Baumgartner WA, Reitz BA. Surgical management of renal cell carcinoma with intracaval neoplastic extension above the hepatic veins. J Urol. 1988;139:1166–72.

14. Novick AC, Kaye MC, Cosgrove DM, Angermeier K, Pontes JE, Montie JE, Streem SB, Klein E, Stewart R, Goormastic M. Experience with cardiopulmonary bypass and deep hypothermic circulatory arrest in the management of retroperitoneal tumors with large vena caval thrombi. Ann Surg. 1990;212:472–6. discussion 476-477

15. Chen YH, Wu XR, Hu ZL, Wang WJ, Jiang C, Kong W, Chen W, Xue W, Liu DM, Huang YR. Treatment of renal cell carcinoma with a level III or level IV inferior vena cava thrombus using cardiopulmonary bypass and deep hypothermic circulatory arrest. World J Surg Oncol. 2015;13:159.

16. Orihashi K, Sueda T, Usui T, Shigeta M. Deep hypothermic circulatory arrest for resection of renal tumor in the inferior vena cava: beneficial or deleterious? Circ J. 2008;72:1175–7.

17. Akchurin RS, Davidov MI, Partigulov SA, Brand JB, Shiriaev AA, Lepilin MG, Dolgov IM. Cardiopulmonary bypass and cell-saver technique in combined oncologic and cardiovascular surgery. Artif Organs. 1997;21:763–5.

27

Feasibility of a novel, synthetic, self-assembling peptide for suture-line haemostasis in cardiac surgery

Suresh Giritharan[1,2]*, Kareem Salhiyyah[1], Geoffrey M. Tsang[1] and Sunil K. Ohri[1]

Abstract

Background: To assess the feasibility and efficacy of PuraStat®, a novel haemostatic agent, in achieving suture line haemostasis in a wide range of cardiac surgical procedures and surgery of the thoracic aorta.

Methods: A prospective, non-randomised study was conducted at our institution. Operative data on fifty consecutive patients undergoing cardiac surgery where PuraStat® was utilised in cases of intraoperative suture line bleeding was prospectively collected. Questionnaires encompassing multiple aspects of the ease of use and efficacy of PuraStat® were completed by ten surgeons (five consultants and five senior registrars) and analysed to gauge the performance of the product.

Results: No major adverse cardiac events were reported in this cohort. Complications such as atrial fibrillation, pacemaker requirement and pleural effusions were comparable to the national average. Mean blood product use of packed red cells, platelets, fresh-frozen plasma (FFP) and cryoprecipitate was below the national average. There was one incidence of re-exploration, however this was due to pericardial constriction rather than bleeding. Analysis of questionnaire responses revealed that surgeons consistently rated PuraStat® highly (between a score of 7 and 10 in the various subcategories). The transparent nature or PuraStat® allowed unobscured visualisation of suture sites and possessed excellent qualities in terms of adherence to site of application. The application of PuraStat® did not interfere with the use of other haemostatic agents or manipulation of the suture site by the surgeon.

Conclusion: PuraStat® is an easy-to-use and effective haemostatic agent in a wide range of cardiac and aortic surgical procedures.

Keywords: Cardiac surgery, Bleeding, Haemostasis, Haemostatic agents, Blood loss, Blood products, Transfusion

Background

Meticulous haemostasis remains a core principal in surgical practice, both for patient safety and for preserving the integrity of surgical repair [1]. The challenge of cardiac surgery involves operating on patients who are receiving single and dual antiplatelet or anticoagulant therapy, systemic heparinization and the effects of hypothermia on the clotting cascade [2]. The consequences of massive haemorrhage are well recognised and rare in modern practice as bleeding into the pericardial space can lead to haemodynamic compromise by cardiac tamponade.

The search for an ideal haemostatic adjunct to complement suturing of cardiac and aortic tissue and in fashioning anastomoses is ongoing, as the agent must possess a comprehensive catalogue of qualities such as ease of application, good adherence to site of use, cause minimal tissue reaction and prove robust in withstanding volume and pressure changes generated from the beating heart [3]. Currently there are many established haemostatic agents on the market with varying mechanisms of action, which attests to the fact that there is no one ideal agent (Figs. 1 and 2).

In this study we report our experience using PuraStat® (3-D Matrix Europe SAS, Caluire et Cuire, France) a

---

* Correspondence: suresh.giritharan@gmail.com
[1]Wessex Cardiac Centre, University Hospitals Southampton, Tremona Road, Southampton SO16 6YD, UK
[2]Southampton, UK

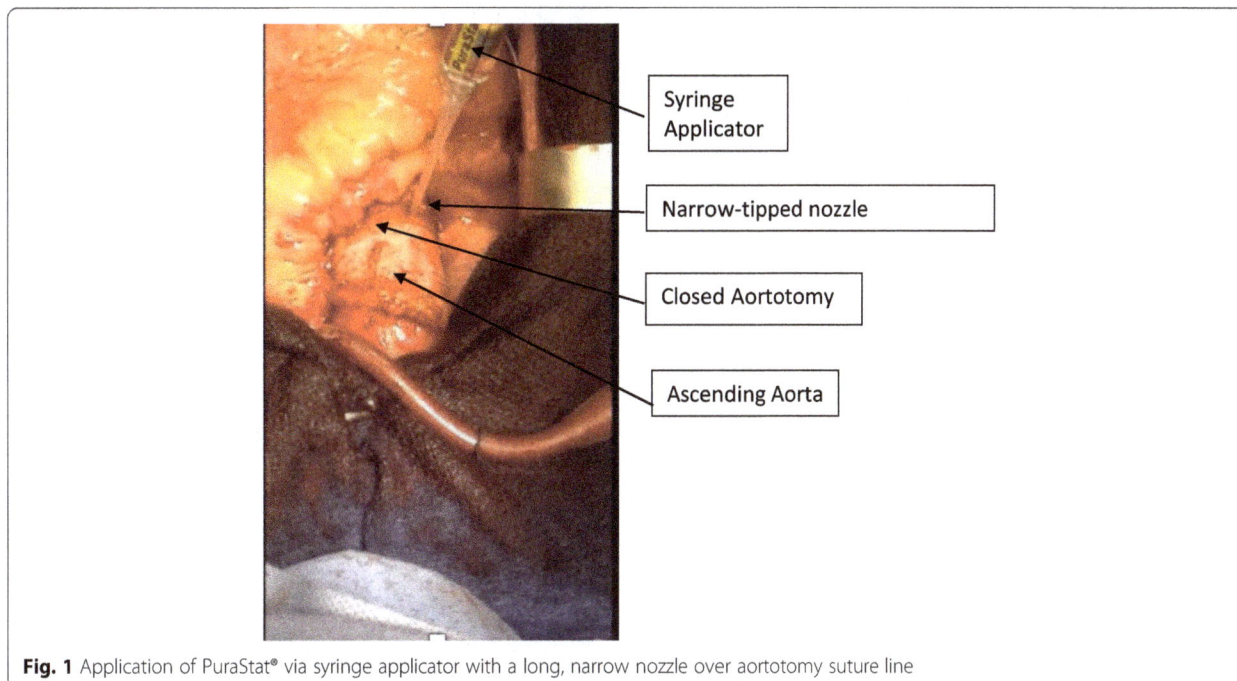

Fig. 1 Application of PuraStat® via syringe applicator with a long, narrow nozzle over aortotomy suture line

novel synthetic haemostat. It relies upon nanotechnology with the self-assembling of constituent peptides, which is triggered by sodium ions within the blood to form a synthetic, non-biogenic, biocompatible, resorbable peptide hydrogel with no risk of transmissible spongiform encephalopathies [4]. It is CE-marked for haemostatic use in humans and is currently being used successfully as a standalone haemostatic agent in endoluminal gastrointestinal procedures, among other applications [5]. Our aim was to investigate the haemostatic efficacy of PuraStat® for cardiac and aortic anastomoses and suture lines.

Methods

A prospective, non-randomised study was conducted at our institution between February 2017 and September 2017. A total of fifty patients undergoing cardiac surgery at the Wessex Cardiothoracic Centre (Southampton, UK) and The Spire Hospital (Southampton, UK) were recruited. The inclusion criteria encompassed all adult cardiac surgery cases where the intraoperative use of a haemostatic agent was deemed necessary. A comprehensive case-mix including coronary artery bypass surgery, aortic valve surgery, mitral valve surgery, surgery on the thoracic aorta and other concomitant procedures (e.g. atrial fibrillation ablation procedures) were included, encompassing elective, urgent and emergency presentations. Patients whom exhibited preoperative derangements in haematological and coagulation profiles, and baseline derangements in liver function were excluded. Baseline demographic data such as age, gender, BMI, hypertension, diabetes, hypercholesterolaemia, previous myocardial infarction (MI), left ventricular (LV) function, smoking status, asthma or chronic obstructive pulmonary disease (COPD), renal impairment, neurological

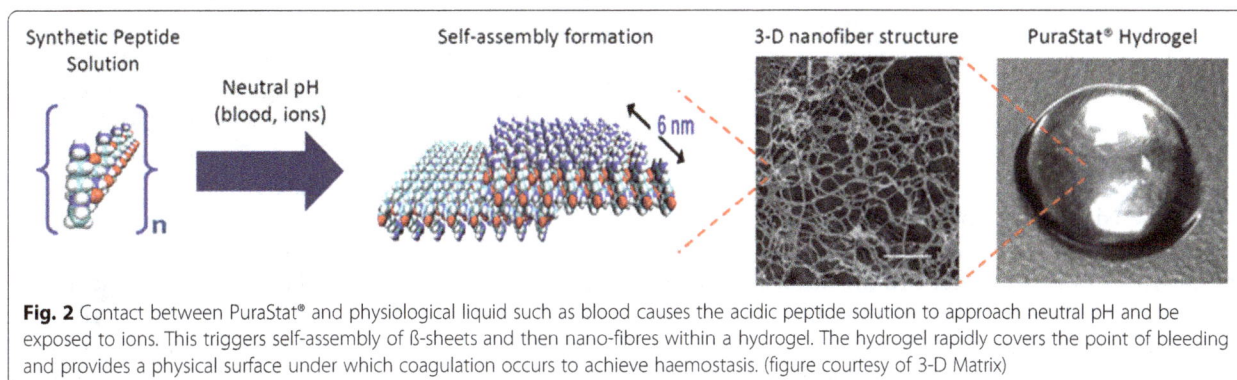

Fig. 2 Contact between PuraStat® and physiological liquid such as blood causes the acidic peptide solution to approach neutral pH and be exposed to ions. This triggers self-assembly of ß-sheets and then nano-fibres within a hydrogel. The hydrogel rapidly covers the point of bleeding and provides a physical surface under which coagulation occurs to achieve haemostasis. (figure courtesy of 3-D Matrix)

impairment and peripheral vascular disease was collected from pre-admission clerking sheets. Additional data included the use of preoperative antiplatelet or anticoagulant therapy. Preoperative blood results for haemoglobin, platelet count, INR, APTR and fibrinogen were also noted.

Intraoperative data included details of the operation, cardiopulmonary bypass time, aortic cross-clamp time and site of use of PuraStat® and if additional haemostatic agents were required to achieve haemostasis. In all cases, the application of PuraStat® was done following reversal of systemic heparinization with Protamine Sulfate.

As the purpose of this study was to evaluate feasibility and efficacy, a questionnaire was developed with a view of gaining detailed observation and feedback on the use of PuraStat® in various scenarios. These questionnaires were given to the operating surgeon to complete following use of the product. The surgeons were asked to score the product on a scale of 1–10 for various factors. These were site of application, grade of bleeding, ease of preparation, time of preparation, ease of delivery to the sterile field, ease of use, delivery to the sterile field, application, conformation to irregular surfaces, compatibility with other haemostatic agents (when used), and reduction in haemostatic time. The questionnaire paid particular emphasis on the efficacy of PuraStat® alone in achieving haemostasis, and if not, what other haemostatic agent was used in conjunction with PuraStat®. Surgeons were also asked about their overall satisfaction with PuraStat®. A total of ten surgeons (five consultants and five senior registrars) provided feedback.

Chest drain output over the first 24 h was recorded along with the total use of blood products (packed red blood cells, platelets, fresh frozen plasma (FFP) and cryoprecipitate). Postoperative complications such as death, postoperative myocardial infarction, stroke, re-exploration for bleeding, atrial fibrillation, other arrhythmia, pleural effusion and reintubation were collated from a review of contemporaneously-completed inpatient notes. The results were then tabulated, with categorical variables expressed as a percentage of the total patient population and continuous variables expressed as the mean value with standard deviations. The mean rating for each criterion gauged in the questionnaire was calculated.

Results
Baseline demographics
Within the seven-month period, a total of fifty patients were recruited, and their baseline demographics are displayed below (Table 1) The mean age was 71.9 ± 10.4 years and the mean body mass index (BMI) was 28.7 ± 4.8 kg/m². Thirty (60%) of participants were male and twenty (40%) were female. In terms of preoperative comorbidities, twenty-eight (56%) had hypertension (defined as patients

Table 1 Baseline Demographics of Patients

Variable	number (% of total)	mean	SD
Age		71.9	10.4
Gender			
Male	30 (60%)		
Female	20 (40%)		
BMI (kg/m²)		28.7	4.8
Hypertension	28 (56%)		
Diabetes	11 (22%)		
Myocardial Infarction?	5 (10%)		
Asthma/COPD	3 (6%)		
Peripheral Vascular Disease	5 (10%)		
Never smoked	36 (72%)		
Left Ventricular Function			
Good	45 (90%)		
Moderate	4 (8%)		
Poor	1 (2%)		
Preoperative Blood Results			
Haemoglobin		130.5	14.3
Platelets		240.2	71.6
INR		1.06	0.12
APTR		1.05	0.2
Fibrinogen		4.54	1.18

Values are total number of patients, n (% of n), mean and standard deviation (SD). BMI, body mass index; MI, myocardial infarction; COPD, chronic obstructive pulmonary disease; INR, international normalized ratio; APTR, activated partial thromboplastin time ratio

receiving antihypertensive medications or having known but untreated hypertension [blood pressure > 140/90 mmHg]), eleven patients (22%) had diabetes (fasting glucose > 7 mmol/L), five patients had preoperative myocardial infarction (10%), three patients (6%) had chronic obstructive pulmonary disease (COPD) and four patients (8%) had peripheral vascular disease (PVD). Thirty-six (72%) of the participants had never smoked.

All patients in this cohort underwent preoperative transthoracic echocardiographic examination. Forty-five (90%) of patients had good left ventricular function, four patients (8%) had moderate left ventricular function and one patient (2%) had poor left ventricular function. Blood results taken prior to surgery demonstrated mean values for haemoglobin level (130.5 ± 14.3 g/dL), platelet count (240.2 ± 71.6 × 10e9/L), INR (1.05 ± 0.12), APTR (1.05 ± 0.2) and fibrinogen (4.54 ± 1.18 g/L).

Type of operation and site of use
Figures 3 and 4 illustrate the type of operations performed as well as the site of PuraStat® use. In all cases, the application of PuraStat® was done following reversal of systemic heparinization with Protamine Sulfate.

Type of Operation

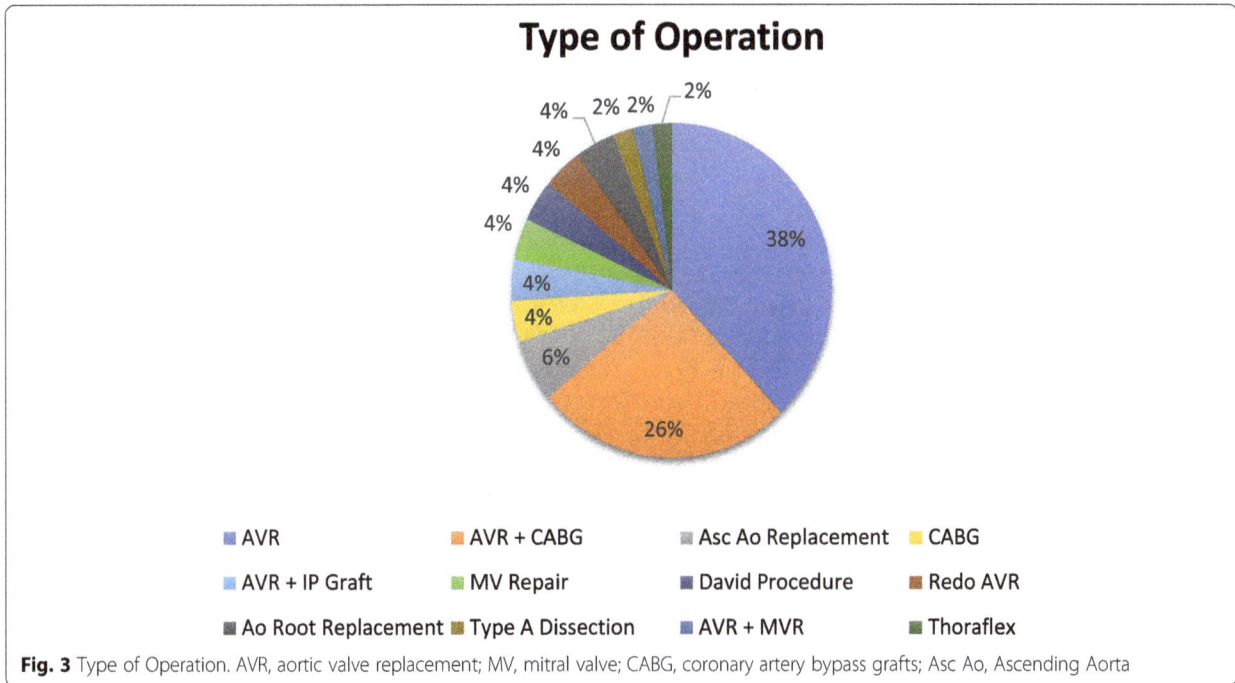

Fig. 3 Type of Operation. AVR, aortic valve replacement; MV, mitral valve; CABG, coronary artery bypass grafts; Asc Ao, Ascending Aorta

Thirty eight percent of patients underwent aortic valve replacement, 26% underwent aortic valve replacement and concomitant coronary artery bypass surgery and 6% of patients had replacement of the ascending aorta with a prosthetic graft. Four percent of patients each had aortic valve replacement with concomitant interpositional graft placement, isolated coronary artery bypass graft surgery, mitral valve repair, valve-sparing aortic root replacement (David Procedure), redo aortic valve replacement and aortic root replacement. Two percent of patients each had emergency repair of a Type A dissection, concurrent aortic and mitral valve replacement and aortic hemiarch replacement with a Thoraflex graft. PuraStat® was most frequently used at the site of aortotomy closure (62%), followed by haemostasis of graft suture lines (18%). It was used to aid haemostasis on closure of the site in 6% of cases, and for 4% of cases each was applied to aortic and right atrial cannulation sites, to needle hole bleeds from prosthetic grafts and to the top ends of vein grafts during CABG surgery. In one

Site of PuraStat® Application

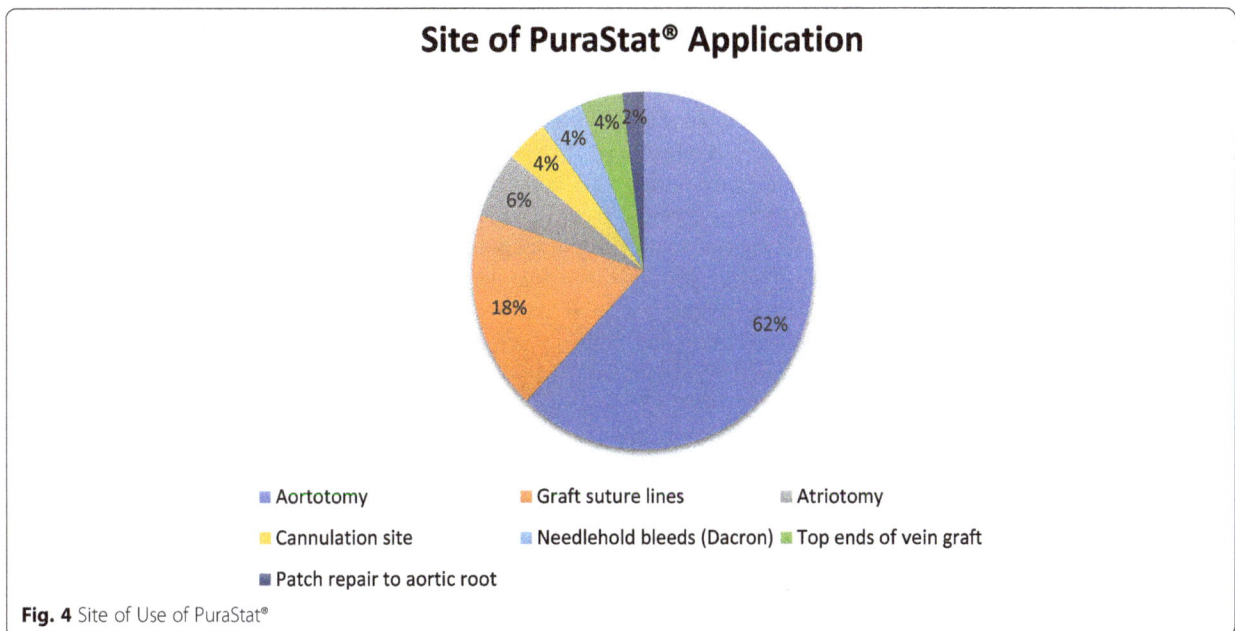

Fig. 4 Site of Use of PuraStat®

case (2%) it was used to aid the fashioning of a pericardial patch which was implanted onto the aortic root.

Total blood product use and 24-h blood lost via intercostal drain output

Table 2 details the mean number of units for blood products such as packed red blood cells (blood), platelets, fresh frozen plasma (FFP) and cryoprecipitate. Additionally, the average number of units of Prothrombin Complex Concentrate (Octaplex®) is included. These results were compared to those of the 2011 Audit of Blood Transfusion in Adult Cardiac Surgery (National Comparative Audit of Blood Transfusion) [6]. Mean values for units of packed redcells (1.45 ± 1.99), platelets (1.22 ± 1.07), fresh frozen plasma (0.94 ± 1.36) and cryoprecipitate (1.33 ± 1.73) were lower than the national average. Mean units of Octaplex use was 1.19 ± 1.54. The percentage reduction of use of blood products in this cohort as compared to the national average was 51.34% for packed red cells, 34.05% for platelets, 52.5% for fresh-frozen plasma and 16.35% for cryoprecipitate.

Table 3 highlights the mean blood loss via intercostal drain output for the first 24 h following surgery and the total cell-salvaged volume transfused following surgery. All patients were infused with the total volume of cell-salvaged blood from cardiopulmonary bypass within the first 24 h following surgery.

Questionnaire results

Table 4 lists the mean scores given by ten surgeons on their experience when using PuraStat®. Every surgeon surveyed has had considerable experience performing the operations in which they used the product, has had the opportunity to use the product more than once and has had experience using similar products from other manufacturers. All theatre scrub staff received training on the product prior to use. PuraStat® scored very highly on pre-application factors such as preparation of the product and dispensation from the applicator. A mean score of 9.7 was assigned for ease of application to the target site. Scores of 8.5, 8.3 and 8.9 respectively were assigned for application to hard-to-reach surfaces, conformation to irregular surfaces and ease of removal (of excess material) from the surgical field. Surgeons found PuraStat® worked well with other agents, reporting no

issues such as smudging, sticking or impaired adherence to the target site when used with Fibrillar®(classified as a haemostat) or BioGlue®(classified as a sealant/glue). It was thought to be valuable in reducing haemostasis time (mean score = 7.5), and subsequently operating time (mean score = 7.3), and in 84% of the cases was adequate in achieving haemostasis without the aid of other haemostatic agents (8% used concurrently with Fibrillar®, 6% used with both Fibrillar® and BioGlue® and 2% used concurrently with BioGlue®).

Postoperative complications

Table 5 lists the inpatient postoperative complications for this cohort of patients. No deaths, cerebrovascular accidents (CVA) or myocardial infarctions (MI) were reported. Fourteen patients (28%) experienced new postoperative atrial fibrillation while ten patients (20%) had pleural effusions confirmed on a chest radiograph. None of the patients were re-explored for bleeding; one patient required surgical re-exploration due to a presentation mimicking cardiac tamponade, however this turned out to be pericardial constriction causing a low cardiac output status. No bleeding was reported from this event.

Discussion

A major challenge when confronted with small-volume, persistent oozing from vascular structures is the limited role of suturing, as every additional bite taken will result in more needle-hole bleeding points. The aforementioned insults to the intrinsic physiological clotting mechanisms from antiplatelet therapy, systemic heparinization and cooling further exacerbate this problem [7, 8]. The current selection of topical haemostatic agents on the market have demonstrated satisfactory haemostatic properties, but has the potential pitfall of enabling transmission of viral and prion diseases (in the case of human blood component-derived substances), and instigating a systemic inflammatory response syndrome to animal-derived peptide-based products [9, 10]. The risk of such complications is negated by the use of a completely synthetic agent like PuraStat®.

In this consecutive case series surgeons reported several distinct qualities of PuraStat® which were felt to be advantageous. The transparent nature provided surgeons

Table 2 Total blood product use compared to the national average

Blood Products Used	Mean units, n	SD	UK Average (CABG)	reduction (%)
Packed Red Cells	1.45	1.99	2.98	51.34%
Platelets	1.22	1.07	1.85	34.05%
FFP	0.94	1.36	1.98	52.50%
Cryoprecipitate	1.33	1.73	1.59	16.35%
Octaplex	1.19	1.54	n/a	n/a

Table 3 Mean cell-salvaged blood infused and 24-h chest drain output

Cell-salvaged blood and Chest Drain Output	Mean Volume, ml	SD
Cell-salvaged blood infused	668.73	280.8
Chest Drain output (24 h)	362.07	287.06

with the novel opportunity to maintain visualisation of the suture line after application of the haemostat. This allowed the opportunity for surveillance of the operative field for slow accumulation of haematoma sandwiched between the vessel and the haemostat layer during the course of the remainder of the operation. A threatened or suboptimal suture repair can then be revised if needed, potentially preventing the need for postoperative re-exploration. The method of delivery and application as a viscous gel rather than a spray applicator was an essential feature when operating within a tight surgical field, enhancing precision (i.e. application over the aortotomy with multiple vein grafts invading the field of view).

The viscosity profile of PuraStat® which demonstrates a more cohesive rather than adhesive characteristic, makes it ideal for concomitant use with other haemostatic materials (in this case, BioGlue® and Fibrillar®). Cross-compatibility with such products is essential, especially in complex aortic procedures in which deep hypothermic circulatory arrest (DHCA) is utilised as the

Table 4 Mean user evaluation scores on the feasibility and efficacy of PuraStat®

Surgeons' Rating of PuraStat®	Average score (1–10)
Ease and efficiency of preparation prior to use	10
Easy to dispense from applicator	10
Ease of application to site of bleed	9.7
Application to hard-to-reach surfaces	8.5
Conformation to irregular surfaces	8.3
Ease of removal of excess PuraStat® from field	8.9
Concomitant use with other haemostatic agents	9.4
Valuable in reducing haemostasis time?	7.5
Potential in reduction of operating time?	7.3
PuraStat® alone enough to achieve haemostasis?	**YES = 84%**
	No = 16%
Other products used concomitantly	None = 84%
	Fibrillar® = 8%
	BioGlue + Floseal = 6%
	BioGlue = 2%

Table 5 Postoperative Complications

Postoperative Complications	Number
AF	14 (28%)
Pleural effusion	10 (20%)
CVA	0
Re-exploration for bleeding	0
MI	0
Other arrhythmias	3
Death	0

dysregulation of coagulative mechanisms is even more pronounced.

Limitations

Our primary aim in this study was to determine feasibility of PuraStat® in aiding haemostasis in cardiac surgery. By evaluating the use this product in fifty consecutive cases, we have established that in a wide variety of surgical scenarios, PuraStat® is shown to be effective in achieving haemostasis. Patients in this study were not stratified according to preoperative risk factors for general morbidity and mortality from cardiac surgery. Neither were they stratified for their individual risks of bleeding and poor tissue healing (i.e. preoperative antiplatelet therapy, type 2 diabetes, corticosteroid use, congestive heart failure and chronic renal failure). The type, length and urgency of the operation would also influence major adverse cardiac events and postoperative bleeding. We propose a follow-up study where patients are propensity-score matched for these criteria [11].

The variation of surgical practice and experience between the ten surgeons resulted in variations in the strategy of application of PuraStat® (i.e. precise location of application and quantity) as well as judgement on how quickly haemostasis was achieved. The point at which different surgeons deemed the product insufficient for haemostasis (and subsequently a different product or change in operative strategy was employed) was not recorded. Previous trials of the efficacy of haemostatic agents have assessed efficacy by standardising the anatomical point of use and time window in achieving bleeding control. Such stringent criteria would provide valuable objective, quantitative data.

Conclusion

Our single-centre, qualitative evaluation found PuraStat® to be a feasible, safe and effective haemostatic agent in a wide range of cardiac and aortic surgical procedures. Specific qualities in terms of the transparent nature and viscosity profile of the product was found to be novel and valuable in our surgical practice. A further randomised-controlled study where patients are propensity-matched for baseline demographics, operative urgency, bleeding risk, tissue integrity factors and operation type is warranted to quantitatively evaluate the performance of PuraStat® in various specific circumstances.

Abbreviations

AF: Atrial Fibrillation; Ao Root: Aortic Root; APTR: Activated Partial Thromboplastin Time Ratio; Asc Ao: Ascending Aorta; AVR: Aortic Valve Replacement; BMI: Body Mass Index; CABG: Coronary Artery Bypass Graft; COPD: Chronic Obstructive Pulmonary Disease; CVA: Cerebrovascular Accident; DHCA: Deep Hypothermic Circulatory Arrest; FFP: Fresh Frozen Plasma; INR: International Normalised Ratio; IP: Interposition; LV: Left Ventricle; MI: Myocardial Infarction; MV: Mitral Valve; MVR: Mitral Valve Replacement; PVD: Peripheral Vascular Disease; RA: Right Atrium

Acknowledgements

We would like to thank Consultant Surgeons (Mr Clifford Barlow, Mr. Geoffrey Tsang, Mr. Theodore Velissaris and Mr. Szabolcs Miskolczi), Senior Surgical Fellows (Mr Syed Sadeque and Mr. Hassan Kattach) and Specialist Registrars (Mr Mano Navaratnarajah, Mr. Simon Duggan and Mr. Aiman Alassar) for completing the questionnaires.

Funding

This research received no specific grant from any funding agency in the public, commercial, or not-for-profit sectors.

Author's contributions

Sunil Ohri and Geoffrey Tsang were responsible for the conceptualization of the study and reviewing the final manuscript. Kareem Salhiyyah was responsible for designing the data capture proforma. Geoffrey Tsang was responsible for access to blood transfusion data and final critical revision of the data. Suresh Giritharan was responsible for data collection, analysis and preparation the manuscript.

Competing interests

Sunil Ohri has received speaker's fees from 3-D Matrix Europe SAS, Caluire et Cuire, France. Suresh Giritharan and Kareem Salhiyyah and Geoffrey Tsang have no declarations.

References

1. Levi M, Cromheecke ME, de Jong E, Prins MH, de Mol BJM, Briët E, et al. Pharmacological strategies to decrease excessive blood loss in cardiac surgery: a meta-analysis of clinically relevant endpoints. Lancet. 1999;354:1940–7.
2. Oz MC, et al. Controlled clinical trial of a novel hemostatic agent in cardiac surgery. Ann Thorac Surg. 2000;69:1376–62.
3. Masuhara H, MD FT, Watanabe T, Koyama N, Tokuhiro K. Novel infectious agent-free hemostatic material (TDM-621) in cardiovascular surgery. Ann Thorac Cardiovasc Surg. 2012;18:444–51.
4. Shander A, Kaplan L, Harris M, Gross I, Nagarsheth N, Nemeth J, et al. Topicral hemostatic therapy in surgery: bridging the knowledge and practice gap. J Am Coll Surg. 2014;219:570–9.
5. Subramaniam S, Kandiah K, Thayalasekaran S, Longcroft-Wheaton G, Bhandari P. Bleeding during endoscopic resection: a novel extracellular scaffold matrix is a safe and effective haemostatic agent. Gut. 2017;66:214–5.
6. Murphy M, Murphy G, Gill R, Herbertson M, Allard S, Grant-Casey J. 2011 Audit of Blood Transfus in Adult Cardiac Surgery Oxford: NHS Blood and Transplant, National Comparitive Audit of Blood Transfusion; 2011.
7. Hartmann M, Sucker C, Boehm O, Koch A, Loer S, Zacharowski K. Effects of cardiac surgery on hemostasis. Transfus Med Rev. 2006;20:230–41.
8. Nasso G, Piancone F, Bonifazi R, Romano V, Visicchio G, De Filippo C, et al. Prospective, randomized clinical trial of the FloSeal matrix sealant in cardiac surgery. Ann Thorac Surg. 2009;88:1520–6.
9. Despotis G, Avidan M, Eby C. Prediction and Bleeding Management in Cardiac Surgery. J Thromb Haemost. 2009;7:111–7.
10. Ibrahim M, Aps C, Young C. A foreign body reaction to Surgicel mimicking an abcess following cardiac surgery. Eur J Cardiothorac Surg. 2002;22:489–90.
11. Ortel T, Mercer M, Thames E, Moore K, Lawson J. Immunologic Impact and Clinical outcomes after surgical exposure to bovine thrombin. Ann Surg. 2001;233:88–96.

28

Detection of patients at high risk for nonocclusive mesenteric ischemia after cardiovascular surgery

Hiroshi Sato[1*], Masanori Nakamura[2], Takeshi Uzuka[2] and Mayo Kondo[2]

Abstract

Objectives: Nonocclusive mesenteric ischemia (NOMI) is a rare but life-threatening complication after cardiovascular surgery. Early diagnosis and treatment is essential for a chance to cure. The aim of this study is to identify the independent risk factors for NOMI based on the evaluation of 12 cases of NOMI after cardiovascular surgery.

Methods: We retrospectively analyzed 12 patients with NOMI and 674 other patients without NOMI who underwent cardiovascular surgery in our hospital. We reviewed the clinical data on NOMI patients, including their characteristics and the clinical course. In addition, we performed a statistical comparison of each factor from both NOMI and non-NOMI groups to identify the independent risk factors for NOMI.

Results: The median duration between the cardiac surgery and the diagnosis of NOMI was 14.0 (10.3–20.3) days. The in-hospital mortality of NOMI patients was 75.0%. Age ($p < 0.05$), peripheral arterial disease ($p < 0.001$), postoperative hemodialysis ($p < 0.001$), intraaortic balloon pump ($p < 0.05$), norepinephrine (NOE) $> 0.10\gamma$ ($p < 0.0001$), percutaneous cardiopulmonary support ($p < 0.001$), sepsis ($p < 0.05$), loss of sinus rhythm ($p < 0.05$), prolonged ventilation ($p < 0.0001$), and resternotomy for bleeding ($p < 0.05$) showed significant differences between NOMI and non-NOMI groups. In the multivariate logistic regression model, prolonged ventilation [odds ratio (OR) = 18.1, $p < 0.001$] and NOE > 0.10 μg/kg/min (OR = 130.0, $p < 0.0001$) were detected as independent risk factors for NOMI.

Conclusions: We have identified the risk factors for NOMI based on the evaluation of the 12 cases of NOMI after cardiovascular surgery. This result may be useful in predicting NOMI, which is considered difficult in clinical practice. For the patient with suspected of NOMI who has these risk factors, early CT scan and surgical exploration should be performed without delay.

Keywords: Nonocclusive mesenteric ischemia, Cardiovascular surgery, Risk model

Introduction

Nonocclusive mesenteric ischemia (NOMI) is a rare complication after cardiovascular surgery, and its incidence rates were reported to be about 0.4 to 9.0% [1–4]. Although the exact pathophysiology is currently unclear, it is assumed that the vasospasm of mesenteric artery results from the low perfusion during cardiopulmonary bypass (CPB) or the various intra/postoperative therapeutic medications [5]. NOMI is a serious complication with a reported 30 to 90%

mortality rate [2, 4, 5]. Clinical signs, such as abdominal pain, vomiting, and hematochezia, can be seen but are not very specific. Also, the abnormal elevation of laboratory data has low specificity. The clinical sign is likely masked because the patient is often sedated and ventilated at the onset of NOMI; therefore, the diagnosis of NOMI is frequently difficult and delayed. In computed tomography (CT) scan findings, absence of bowel wall enhancement, pneumatosis intestinalis, and portal venous gas are specific radiological signs but do not necessarily appear in ischemic conditions. Therefore, constant monitoring of the possibility of intestinal ischemia for the high-risk patient and surgical

* Correspondence: h.sato0229@gmail.com
[1]Department of Cardiovascular Surgery, Sapporo Medical University School of Medicine, S1W16, Chuo-ku, Sapporo 060-8543, Japan
Full list of author information is available at the end of the article

exploration without delay are the only ways for the improvement of survival rate. [6–8]

However, there are few studies that have detected the risk factor of NOMI after cardiovascular surgery [2, 5]. In this study, we reviewed the clinical data of 12 cases of NOMI after cardiovascular surgery in our hospital. Then, we investigated each factor between the two groups and detected the independent risk factors for NOMI.

Materials and methods

Patients

From March 1, 2010 to December 31, 2018, among the patients who underwent cardiovascular surgery in our institution, we conducted a retrospective case-control study for 12 (1.74%) patients who developed NOMI after surgery and 674 (98.3%) other patients. We also included emergent surgical cases and off-pump cases. Excluded cases were the patients with type A aortic dissection who had mesenteric ischemia before surgery, thoracic endovascular aortic repair, and pericardial fenestration.

Diagnosis of NOMI

After cardiovascular surgery, the patients with suspected NOMI because of abdominal distension with absence of bowel sounds, acute abdominal pain, vomiting, hematochezia, or abnormal laboratory data underwent urgent abdominal CT scans. NOMI was diagnosed by the confirmation of the presence of ischemic bowel signs (absence of bowel wall enhancement, pneumatosis intestinalis, or portal venous gas; (Fig. 1) without the occlusion or thrombus of the superior mesenteric artery in the CT scan findings and undisputed mesenteric ischemia by surgical exploration. All radiological signs in the CT scans were reviewed by the radiologist. The CT scan and surgical laparotomy were performed by the judgment of each operator to confirm the diagnosis.

Definition of each analyzed data

Valve surgery included aortic valve replacement /aortic valve plasty, mitral valve replacement (MVR)/mitral valve plasty (MVP), and tricuspid annulus plasty. Thoracic aortic surgery included ascending aortic replacement (AAR)/total arch replacement (TAR)/hemi-arch replacement, and aortic root replacement/remodeling. Each analyzed factor was defined using the following criteria. Norepinephrine (NOE) > 0.10 µg/kg/min was defined as using NOE more than 0.10 µg/kg/min for more than 1 h after surgery. Low output syndrome (LOS) was defined as using mechanical support, that is, intraaortic balloon pump (IABP) support and percutaneous cardiopulmonary support (PCPS). Prolonged ventilation was defined as mechanical ventilation time after surgery of more than 24 h. Loss of sinus rhythm was defined as the documented loss of sinus rhythm for at least 6 h after surgery. Hyperlactatemia was defined as having a serum lactate level of > 5.0 mmol/L.

Statistical analysis

Statistical analysis was performed using Mann-Whitney U test for continuous variables and χ^2 test and Fisher's exact test for categorical variables. Variables found associated with $P < 0.05$ in the univariate analysis were entered into a multivariate logistic regression analysis, using the stepwise selection method, to identify the factors independently associated with a definite risk factor of NOMI. All results were expressed as median (interquartile range). Statistical significance was set at $P < 0.05$ (two-sided). All data analyses were performed using the statistical program R version 3.2.1 (R Foundation for Statistical Computing, http://www.r-project.org/).

Results

Among patients who underwent cardiovascular surgery in our institution, 12 (1.74%) cases developed NOMI. The background of NOMI cases, including patient characteristics, surgery type, and state at the onset of

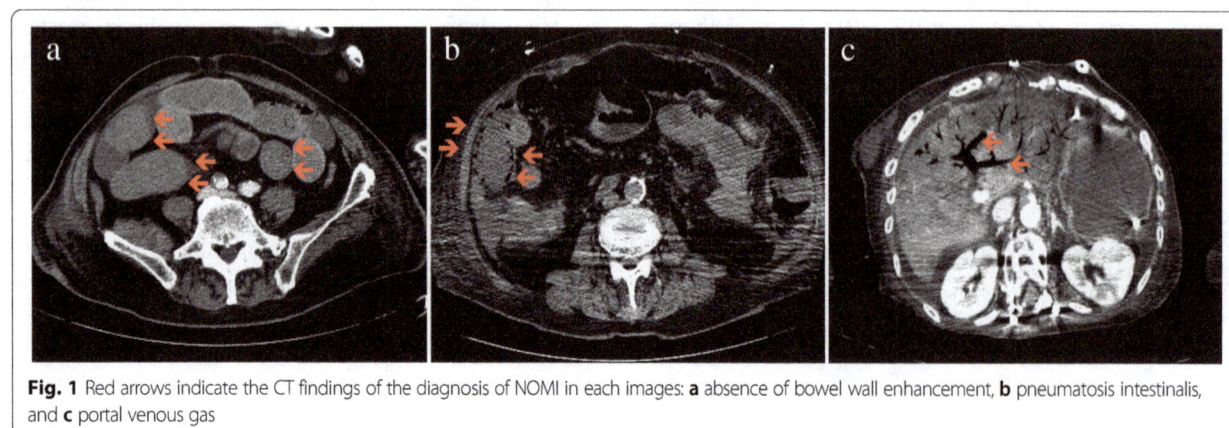

Fig. 1 Red arrows indicate the CT findings of the diagnosis of NOMI in each images: **a** absence of bowel wall enhancement, **b** pneumatosis intestinalis, and **c** portal venous gas

NOMI, is displayed in Table 1. The mean age of patients was 74.67 ± 7.6 years, and 8 (66.7%) patients were male and 4 (33.3%) patients were female. The details of the cardiovascular surgery were 5 (41.7%) off-pump coronary artery bypass graft surgery (OPCABG), 4 (33.3%) CABG, 2 (16.7%) valve surgery, and 2 (16.7%) thoracic aortic surgery. As initial symptoms and findings of NOMI, abdominal pain, vomiting, fever, hematochezia, hypotension, or hyperlactatemia were noted. At the onset of NOMI, 8 of 12 cases were under sedation due to mechanical ventilation. Nine (75.0%) cases died in the hospital and 3 (25.0%) survived. The median duration between the cardiovascular surgery and the onset of NOMI was 14.0 (10.3–20.3) days, and the onset of NOMI for 6 of 12 cases (50.0%) was between 15 and 20 days (Fig. 2).

NOE > 0.10 µg/kg/min was used for 7 of 12 cases within 24 h before the onset of NOMI. Cases 5 to 7 and 11 were in a state of LOS; furthermore, case 11 also had sepsis and underwent hemodialysis. Cases 5 and 7 underwent hemodialysis too, and Case 6 did not. Cases 1, 8, and 9 were not at a state of LOS and had sepsis but underwent hemodialysis while using NOE. NOE was not used for Cases 2 to 4, 10, and 12. Cases 2 and 4 had sepsis, and Case 12 was at a state of LOS and underwent hemodialysis. Cases 3 and 10 were not in any condition. As initial findings/symptoms, 7 of 12 cases showed hyperlactatemia. In others, 1 hypotension, 2 abdominal pain, 1 vomiting, and 1 hematochezia were found.

Between NOMI and non-NOMI groups, pre/intra/postoperative factors were summarized and subjected to statistical comparison (Tables 2 and 3). There was a significant difference in 10 factors: age ($p < 0.05$), peripheral arterial disease (PAD; $p < 0.001$), postoperative hemodialysis ($p < 0.001$), IABP ($p < 0.01$), NOE > 0.10 µg/kg/min ($p < 0.0001$), PCPS ($p < 0.0001$), sepsis ($p < 0.01$), loss of sinus rhythm ($p < 0.01$), prolonged ventilation ($p < 0.0001$), and resternotomy for bleeding ($p < 0.01$). Finally, these 10 factors were introduced for the multivariate logistic regression model as covariates and adjusted odds ratio (OR) were calculated. As a result, prolonged ventilation (OR = 18.1, $p < 0.001$) and NOE > 0.10 µg/kg/min (OR = 130.0, $p < 0.0001$) were detected as independent risk factors for NOMI (Table 4).

Further analysis for these two variables showing significant difference in the multivariate logistic model has proceeded. Among the total 26 cases corresponding to NOE > 0.10 µg/kg/min, total quantity (µg/kg), duration (h), and maximum dose of NOE (µg/kg/min) were statistically compared between NOMI (9 cases) and non-NOMI (17 cases) groups. Similarly, among the total 117 cases corresponding to prolonged ventilation, maximum PEEP (cmH_2O), total ventilation time (h), and index calculated from PEEP * ventilation time/body weight (BW) (cmH_2O * h/kg) were statistical compared between NOMI (9 cases) and non-NOMI (108 cases) groups. As a result, all variables were higher in the NOMI group, but no significant difference was found between the two groups (Table 5).

Discussion

NOMI is a rare but life-threatening complication after cardiovascular surgery. Although it is assumed to be the result of microcirculatory alterations initiated during CPB and the vasospasm of mesenteric artery, its pathomechanism is as yet unclear. It is considered

Table 1 Background of 12 NOMI patients

No	Age	Sex	Surgery	Emergency	Initial symptoms/findings	Duration between Surgery and NOMI(days)	Patient state at the onset of NOMI					Result
							NOE > 0.10 µg/kg/min	LOS	Sepsis	HD	Sedation	
1	83	Male	TAR	No	Hyperlactatemia	13	Yes	No	No	Yes	Yes	Death
2	81	Male	OPCABG	No	Hematochezia	64	No	No	Yes	Yes	Yes	Death
3	67	Male	OPCABG	No	Abdominal pain	13	No	No	No	No	No	Survival
4	66	Male	OPCABG	No	Abdominal pain	34	No	No	Yes	No	No	Survival
5	77	Female	AAR	Yes	Hyperlactatemia	17	Yes	Yes	No	Yes	Yes	Death
6	81	Male	CABG	No	Hyperlactatemia	30	Yes	Yes	No	No	No	Death
7	86	Male	OPCABG	Yes	Hyperlactetamia	8	Yes	Yes	No	Yes	Yes	Death
8	69	Female	OPCABG	No	Hyperlactetamia	11	Yes	No	No	Yes	Yes	Death
9	67	Female	CABG	No	Hyperlactatemia	2	Yes	No	No	Yes	Yes	Death
10	76	Female	MVP, TAP	No	Vomiting	15	No	No	No	No	No	Survival
11	79	Male	CABG, MVR	No	Hypotension	15	Yes	Yes	Yes	Yes	Yes	Death
12	64	Male	CABG	Yes	Hyperlactatemia	5	No	Yes	No	Yes	Yes	Death

NOMI non-occlusive mesenteric ischemia, *NOE* norepinephrine, *LOS* low output syndrome, *HD* hemodialysis, *TAR* Total Arch Aortic Replacement, *OPCABG* off-pump coronary artery bypass graft surgery, *AAR* Ascending Aortic Replacement, *CABG* coronary artery bypass graft surgery, *MVP* mitral valve plasty, *TAP* tricuspid annuloplasty, *MVR* mitral valve replacement

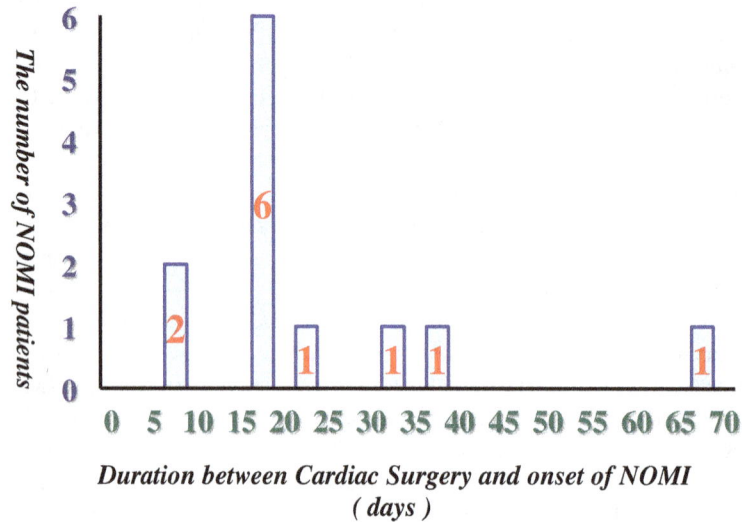

Fig. 2 Relationship of the number of NOMI patients and duration between cardiovascular surgery and onset of NOMI

that it is caused by not only the invasion with cardiovascular surgery itself but also various factors such as the exacerbation of general conditions and using each therapeutic medication for it after surgery [8, 9]. In previous studies, its incidence rate was reported to be about 0.4 to 9.0%, and mortality was 30 to 93% [1–5]. In the present study, the incidence rate was 1.91% and in-hospital mortality was 75.0%, which was a similar result.

We have reviewed the clinical data of 12 NOMI cases and assumed the mechanism and the cause at the onset. Almost all the patients used high-dose NOE after surgery because of their condition of LOS, sepsis, or need for hemodialysis. When we investigated their clinical course in detail, it turned out that there were several factors that developed in combination at the onset of NOMI. In some cases, NOE was dose up just before the onset of NOMI due to the deterioration of LOS and sepsis or at the beginning of dehydration by hemodialysis. The effect of

NOE, which induces vasoconstriction, increases resistance in peripheral splanchnic vessels, and stimulates β receptors in a dose-dependent manner to increase intestinal oxygen consumption, is likely to cause mesenteric ischemia [2, 5, 10]. As the result of the multivariate analysis of this study, the use of NOE > 0.10 µg/kg/min has shown significantly high OR and may have a strong association with the development of NOMI. It is difficult to detect the definite cause of NOMI because this cannot be explained by only the use of NOE and several factors may be related in complicated. However, the status of NOE and the presence of LOS, sepsis, and hemodialysis, which may be the reason for the use of NOE, can be the important factor in the pathogenic mechanism of NOMI.

Selective catheter angiography for mesenteric artery remains the gold standard for the diagnosis of NOMI. In previous studies, angiography was performed for all patients with suspected mesenteric ischemia because of the decreased intestinal peristalsis after cardiovascular

Table 2 Preoperative characteristics

Variables	NOMI (n = 12)	Non-NOMI (n = 674)	P value
Age, median (IQR) (years)	67 (64–74.5)	63 (29–70)	< 0.05
Age > 75, n (%)	7 (58.3)	193 (28.1)	< 0.05
Sex: Male, n (%)	8 (66.7)	430 (62.7)	0.99
COPD, n (%)	2 (16.7)	138 (20.4)	0.95
Diabetes, n (%)	5 (41.7)	248 (36.9)	0.77
Hemodialysis, n (%)	4 (33.3)	115 (16.8)	0.138
Hypertension, n (%)	8 (66.7)	421 (61.4)	0.775
Peripheral Arterial Disease, n (%)	5 (41.7)	43 (6.3)	< 0.001
Stroke, n (%)	1 (8.3)	20 (2.9)	0.314

IQR interquartile range, *COPD* chronic obstructive pulmonary disease

Table 3 Operative and postoperative characteristics and in-hospital mortality

Variables	NOMI (n = 12)	Non-NOMI (n = 674)	P value
Operative			
Operation types			
OPCABG, n (%)	5 (41.7)	136 (19.8)	0.078
CABG, n (%)	4 (33.3)	180 (26.2)	0.742
Valve surgery, n (%)	2 (16.7)	251 (36.6)	0.227
Thoracic Aortic, n (%)	2 (16.7)	121 (17.6)	0.95
Others, n (%)	0 (0)	37 (5.4)	0.95
Emergency, n (%)	3 (25.0)	77 (11.2)	0.155
CPB, n (%)	7 (58.3)	425 (62.0)	0.768
Operation time, median (IQR) (min)	422.8 (255–480)	340 (40–420)	0.139
ACC time, median (IQR) (min)	139 (112–140)	120.8 (28–160)	0.951
CPB time, median (IQR) (min)	195.5 (158–240)	188.8 (50–239)	0.889
Postoperative			
Hemodialysis, n (%)	8 (66.7)	123 (17.9)	< 0.001
IABP, n (%)	5 (41.7)	71 (10.3)	< 0.05
Loss of sinus rhythm, n (%)	9 (75.0)	201 (29.3)	< 0.05
Sepsis, n (%)	2 (16.7)	13 (1.9)	< 0.05
NOE > 0.10 µg/kg/min, n (%)	9 (75.0)	17 (2.5)	< 0.0001
PCPS, n (%)	4 (33.3)	20 (2.9)	< 0.001
Prolonged ventilation, n (%)	9 (75.0)	108 (15.7)	< 0.0001
Resternotomy for bleeding, n (%)	3 (25.0)	33 (4.8)	< 0.05
In-hospital mortality, %	75	5.4	< 0.0001

IQR interquartile range, OPCABG off-pump coronary artery graft bypass surgery, CABG coronary artery graft bypass surgery, ACC aortic cross-clamp, CPB cardiopulmonary bypass, IABP intra-aortic balloon pump, NOE Norepinephrine, PCPS percutaneous cardiopulmonary support

surgery [2, 3]. In addition to the detection of the mesenteric arterial vasospasm, the inserted catheter allows the selective mesenteric intraarterial infusion of vasodilatative drugs. Using this diagnosis and treatment method, the result of low mortality was reported [3]. However, there were also reported cases that required surgical exploration and intestinal resection eventually,

so its therapeutic effects are not clear yet [3, 11]. Angiography is an invasive procedure that cannot be applied for all patients with suspected symptoms.

In CT scan findings, pneumatosis intestinalis and portal venous gas are specific radiological signs, but both may be seen as nonischemic conditions [12]. Hasan et al. have reported that, among 26 patients with suspected NOMI

Table 4 Univariate and multivariate logistic regression model

Risk factor	Univariate analysis			Multivariate analysis		
	OR	95% CI	P Value	Adjusted OR	95% CI	P Value
Age > 75	3.52	1.10–11.20	< 0.05			
Peripheral Arterial Disease	10.30	3.12–33.80	< 0.001			
Postoperative hemodialysis	8.88	2.63–30.00	< 0.001			
IABP	5.65	1.75–18.30	< 0.01			
Loss of sinus rhythm	6.92	1.85–25.80	< 0.01			
Sepsis	10.10	1.98–50.90	< 0.05			
NOE > 0.10 µg/kg/min	52.40	15.00–183.00	< 0.0001	130.0	21.4–921.0	< 0.0001
PCPS	15.70	4.34–56.60	< 0.001			
Prolonged ventilation	15.10	4.02–56.70	< 0.0001	18.1	6.64–388.0	< 0.001
Resternotomy for bleeding	7.55	1.93–29.60	< 0.05			

Table 5 NOE and ventilation factors of NOMI and non-NOMI groups

Variables	NOMI ($n = 9$)	Non-NOMI ($n = 17$)	P value
NOE factor			
Quantity, median (IQR) (µg/kg)	1237.2 (853.6–1850.1)	559.6 (331–2821.7)	0.403
Maximum dose, median (IQR) (µg/kg/min)	0.43 (0.28–0.75)	0.37 (0.21–0.56)	0.219
Duration, median (IQR) (h)	106.3 (38–146)	81 (37.3–208.3)	0.9
Variables	NOMI (n = 9)	Non-NOMI ($n = 108$)	P value
Ventilation factor			
Maximum PEEP, median (IQR) (cmH2O)	10 (10–14)	10 (8–10)	0.157
Total ventilation time, median (IQR) (h)	226 (116–308)	87 (51.5–189.5)	0.077
PEEP * ventilation time/BW index, median (IQR) (cmH$_2$O * h/kg)	24.2 (15.6–36.9)	11.7 (6.5–28.7)	0.051

IQR interquartile range, *NOE* Norepinephrine, *PEEP* positive end expiratory pressure, *BW* body weight

from CT scan findings, 13 (50%) patients have confirmed bowel ischemia by surgical exploration and definite diagnosis of NOMI [7]. They have indicated the inaccuracy of the diagnosis by CT scan findings and necessity of surgical exploration without delay. A surgical exploration is only reliable way to provide an accurate assessment of bowel viability and necrotic sections requiring segmental intestinal resection [7, 10, 12]. Therefore, when we suspected the presence of intestinal ischemia from the comprehensive evaluation of the clinical course and laboratory data, we make it a rule to perform the CT scan and surgical exploration without hesitation.

In previous studies, the analysis for each laboratory data to predict and detect NOMI has been reported. In particular, there are several studies that indicate the elevation of lactate at the onset of NOMI [2, 3, 5, 13]. However, because hyperlactatemia can be found in various conditions, it is difficult to distinguish whether the cause of hyperlactatemia is NOMI or other factors [6, 14]. Simon et al. provided the results of analyzed laboratory data including lactate, creatine kinase, and lactate dehydrogenase isozyme. There were no significant differences between confirmed and negative diagnoses among patients with suspected NOMI [12].

In the present study, 7 of 12 cases were diagnosed with NOMI with hyperlactenemia as initial findings. However, because the elevation of serum lactate level was thought to be reflected irreversible and lethal mesenteric ischemia, all of 7 cases having shown hyperlactatemia could not be saved. When the serum lactate level has been elevated, it is highly likely to be too late for cure. Thus, lactate has lower usefulness for early diagnosis, and rather nonspecific gastrointestinal symptoms such as abdominal pain or vomiting may be more useful. Also, among the 12 cases in this study, 3 cases who survived were diagnosed early from subjective symptoms such as abdominal pain, not objective laboratory data. However, it was difficult to find subjective symptoms early because almost all

NOMI patients were under sedation for mechanical ventilation. Such a situation is often seen at the onset of NOMI and may impede the early diagnosis.

Although there have been several studies that reported predictive factors for occlusive mesenteric ischemia after cardiovascular surgery or NOMI during intensive care, only a few focused on NOMI after cardiovascular surgery [2, 5, 13–19]. As the result of this analysis, NOE > 0.10 µg/kg/min and prolonged ventilation were identified as isolate risk factors for the onset of NOMI. The prolonged ventilation may be the cause of mesenteric ischemia because of peripheral hypoperfusion under sustained sedation and long-term bedridden condition [2, 15–18]. It is also suggested that PEEP decreases mesenteric blood flow and lung injury by mechanical ventilation can spread the pulmonary inflammation to distant organs [20, 21].

In this present study, we have further analyzed the use of NOE and prolonged ventilation as independent risk factors for NOMI, focusing on corresponding cases. This is because we considered that the definite cutoff value of NOE and ventilation factor can be further effective to predict the incidence of NOMI. For the NOE factor, total quantity, duration, and maximum dose of NOE were analyzed. For the prolonged ventilation factor, maximum PEEP, total ventilation time, and index calculated from PEEP * ventilation time/ BW were analyzed. However, between NOMI and non-NOMI groups corresponding to each factor, there were no significant differences and definite cutoff value could not be calculated in both factors (Table 5). This is because each patient status after cardiovascular surgery was individually different, and the threshold of the onset of mesenteric ischemia was varied depending on the patient's general conditions. For example, even between patients who used the same high dose of NOE, there are several factors related to intestinal blood flow. Consequently, the actual dose that can be the cause of mesenteric ischemia for each case is not expected to be the same. If insufficient circulatory dynamics or severe arteriosclerotic change is present, mesenteric ischemia can be caused by an even lower dose of NOE. The same applies to the ventilation factor. Hence, the use of high dose of NOE and prolonged ventilation are important for the onset of NOMI; however, it is very difficult to detect the definite and detailed cutoff value.

There are several limitations to our study. Because this is a retrospective and single-center database study, the reliability of each data is insufficient. In particular, suspecting the onset of NOMI and judging to perform the CT scan and laparotomy are dependent on the surgeon's judgment. Furthermore, we have detected the independent risk factors from the multivariate regression model, but statistical reliability does not seem to be high because of a small number of NOMI cases.

There may be patients with mesenteric ischemia who were excluded from the NOMI group as we did not confirm mesenteric ischemia with surgical exploration. We confirmed no occlusion of mesenteric vessels from the CT scan findings instead of the selective mesenteric angiography. The cause of mesenteric ischemia may have been the occlusion or thrombosis.

Conclusions

We have reviewed 12 cases who developed NOMI after cardiovascular surgery in our institution. Rapid prediction and diagnosis are essential to lower mortality. However, they are very difficult in practice because almost all patients with NOMI were under sedation and mechanical ventilated; thus, their prognosis was extremely poor.

In the multivariate logistic regression model, we have detected the use of NOE > 0.10 μg/kg/min and prolonged ventilation as independent risk factors of NOMI after cardiovascular surgery. In particular, we consider that the status of NOE and the presence of the factor, which can be the reason for the use of NOE, are strongly associated with the onset of NOMI. For the patient with suspected NOMI who have these risk factors, early CT scan and surgical exploration should be performed without delay.

Abbreviations

AAR: Ascending aortic replacement; BW: Body weight; CPB: Cardiopulmonary bypass; CT: Computed tomography; IABP: Intraaortic balloon pump; LOS: Low output syndrome; MVP: Mitral valve plasty; MVR: Mitral valve replacement; NOE: Norepinephrine; NOMI: Nonocclusive mesenteric ischemia; OPCABG: Off-pump coronary artery bypass graft surgery; OR: Odds ratio; PCPS: Support and percutaneous cardiopulmonary support; SD: Standard deviation; TAR: Total arch replacement

Acknowledgements
Not applicable.

Funding
Not applicable.

Authors' contributions
All authors read and approved the final manuscript.

Competing interests
The authors declare that they have no competing interests.

Author details
[1]Department of Cardiovascular Surgery, Sapporo Medical University School of Medicine, S1W16, Chuo-ku, Sapporo 060-8543, Japan. [2]Department of Cardiovascular Surgery, Sapporo City General Hospital, N11W13, Chuo-ku, Sapporo 060-8604, Japan.

References
1. Hajjar LA, Vincent JL, Barbosa Gomes Galas FR, Rhodes A, Landoni G, Osawa EA, et al. Vasopressin versus norepinephrine in patients with Vasoplegic shock after cardiac surgery: the VANCS randomized controlled trial. Anesthesiology. 2017;126:85–93.
2. Groesdonk HV, Klingele M, Schlempp S, Bomberg H, Schmied W, Minko P, et al. Risk factors for nonocclusive mesenteric ischemia after elective cardiac surgery. J Thorac Cardiovasc Surg. 2013;145:1603–10.
3. Klotz S, Vestring T, Rötker J, Schmidt C, Scheld HH, Schmid C, et al. Diagnosis and treatment of nonocclusive mesenteric ischemia after open heart surgery. Ann Thorac Surg. 2001;72:1583–6.
4. Suguru W, Genya Y, Azumi H, Shunichi K. Early diagnosis and therapy of non-occlusive mesenteric ischemia after open heart surgery. Jpn J Cardiovasc Surg. 2008;37:69–73.
5. Lim JY, Kim JB, Jung SH, Choo SJ, Chung CH, Lee JW. Risk factor analysis for nonocclusive mesenteric ischemia following cardiac surgery: a case-control study. Medicine (Baltimore). 2017;9:e8029.
6. Edwards M, Sidebotham D, Smith M, Leemput JV, Anderson B. Diagnosis and outcome from suspected mesenteric ischaemia following cardiac surgery. Anaesth Intensive Care. 2005;33:210–7.
7. Hasan S, Ratnatunga C, Lewis CT, Pillai R. Gut ischaemia following cardiac surgery. Interact Cardiovasc Thorac Surg. 2004;3:475–8.
8. Ghosh S, Roberts N, Firmin RK, Jameson J, Spyt TJ. Risk factors for intestinal ischaemia in cardiac surgical patients. Eur J Cardiothorac Surg. 2002;21:411–6.
9. Trompeter M, Brazda T, Remy CT, Vestring T, Reimer P. Non-occlusive mesenteric ischemia: etiology, diagnosis, and interventional therapy. Eur Radiol. 2002;12:1179–87.
10. O'Dwyer C, Woodson LC, Conroy BP, Lin CY, Deyo DJ, Uchida T, et al. Regional perfusion abnormalities with phenylephrine during normothermic bypass. Ann Thorac Surg. 1997;63:728–35.
11. Mitsuyoshi A, Obama K, Shinkura N, Ito T, Zaima M. Survival in nonocclusive mesenteric ischemia: early diagnosis by multidetector row computed tomography and early treatment with continuous intravenous high-dose prostaglandin E(1). Ann Surg. 2007;246:229–35.
12. Bourcier S, Oudjit A, Goudard G, Charpentier J, Leblanc S, Coriat R. Diagnosis of non-occlusive acute mesenteric ischemia in the intensive care unit. Ann Intensive Care. 2016;6:112.
13. Quiroga B, Verde E, Abad S, Vega A, Goicoechea M, Reque J, et al. Detection of patients at high risk for non-occlusive mesenteric ischemia in hemodialysis. J Surg Res. 2013;180:51–5.
14. Abboud B, Daher R, Boujaoude J. Acute mesenteric ischemia after cardio-pulmonary bypass surgery. World J Gastroenterol. 2008;14: 5361–70.
15. Spotnitz WD1, Sanders RP, Hanks JB, Nolan SP, Tribble CG, Bergin JD et al. General surgical complications can be predicted after cardiopulmonary bypass. Ann Surg 1995;22:489–496.

16. Aouifi A, Piriou V, Bastien O, Joseph P, Blanc P, Chiari P, et al. Severe digestive complications after heart surgery using extracorporeal circulation. Can J Anaesth. 1999;46:114–21.

17. D'Ancona G, Baillot R, Poirier B, Dagenais F, de Ibarra JI, Bauset R, et al. Determinants of gastrointestinal complications in cardiac surgery. Tex Heart Inst J. 2003;30:280–5.

18. Chaudhuri N, James J, Sheikh A, Grayson AD, Fabri BM. Intestinal ischaemia following cardiac surgery: a multivariate risk model. Eur J Cardiothorac Surg. 2006;29:971–7.

19. Rastan AJ, Tillmann E, Subramanian S, Lehmkuhl L, Funkat AK, Leontyev S, et al. Visceral arterial compromise during intra-aortic balloon counterpulsation therapy. Circulation. 2010;122:92–9.

20. Love R, Choe E, Lippton H, Flint L, Steinberg S. Positive end-expiratory pressure decreases mesenteric blood flow despite normalization of cardiac output. J Trauma. 1995;39:195–9.

21. Badenes R, Lozano A, Belda FJ. Postoperative pulmonary dysfunction and mechanical ventilation in cardiac surgery. Crit Care Res Pract 2015;2015:420513.

Radiofrequency ablation of stage IA non–small cell lung cancer in patients ineligible for surgery: results of a prospective multicenter phase II trial

J. Palussière[1][*], F. Chomy[2], M. Savina[3], F. Deschamps[4], J. Y. Gaubert[5], A. Renault[6], O. Bonnefoy[6], F. Laurent[7], C. Meunier[8], C. Bellera[3], S. Mathoulin-Pelissier[3] and T. de Baere[4]

Abstract

Background: A prospective multicenter phase II trial to evaluate the survival outcomes of percutaneous radiofrequency ablation (RFA) for patients with stage IA non-small cell lung cancer (NSCLC), ineligible for surgery.

Methods: Patients with a biopsy-proven stage IA NSCLC, staging established by a positron emission tomography-computed tomography (PET-CT), were eligible. The primary objective was to evaluate the local control of RFA at 1-year. Secondary objectives were 1- and 3-year overall survival (OS), 3-year local control, lung function (prior to and 3 months after RFA) and quality of life (prior to and 1 month after RFA).

Results: Of the 42 patients (mean age 71.7 y) that were enrolled at six French cancer centers, 32 were eligible and assessable. Twenty-seven patients did not recur at 1 year corresponding to a local control rate of 84.38% (95% CI, [67.21–95.72]). The local control rate at 3 years was 81.25% (95% CI, [54.35–95.95]). The OS rate was 91.67% (95% CI, [77.53–98.25]) at 1 year and 58.33% (95% CI, [40.76–74.49]) at 3 years. The forced expiratory volume was stable in most patients apart from two, in whom we observed a 10% decrease. There was no significant change in the global health status or in the quality of life following RFA.

Conclusion: RFA is an efficient treatment for medically inoperable stage IA NSCLC patients. RFA is well tolerated, does not adversely affect pulmonary function and the 3-year OS rate is comparable to that of stereotactic body radiotherapy, in similar patients.

Keywords: Ablation, Non-small cell lung cancer, Radiofrequency ablation, Stereotactic body radiotherapy

Background

Lobectomy and lymph node resection remains the first-line treatment and the best option for stage I non-small-cell lung cancer (NSCLC) [1]. Despite the development of sub-lobular resection [2] to limit the functional damage of lobectomy, approximately 20% of patients remain ineligible for surgery (mostly due to co-morbidities). The 5-year overall survival (OS) without treatment ranges from 6 to 14% for these patients [3].

Until recently, these 'non-surgical' patients were treated with conventional radiotherapy [4]. However, current treatments such as stereotactic body radiotherapy (SBRT) [5–8] and thermal ablation [9–15] are increasingly offered as alternative therapies for non-surgical candidates. Radiofrequency ablation (RFA) has been the most commonly used and evaluated image-guided thermal ablation technique. RFA was shown to be feasible and safe in highly selected patients [9–14]. One of the advantages of RFA is that it is a stand-alone therapy which can be repeated in case of local failure. RFA has the ability to eradicate a tumor with heat while causing minimal damage to the surrounding normal lung tissue.

* Correspondence: j.palussiere@bordeaux.unicancer.fr
[1]Department of Interventional Radiology, Institut Bergonié, 229 Cours de l'Argonne, 33000 Bordeaux, France
Full list of author information is available at the end of the article

The objectives of this multicenter study were to prospectively analyze the efficacy and the tolerance of RFA in stage I NSCLC for non-surgical patients.

Methods

The study was approved by the ethics committee and was funded by the Programme Hospitalier de Recherche Clinique (PHRC, grant number A00812–53) and was conducted in six French institutions. This study followed Consolidated Standards of Reporting Trials guidelines.

Objectives

The main objective was to evaluate the local control of RFA at 1 year. Secondary objectives were to estimate the overall survival (OS) at one and 3 years, local control at 3 years, lung function and quality of life (QoL) after RFA.

Patients

Inclusion and exclusion criteria

Patient, clinical and follow-up data were prospectively registered. Prior to participation, all patients provided written informed consent. Eligible patients had biopsy-proven stage IA NSCLC with a maximum tumor diameter ≤ 3 cm; staging was established by a positron emission tomography-computed tomography (PET-CT) and contrast-enhanced CT. Fluorine-18 fluorodeoxyglucose PET-CT was performed no more than 8 weeks prior to inclusion. RFA was considered technically feasible following a discussion by the local thoracic tumor board. Tumor location < 1 cm from the hilum was the main technical contraindication for RFA. Patients with a tumoral standardized uptake value ≤2.5 on PET-CT were excluded. Patients were required to have an Eastern Cooperative Oncology Group (ECOG) performance status of 0 to 2. Lung insufficiency with forced expiration volume in the first second of expiration (FEV1) < 1 l was not an absolute contraindication.

RFA treatment

CT guidance was used to treat tumors under general anesthesia. Thoracic epidural anesthesia was administered in case of contraindication to general anesthesia mostly due to poor respiratory function. All patients were treated with the same multitine electrodes (LeVeen; Boston Scientific, Nattick. MA) measuring 3, 3.5, or 4 cm in diameter and at least 10 mm larger than the diameter of the target tumor. Multiple overlapping ablations were performed, when needed, in different parts of the tumor in order to cover the entire volume.

Imaging follow-up and complications

Patients were followed-up with a thoracic contrast enhanced CT imaging at 1, 3, 6, 9 and 12 months and a whole body contrast enhanced CT every 6 months. A PET-CT was performed at 3 months and 1 year. Whilst any decrease or stable size in CT images was considered as complete treatment, local control was deemed incomplete in case of > 20% increase in the size of the ablation zone in the largest diameter between two follow-up CTs, or appearance of any irregular, nodular foci at the margin of the ablation zone. On PET-CT, if the ablation zone uptake was greater than the mediastinal background, it was considered as a local recurrence [16]. All images have been remotely reviewed by an independent re-interpretation committee.

In case of a local recurrence, the patient file was reviewed by the tumor board to determine the best option. After 1 year, a PET-CT was proposed to evaluate local control or systemic progression. Complications observed during follow-up, either clinically relevant or observed in imaging, were noted for each patient. Adverse events, based on CTCAE 3.0 [17], were noted and attributed to the study treatment if the physician believed so. Any patient death within 30 days after RFA was considered a grade 5 adverse event. Grade 3 or 4 adverse events were defined as major complications and grade 1 or 2 as minor complications.

Evaluation criteria/ analysis

The main objective was to evaluate local tumor control rate at 1 year, local control defined as the absence of progression of the ablated site. In case of discordance between CT and PET-CT at 1 year, a biopsy was performed. In order to obtain a homogeneous interpretation and to validate the results, one-year imaging data were reviewed at the end of the study by an independent committee composed of a radiologist, a nuclear physicist and a thoracic oncologist. The local control rate was calculated as the ratio of the number of patients alive without local progression at 1 year. A sensitivity study was performed by including eligible patients who had received the RFA treatment and lost to follow-up or deceased before their 1-year evaluation. Based on their last follow-up evaluation before 1 year, patients were deemed locally progressive or not, and the corresponding local control rate was calculated. Confidence intervals of the local control rates were estimated by the Fisher approximation method based on the sample size.

Survival endpoints were defined according to the DATECAN guidelines [18]. OS was defined as the time from RFA treatment to death, whatever the cause. If the patient was still alive at the end of study or lost to follow-up, the patient was censored at the date of last news. PFS was defined as the time from RFA treatment to disease progression or death, whatever the cause. If the patient was still alive with no progression at the end of study or lost to follow-up before observation of a progression, the patient was censored at the date of last news.

Survival endpoints were evaluated using the Kaplan-Meier method and survival rates are reported with their standard error (SE).

Lung function tests including FEV1, forced vital capacity (FVC), total lung capacity (TLC), were performed prior to and 3 months following RFA. A 10% decrease in FEV1 and FVC, and a 20% TLC decrease were considered significant. QoL was measured prior to and 1 month following RFA with the QLQ C 30 questionnaire, developed by the EORTC [19]. The questionnaire consists of 30 items that allow estimating 5 functional and 5 symptomatic scores as well as a global health status score (between 0 and 100). A score of 100 corresponds to a perfect QoL, whereas a score of 0 reflects a very poor QoL. On the contrary, on the symptomatic scale, a score of 100 corresponds to a very poor QoL and a score of 0 reflects a perfect QoL. A 10 point increase or decrease between the pre- and the post-RFA evaluations were considered significant.

Statistical analysis

The number of patients to include was assessed following a binomial law, considering a 5% type-one error and 85% statistical power. In order to observe a 1-year local control rate statistically superior to 65%, with the hypothesis that it will reach 85% in the experimental RFS arm, 33 assessable patients were necessary. Taking into account eventual losses (patients lost to follow-up or deceased before 1 year), at least 40 patients needed to be included.We reported confidence intervals for a 95% two-sided confidence-level (95% CI), estimated using the binomial approach. All statistical analyses were performed using SAS software v9.3 and figures were generated using STATA software and Microsoft Excel software.

Results

Patient characteristics are given in Table 1. A total of 42 patients were included in the study out of which 36 patients were eligible and 32 patients were eligible and assessable for the main criteria (Fig. 1). Majority of patients were ECOG1 and the tumor characteristics (pathology, dimensions etc.) are presented Table 1. Histological analysis revealed an adenocarcinoma in 60% of the patients. T1a and T1b tumors were almost equally distributed. PET-CT at inclusion revealed that SUVmax ranged from 2.7 to 22.2 (mean = 6.9; median = 6.7) for all patients and from 2.7 to 14.5 (mean = 6.3; median = 5.4) for assessable patients. RFA treatments were performed under general anesthesia, except for 4 interventions where thoracic epidural anesthesia was administered. A 4 cm electrode was used in 60% of patients, even though half of the tumors were T1a. Moreover, overlapping ablations were frequent and were performed in more than half of the tumors. A 48 h hospitalization was systematically planned for every patient as part of the

Table 1 Patient characteristics

	Population $n = 42$	Eligible population $n = 36$	Eligible and assessable population $n = 32$
Men	29	23	21
Women	13	13	11
Mean Age (years)	71.7	72.8	72.7
ECOG Status			
0	11	10	9
1	23	20	17
2	1	0	0
Non-documented	7	6	6
Smoking			
No	5	5	5
Yes	23	18	16
Non-documented	14	13	11
Histological analysis			
Squamous cell carcinoma	10	9	8
Adenocarcinoma	26	23	21
Large cell carcinoma	4	3	3
Undifferentiated non-small cell	1	1	0
Neuroendocrine	1	0	0
Tumor size (mm)			
Max.	37	29	29
Min.	13	13	13
Average	21.1	20.4	20.7
STD	6.34	5.04	5.0
Tumor stage			
T1a	24 (57%)	21 (58%)	18 (56%)
T1b	15 (36%)	15 (42%)	14 (44%)
T2	3 (7%)	0 (0%)	0 (0%)

protocol for this old and fragile population with multiple comorbidities. Hospitalization duration ranged from 2 to 19 days (mean = 4 days; median = 3 days). An X-ray for pneumothorax was performed during ablation in 26 treatments (83.87%), with the need for a chest tube in 17. Chest tubes were always removed within 2 days. Other CT findings were pleural effusion (n = 4; 1 mild and 3 minimal), alveolar hemorrhage (n = 2; subsegmental), hemothorax (n = 1); however, no clinical symptoms were noted in relation to these findings. Two major adverse events were recorded in 2 patients (4.7% of the overall population) and 3 delayed minor adverse events were noted (Table 2).

Local control (Table 3)

Local control was observed in 27 of the 32 eligible patients assessable for efficacy corresponding to a local

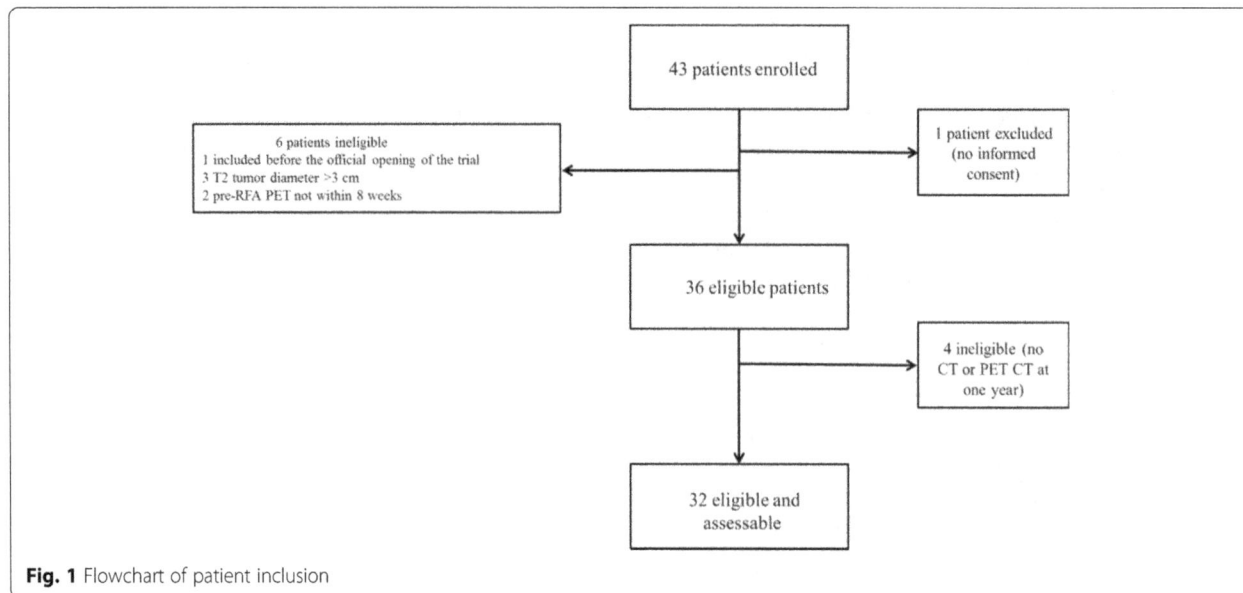

Fig. 1 Flowchart of patient inclusion

control rate of 84.38% (95% CI, [67.21–95.72]). Among the 5 diagnosed with local progression, 1 required biopsy to prove the local failure due to a discrepancy in the interpretations of PET-CT and CT. A second RFA was performed in two of the 5 local progression cases. The local control rate at 3 years was 81.25% (95% CI, [54.35–95.95]). A sensitivity study was performed including all eligible patients and the local control rate was 86.11% [95% CI, [70.50–95.33]) at 1 year and 77.78% [95% CI, [60.85–89.88]) at 3 years.

Secondary objectives

OS and progression free survival (PFS)

The OS was 91.67% (95% CI, [77.53–98.25]) at 1 year and 58.33% (95% CI, [40.76–74.49]) at 3 years (Fig. 2). PFS was 71.76% (95% CI, [42.25–88.00]) at 1 year and 25% (95% CI, [12.12–42.20]) at 3 years. Fifteen patients died within the 3 years follow-up (7 from cancer progression and 8 from other causes) and two patients died before 1 year (1 from cancer progression).

Lung function

Of the 36 eligible patients, FEV1 was available for 21 patients prior to treatment and for 18 patients at 3 months. Prior to treatment, FEV1 ranged from 0.6 to 35.7 (mean = 3.2; median = 1.6) whereas at 3 months FEV1 ranged from 0.6 to 3.2 (mean = 1.6; median = 1.6).

If we only focus on the 14 patients assessed both prior to and after treatment, pre-treatment FEV1 ranged from 0.9 to 35.7 (mean = 4.2; median = 1.7) and three-month FEV1 ranged from 0.9 to 3.2 (mean = 1.7; median = 1.6). Two patients had 10% decrease and two patients had a 10% increase in FEV1.

Regarding FVC, pre-treatment and three-month assessment was available for 20 and 17 patients, respectively. Prior to treatment, FVC ranged from 1.5 to 4.3 (mean = 2.6; median = 2.3). Three months after RFS, FVC ranged from 1.6 to 4.9 (mean = 2.7; median = 2.3). If we only consider the 13 patients assessed both prior to and 3 months after treatment, pre-treatment FVC ranged from 1.7 to 4.3 (mean = 2.6; median = 2.3) and post-treatment FVC ranged from 1.6 to 4.9 (mean = 2.8; median = 2.3). Lung function test was available for 14 of

Table 2 Adverse Events

Description	Grade CTCAE	Nb	Evolution	Imputability
Pulmonary embolism	4	1	Healing without sequelae	Non-attributable
Acute lung insufficiency	5	1	Death	Attributable
Dyspnea	2	1	Healing without sequelae	Non-attributable
Dyspnea	2	1	Healing with sequelae	Attributable
Rib lysis and fracture	1	1[a]	Healing	Attributable

[a]2nd right rib was concerned and the fracture occurred 6 months after RFA, the ablation zone was in contact with the chest wall

Table 3 Different recurrences

Type of recurrence	Number
Local failure (ablation area)	5
Lymph node (hilar)	2
Lymph node N2	2
Lymph node N3	1
Metastatic disease	1
Lymph node + metastatic disease	1
Recurrence within another lobe + Lymph node	1

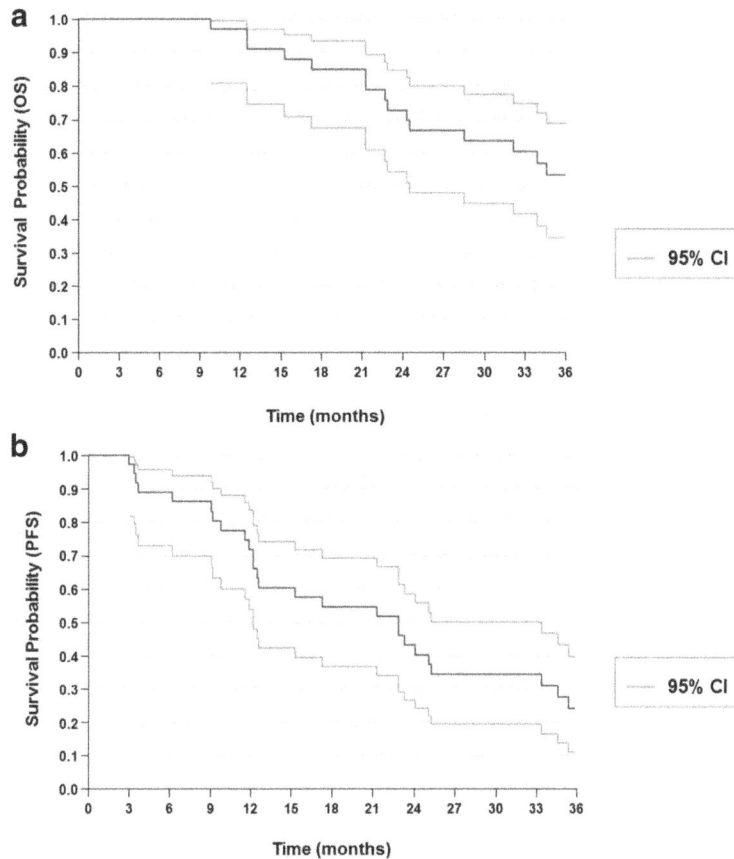

Fig. 2 a Overall survival and (**b**) Progression-free survival curves

the 36 eligible patients, with a 10% decrease in FEV1 in two patients and a 10% increase in two patients. A 20% decrease was observed in one patient and a 20% increase in two patients. TLC was available for nine patients and a 20% decrease was observed in one patient.

Quality of life

QLQ C 30 questionnaires were available for 34 of the 36 eligible patients and the results are presented in Fig. 3. Between inclusion and 1 month, a significant deterioration of cognitive functions (decrease of 17.67 points) and fatigue (increase of 11.11 points) were observed, whereas insomnia significantly decreased (down by 33.33 points). It is worth noting that no significant modification of the median global health status, physical functioning, pain and dyspnea occurred.

Discussion

This multicenter study is the second prospective study on RFA and non-surgical patients with stage I NSCLC. Dupuy et al. have published [20] the results of American College of Surgeons oncology group Z4033 trial, with a local recurrence-free rate of 68.9 and 59.8% at 1 and 2 years, respectively. In our study, the local control rate

was 84.38% (95% CI, [67.21–95.72]) at 1 year and 81.25% (95% CI, [54.35–95.95]) at 3 years. In our study, local recurrence refers to a recurrence in the RFA zone (Fig. 4) whereas in the Z4033 trial it refers not only to a recurrence in the RFA site but also in the primary tumor lobe and the hilar lymph node. Our results are in accordance with our previously published retrospective study, with local control rates of 88.5 and 78.9% at 1 and 3 years, respectively [21].

In this study, expandable multitined electrodes were used with an electrode array diameter of the at least 10 mm larger than the tumor, such oversizing the ablation volume was previously reported to increase the success rate of the treatment [22]. Moreover, a pathological study following RFA on NSCLC demonstrated the benefit of oversizing the ablation zone by encompassing the tumor; < 5 mm margins were observed in patients with incomplete ablation whilst a mean margin of 8 mm was noted in complete ablations [23]. This emphasizes the need for an extensive RFA to take into consideration the microscopic extension of NSLCC. Beland et al. [10] recommended an ablation zone *"that includes the primary tumor plus at least an additional 8–10 mm of ablation beyond the visible tumor margin in all directions"*. In our

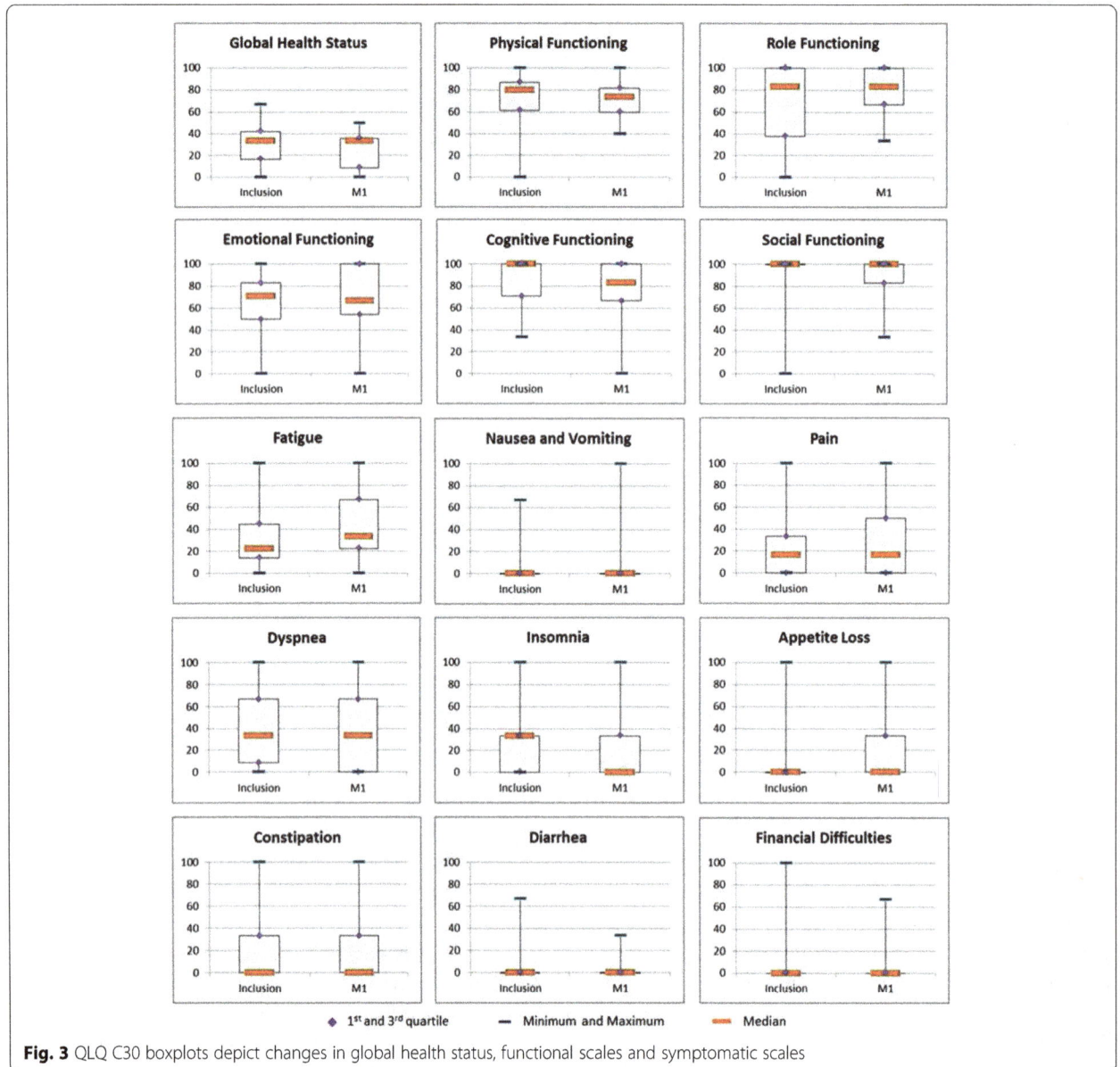

Fig. 3 QLQ C30 boxplots depict changes in global health status, functional scales and symptomatic scales

series, all the patients apart from three were treated with a 3.5 or a 4 cm electrode for a mean tumor size of 20.7 mm, probably explaining the good high rate of local control we report herein. Other ablation techniques such as microwaves may also improve the local control rate by providing a larger ablation volume compared to RFA, as reported in an animal study [24]. Cryotherapy [25], offers the possibility of using multiple probes to obtain a larger ablation volume.

Ever since the use of thermal ablation on lung tumors, different studies [10, 23, 26] have shown that repeated imaging is important to follow the variations in size of the ablation zone, to identify the different imaging patterns of lung tumors after RFA and finally, to distinguish total ablation from local tumor progression. The strength of

this study is the strict prospective continuous imaging follow-up during 3 years, for all patients. Recurrence was determined using CT and PET-CT, as well as the possible use of biopsy. In one case, there was discordance between CT and PET-CT at 1 year, a local recurrence was confirmed by a biopsy. A new RFA was proposed for 2 out of 5 local failures. Moreover, with the possibility of re-treatment, loco-regional progression did not seem to negatively impact the OS [27]. The 1- and 3-year OS rates were of 91.67 and 58.33%, respectively which are similar to the American prospective trial results [20] with an OS rate of 86.3 and 69.8% (at 1 and 2 years, respectively). Furthermore, our patient population was old, frail and contraindicated for surgery. We note that RFA results are difficult to compare with those of sub-lobular

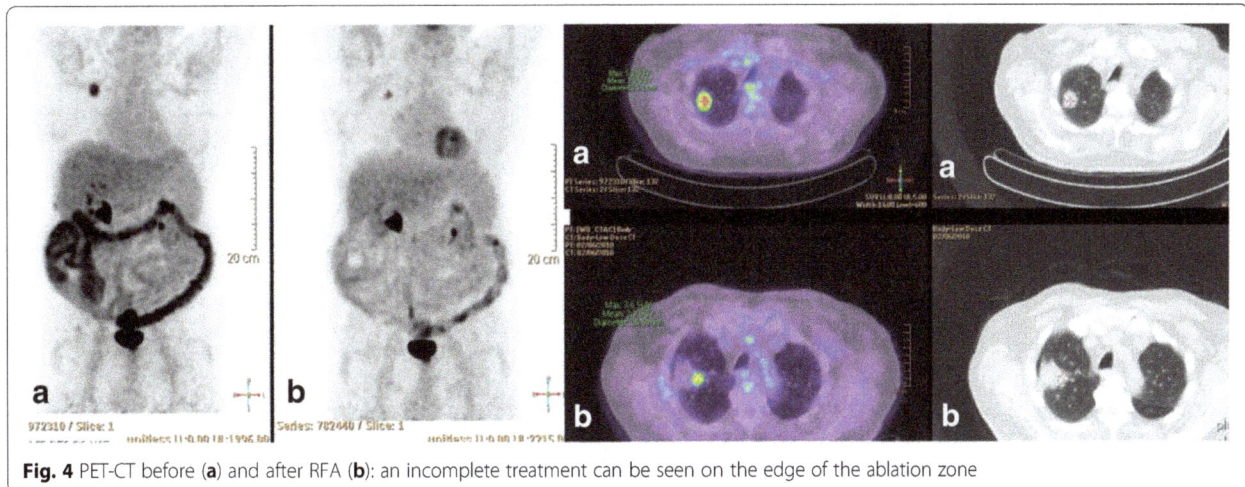

Fig. 4 PET-CT before (**a**) and after RFA (**b**): an incomplete treatment can be seen on the edge of the ablation zone

resection and Stereotactic Body Radiation Therapy (SBRT). Patients for thermal ablation are often the frailest and the oldest [28], in this series all patients were medically inoperable and at 3 years, half of the patients died of causes other than cancer. Nevertheless, SBRT resulted in similar survival rates (86 and 45% at 1 and 3 years, respectively) in an elderly population [6]. The local control rate at 3 years was 89% which is comparable to ours. However, in this series at 12 months of follow-up, imaging (CT scans) was available for 88% of patients, and PET-CT was obtained only when there was suspicion of disease recurrence. Moreover, histological confirmation of malignancy was available only for 39% of patients vs 100% in our series. The absence of pathological confirmation of cancer in a significant number of patients may raise the concern of whether those lung lesions may be benign. This is a weakness of numerous SBRT studies. Comparison with surgery is difficult as patients treated with ablation are not surgical candidates. Nevertheless, using propensity scores to match patient subgroups, Kwan et al. recently demonstrated comparable overall and lung-cancer specific survival between RFA and sub-lobular resection in patients ≥65 years old with stage IA or IB NSCLC [29]. The lack of pathological mediastinal lymph node information, which may impair patient survival compared to surgery, remains a limitation of RFA and SBRT for early stage NSCLC.

RFA seems to have been well tolerated. No delayed pneumothorax occurred and all pneumothoraces cleared rapidly. In a large series of 1000 RFA sessions [30], pneumothorax requiring pleural sclerosis was rare (1.6%). Besides pneumothorax, we observed two major adverse events. An ECOG 2 patient with a FEV of 800 mL died a few weeks later from respiratory decompensation that has been attributed to RFA. Exacerbation of interstitial pneumonia has been mentioned as a major cause of death [30] and has also been reported after lung surgery and radiotherapy. Consequently, the indication of a thermal ablation must be carefully weighted in patients with lung insufficiency, even though it is difficult to propose a clear lower threshold for respiratory function for lung RFA [23]. The stable lung function and the positive impact on QoL in our series also highlight the good tolerance of the RFA. QLQ C 30 tests propose large scale measurements and are not focused on lung disorders. A majority of patients considered that RFA did not modify either their life status perception or their main vital function, including lung function. A significant deterioration of cognitive function and fatigue was observed.

Conclusion

This prospective study confirms that RFA is an effective, safe and well-tolerated option in the treatment of patients presenting stage IA NSCLC who are ineligible for surgery. The 3-year local control rate is encouraging and similar to SBRT results. The survival is comparable to another recent prospective study confirming the place of thermal ablation in this fragile non-surgical population. A prospective trial comparing RFA to other techniques such SBRT is required.

Abbreviations
ECOG: eastern cooperative oncology group; FEV1: first second of expiration; FVC: forced vital capacity; NSCLC: non-small cell lung cancer; OS: overall survival; PET-CT: positron emission tomography-computed tomography; PFS: progression-free survival; QoL: quality of life; RFA: radiofrequency ablation; SBRT: stereotactic body radiotherapy; TLC: total lung capacity

Acknowledgements
The authors would like to thank Dr. Ravi Nookala of Institut Bergonié for the medical writer services.

Funding
The study was approved by the ethics committee and was funded by the Programme Hospitalier de Recherche Clinique (PHRC, grant number A00812–53).

Authors' contributions

Study concepts: JP, FC. Study design: JP, FC, CB, SM. Data acquisition: JP, FD, JYG, AR, OB, FL, CM, TdB. Quality control of data and algorithms: JP, MS, CB, SM. Data analysis and interpretation: JP, FC, MS, CB, SM. Statistical analysis: MS. Manuscript preparation: JP, TdB, MS. Manuscript editing: JP. Manuscript review: JP, MS. All authors read and approved the final manuscript.

Competing interests

The authors declare that they have no competing interests.

Author details

[1]Department of Interventional Radiology, Institut Bergonié, 229 Cours de l'Argonne, 33000 Bordeaux, France. [2]Department of Medical Oncology, Institut Bergonié, 229 Cours de l'Argonne, 33000 Bordeaux, France. [3]Department of Clinical and Epidemiological Research, Institut Bergonié, 229 Cours de l'Argonne, 33000 Bordeaux, France. [4]Department of Interventional Imaging, Institut Gustave Roussy, 114 Rue Edouard Vaillant, 94800 Villejuif, Paris, France. [5]Department of Imaging, CHU Timone, 264 Rue Saint-Pierre, 13385 Marseille, France. [6]Department of Imaging, CHU Pau, 4 Boulevard Hauterive, 64000 Pau, France. [7]Department of Imaging, CHU Haut Lévêque, Avenue Magellan, 33600 Pessac, France. [8]Department of Imaging, CHU Rennes, 2 rue Henri Le Guilloux, 35033 Rennes, France.

References

1. Rami-Porta R, Ball D, Crowley J, Giroux DJ, Jett J, Travis WD, et al. The IASLC lung Cancer staging project: proposals for the revision of the T descriptors in the forthcoming (seventh) edition of the TNM classification for lung cancer. J Thorac Oncol. 2007;2(7):593–602.
2. Rami-Porta R, Tsuboi M. Sublobar resection for lung cancer. Eur Respir J. 2009;33(2):426–35.
3. Raz DJ, Zell JA, Ou SH, Gandara DR, Anton-Culver H, Jablons DM. Natural history of stage I non-small cell lung cancer: implications for early detection. Chest. 2007;132(1):193–9.
4. Qiao X, Tullgren O, Lax I, Sirzen F, Lewensohn R. The role of radiotherapy in treatment of stage I non-small cell lung cancer. Lung Cancer. 2003;41(1):1–11.
5. Fakiris AJ, McGarry RC, Yiannoutsos CT, Papiez L, Williams M, Henderson MA, et al. Stereotactic body radiation therapy for early-stage non-small-cell lung carcinoma: four-year results of a prospective phase II study. Int J Radiat Oncol Biol Phys. 2009;75(3):677–82.
6. Haasbeek CJ, Lagerwaard FJ, Antonisse ME, Slotman BJ, Senan S. Stage I nonsmall cell lung cancer in patients aged > or =75 years: outcomes after stereotactic radiotherapy. Cancer. 2010;116(2):406–14.
7. Onishi H, Araki T, Shirato H, Nagata Y, Hiraoka M, Gomi K, et al. Stereotactic hypofractionated high-dose irradiation for stage I nonsmall cell lung carcinoma: clinical outcomes in 245 subjects in a Japanese multiinstitutional study. Cancer. 2004;101(7):1623–31.
8. Timmerman R, Paulus R, Galvin J, Michalski J, Straube W, Bradley J, et al. Stereotactic body radiation therapy for inoperable early stage lung cancer. JAMA. 2010;303(11):1070–6.
9. Ambrogi MC, Fanucchi O, Cioni R, Dini P, De LA, Cappelli C, et al. Long-term results of radiofrequency ablation treatment of stage I non-small cell lung cancer: a prospective intention-to-treat study. J Thorac Oncol. 2011;6(12):2044–51.
10. Beland MD, Wasser EJ, Mayo-Smith WW, Dupuy DE. Primary non-small cell lung cancer: review of frequency, location, and time of recurrence after radiofrequency ablation. Radiology. 2010;254(1):301–7.
11. Fernando HC, De HA, Landreneau RJ, Gilbert S, Gooding WE, Buenaventura PO, et al. Radiofrequency ablation for the treatment of non-small cell lung cancer in marginal surgical candidates. J Thorac Cardiovasc Surg. 2005;129(3):639–44.
12. Hiraki T, Gobara H, Iishi T, Sano Y, Iguchi T, Fujiwara H, et al. Percutaneous radiofrequency ablation for clinical stage I non-small cell lung cancer: results in 20 nonsurgical candidates. J Thorac Cardiovasc Surg. 2007;134(5):1306–12.
13. Lanuti M, Sharma A, Digumarthy SR, et al. Radiofrequency ablation for treatment of medically inoperable stage I non–small cell lung cancer. J Thorac Cardiovasc Surg. 2009;137:160–6.
14. Pennathur A, Luketich JD, Abbas G, Chen M, Fernando HC, Gooding WE, et al. Radiofrequency ablation for the treatment of stage I non-small cell lung cancer in high-risk patients. J Thorac Cardiovasc Surg. 2007;134(4):857–64.
15. Simon CJ, Dupuy DE, DiPetrillo TA, Safran HP, Grieco CA, Ng T, et al. Pulmonary radiofrequency ablation: long-term safety and efficacy in 153 patients. Radiology. 2007;243(1):268–75.
16. Bonichon F, Palussière J, Godbert Y, Pulido M, Descat E, Devillers A, Meunier C, Leboulleux S, de Baère T, Galy-Lacour C, Lagoarde-Segot L, Cazeau AL. Diagnostic accuracy of 18F-FDG PET/CT for assessing response to radiofrequency ablation treatment in lung metastases: a multicentre prospective study. Eur J Nucl Med Mol Imaging. 2013;40(12):1817–27.
17. Trotti A, Colevas AD, Setser A, Rusch V, Jaques D, Budach V, Langer C, Murphy B, Cumberlin R, Coleman CN, Rubin P. CTCAE v3.0: development of a comprehensive grading system for the adverse effects of cancer treatment. Semin Radiat Oncol. 2003;13:176–81.
18. Bellera CA, Pulido M, Gourgou S, Collette L, Doussau A, Kramar A, Dabakuyo TS, Ouali M, Auperin A, Filleron T, Fortpied C, Le Tourneau C, Paoletti X, Mauer M, Mathoulin-Pélissier S, Bonnetain F. Protocol of the definition for the assessment of time-to-event endpoints in CANcer trials (DATECAN) project: formal consensus method for the development of guidelines for standardised time-to-event endpoints' definitions in cancer clinical trials. Eur J Cancer. 2013;49(4):769–81.
19. Aaronson NK, Ahmedzai S, Bergman B, Bullinger M, Cull A, Duez NJ, Filiberti A, Flechtner H, Fleishman SB, de Haes JCJM, Kaasa S, Klee M, Osoba D, Razavi D, Rofe PB, Schraub S, Sneeuw K, Sullivan M, Takeda F. The European Organization for Research and Treatment of Cancer QLQ-C30: a quality-of-life instrument for use in international clinical trials in oncology. JNCI J Natl Cancer Inst. 1993;85(5):365–76.
20. Dupuy DE, Fernando HC, Hillman S, Ng T, Tan AD, Sharma A, Rilling WS, Hong K, Putnam JB. Radiofrequency ablation of stage IA non-small cell lung cancer in medically inoperable patients: results from the American College of Surgeons oncology group Z4033 (alliance) trial. Cancer. 2015;121(19):3491–8.
21. Palussiere J, Lagarde P, Aupérin A, Deschamps F, Chomy F, de Baere T. Percutaneous lung thermal ablation of non-surgical clinical N0 non-small cell lung cancer: results of eight years' experience in 87 patients from two centers. Cardiovasc Intervent Radiol. 2015 Feb;38(1):160–6.
22. Ihara H, Gobara H, Hiraki T, et al. Radiofrequency ablation of lung tumors using a multitined expandable electrode: impact of the electrode Array diameter on local tumor progression. J Vasc Interv Radiol. 2016;27:87–95.
23. Ambrogi MC, Fontanini G, Cioni R, Faviana P, Fanucchi O, Mussi A. Biologic effects of radiofrequency thermal ablation on non-small cell lung cancer: results of a pilot study. J Thorac Cardiovasc Surg. 2006;131(5):1002–6.
24. Planche O, Teriitehau C, Boudabous S, Robinson JM, Rao P, Deschamps F, Farouil G, de Baère T. In vivo evaluation of lung microwave ablation in a porcine tumor mimic model. Cardiovasc Intervent Radiol. 2013;36(1):221–8.
25. Moore W, Talati R, Bhattacharji P, et al. Five-year survival after cryoablation of stage I non-small cell lung cancer in medically inoperable patients. J Vasc Interv Radiol. 2015;26:312–9.
26. Abtin GA, Eradat J, Gutierrez AJ, Lee C, Fishbein MC, Suh RD. Radiofrequency ablation of lung tumors : imaging features of the post-ablation zone. RadioGraphics. 2012;32:947–69.
27. Lanuti M, Sharma A, Willers H, Digumarthy SR, Mathisen DJ, Shepard JA. Radiofrequency ablation for treatment of stage I non-small cell lung cancer: management of locoregional recurrence. Ann Thorac Surg. 2012;93(3):921–7.
28. Crabtree T, Puri V, Timmerman R, et al. Treatment of stage I lung cancer in high-risk and inoperable patients: comparison of prospective clinical trials using stereotactic body radiotherapy (RTOG 0236), sublobar resection (ACOSOG Z4032), and radiofrequency ablation (ACOSOG Z4033). J Thorac Cardiovasc Surg. 2013;145:692–9.

30

Neutrophil-lymphocyte ratio predicts recurrence in patients with resected stage 1 non-small cell lung cancer

Shinjiro Mizuguchi[*], Nobuhiro Izumi, Takuma Tsukioka, Hiroaki Komatsu and Noritoshi Nishiyama

Abstract

Background: The aim was to determine the prognostic value of the neutrophil-lymphocyte ratio (NLR) in patients with completely resected stage 1 non-small cell lung cancer (NSCLC).

Methods: The study enrolled 382 NSCLC patients, and an optimal NLR cutoff value was determined by ROC analysis. Patients were divided by preoperative NLR into low (< 1.5, $n = 99$), intermediate ($1.5 \leq NLR < 3.5$, $n = 245$), and high (NLR ≥ 3.5, $n = 38$) value groups. Serum diacron-reactive oxygen metabolites (d-ROMs) were assayed in 33 consecutive patients and used as an indicator of oxidative stress.

Results: The mean NLR in patients with high d-ROMs (> 300 U.CARR, $n = 16$) was 1.72 ± 0.67, which was significantly higher than that in patients with low d-ROMs (1.41 ± 0.39, $n = 17$; $P = 0.018$). The 3-, 5- and 10-year survival rates in the three NLR groups were 92, 77, and 59% (low); 82, 70, and 50% (intermediate); and 76, 58, and 32% (high) ($P = 0.034$). The 1-, 3- and 5-year recurrence-free survival rates in the three groups were 98, 90, and 86% (low), 91, 77, and 74% (intermediate); and 92, 77, and 68% (high) ($P = 0.033$). Multivariate analysis found that although NLR was not predictive of overall survival, high NLR was an independent risk factor of recurrence (hazard ratio: 2.03, 95% confidence interval: 1.17–3.79, $P = 0.011$) as were as age, pathological stage, tumor differentiation, and lymph-vascular invasion.

Conclusions: A low preoperative NLR predicted good prognosis, and was associated with low systemic inflammation status in patients with stage 1 NSCLC. It may be helpful when considering intervals of routine follow-up or choice of adjuvant therapy.

Keywords: Non-small cell lung cancer, Prognosis, Recurrence-free survival, Neutrophil-lymphocyte ratio, Surgery

Background

Interest in links between systemic inflammation and the management of cancer is increasing. Many cancers develop at sites of infection, chronic irritation, and inflammation, and regardless of the location, inflammatory cells in the tumor microenvironment are indispensable participants in the neoplastic process, promoting cell proliferation, survival, angiogenesis, and migration [1]. Loss of tissue integrity caused by reduction of cellular adhesion is an early step in metastasis, allowing the spread of tumor cells from the primary tumor [2]. In mammary epithelial cells, malignant transformation and metastasis are stimulated by generation of endogenous reactive oxygen species (ROS) [3]. ROS

contribute to carcinogenesis and the aberrant growth, metastasis, and angiogenesis that are characteristic of malignant tumors [4, 5] and associated with oxidative stress.

The evidence for neutrophil-lymphocyte ratio (NLR) as a novel marker of systemic inflammation, immunological response, and prognosis has been recently reviewed. A systematic review found that the NLR had independent prognostic value in unselected cohorts of more than 12,000 routinely treated patients, operative disease (20 studies), patients receiving neoadjuvant treatment and resection (5 studies), patients receiving chemo/radiotherapy (12 studies), and patients with inoperable disease (6 studies) [6, 7]. In advanced lung cancer patients, both the European Lung Cancer Working Group [8] and the Japan Multinational Trial Organization [9] reported that an elevated neutrophil count was an independent prognostic factor in patients

* Correspondence: m1293795@msic.med.osaka-cu.ac.jp
Department of Thoracic Surgery, Osaka City University Hospital, 1-4-3 Asahimachi, Abeno-ku, Osaka 545-8585, Japan

with advanced non-small cell lung cancer (NSCLC). Several studies have evaluated the prognostic significance of the NLR in patients with completely resected NSCLC [10–17], but, the prognostic value of preoperative NLRs in early stage, completely resected NSCLC is not well known. The study objective was to determine the significance of increased NLR and its relationship to serum ROS generation, survival, and recurrence in patients with stage 1 NSCLC.

Methods
Patients
The medical records of 587 consecutive patients at Osaka City University Hospital, Osaka, Japan, with pulmonary resection for stage I NSCLC between January 1998 and December 2012 were analyzed retrospectively. Patients with partial wedge resection or segmentectomy, those without radical mediastinal lymph node dissection (R0), and those given neoadjuvant therapy were excluded from the study. Patients with hematologic cancers, autoimmune disorders, with recent steroid or immunosuppressive therapy, or preoperative infection were excluded from the NLR analysis. The records of the 382 remaining patients with pathological stage I NSCLC with lobectomy or bilobectomy and R0 were evaluated. Tumor histology was classified following World Health Organization criteria, and postoperative staging was based on the international TNM classification for lung cancer (7th) [18]. Patients were followed at 1–6-month intervals postoperatively. Follow-up evaluation included physical examination, chest X-ray, and blood examination, including for tumor markers. Chest, brain and abdominal computed tomography were performed at 6–12 month intervals. Bone scanning was not routinely performed in asymptomatic patients. Whenever any symptoms or signs of recurrence were detected, magnetic resonance imaging of the brain and bone scintigraphy was performed. Of the 382 patients, 264 had adenocarcinoma, 92 had squamous cell carcinoma, 12 had adenosquamous carcinoma, 14 had large-cell neuroendocrine carcinoma; 212 were pathological stage IA and 170 were stage IB. Fifty-one of 140 patients (36%) with stage 1A (T1b) and 1B adenocarcinoma received oral fluoropyrimidine for 2 years. Dosage escalation or schedule modification was at the discretion of the clinician. Patients underwent chemotherapy, radiotherapy, or the best available supportive care when recurrence was detected. This study was conducted following Helsinki Declaration guidelines and was approved by the institutional review board of Osaka City University (reference number 3361).

NLR
Preoperative NLRs were calculated from routine blood counts performed on admission. The optimal NLR cutoff value for predicting recurrence within 3 years, as identified by receiver operating characteristic (ROC) curves, was 1.5

(Youden index = 0.154), the sensitivity was 30.6%, specificity was 84.8%, and area under the curve (AUC) = 0.572; 95% CI: 0.503–0.638). The patients were stratified by their preoperative NLR to three groups: low (< 1.5, $n = 99$), intermediate ($1.5 \leq NLR < 3.5$, $n = 245$), and high (≥ 3.5, $n = 38$). The clinicopathological features, clinical course, and postsurgical survival of the groups were compared.

Assay of reactive oxygen metabolites (ROM) in serum
Serum diacron (d)-ROM levels of 33 consecutive patients were measured as an indicator of oxidative using a spectrophotometric method using a commercial free radical analysis system (FRAS; Diacron, Grossto, Italy) as previously described [19]. As hydroperoxides are an intermediate oxidation product of lipids, peptides, and amino acids, overall oxidative stress can be spectrophotometrically estimated by measuring total hyperperoxide level [20]. Serum samples were collected just before surgery and stored at −80 °C until they were assayed. Briefly, 10 µL of serum were added to 1 mL of assay mixture, gently agitated for 1 min at 37 °C, and the optical density (OD) was measured at 505 nm using a spectrophotometer. The results were expressed in Carratelli (CARR) units, where 1 U. CARR corresponds to 0.08 mg H_2O_2/100 mL serum [20].

Statistical analysis
Values of continuous and dichotomous variables were compared using Kruskal–Wallis one-way analysis, the Mann–Whitney U test, the χ^2 test, or Fisher's exact test. The Kaplan–Meier method and log-rank test were used to analyze survival. To determine the independent prognostic factors, multivariate analysis was conducted using the Cox proportional hazard model. P-values < 0.05 were considered statistically significant. Statistical analysis was performed using JMP 10 software (SAS Institute, Cary, NC, USA).

Results
Relation between serum d-ROM and NLR
The mean d-ROM value of the 33 patients tested was 297 U.CARR (range, 215–434). As shown in Fig. 1, the mean NLR in patients with high (> 300 U.CARR, $n = 16$) d-ROM levels was 1.72 ± 0.67, which was significantly higher than that in patients with low (< 300 U.CARR, $n = 17$) d-ROM levels (1.41 ± 0.39, $P = 0.018$).

Clinicopathological characteristics and NLR
Of the 382 patients, there were 264 with adenocarcinoma, 92 with squamous cell carcinoma, 12 with adenosquamous carcinoma, and 14 with large cell neuroendocrine carcinoma. Twelve patients were pathological stage IA, and 170 were stage IB. Table 1 shows the characteristics of patients stratified by NLR into low-, intermediate- and high-value groups). There were no significant differences in age, sex, smoking history, Eastern Cooperative Oncology Group

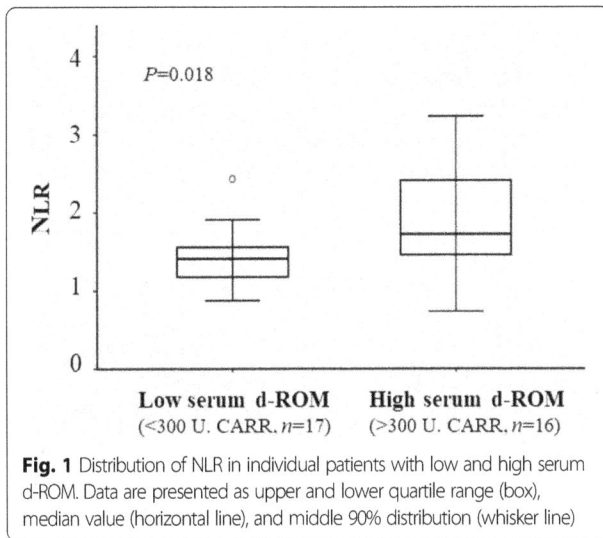

Fig. 1 Distribution of NLR in individual patients with low and high serum d-ROM. Data are presented as upper and lower quartile range (box), median value (horizontal line), and middle 90% distribution (whisker line)

performance status (PS), postoperative predicted pulmonary function tests (PFTs), differentiation of the resected tumor, pathological stage, Child-Pugh score, estimated glomerular filtration rate (eGFR), or serum albumen concentration among the groups. Patients with high NLRs had a significantly lower body mass index (BMI) and higher concentration of serum C-reactive protein (CRP) than those in the other two groups ($P = 0.049$ and < 0.001, respectively).

Postoperative outcome

The overall mean duration of follow-up was 5.6 years (range 0.1–16.2 years), a total of 2146 patient-years. There were 63 deaths from lung cancer and 73 from other diseases, including 23 from other cancers; 246 patients were still alive, including 16 with a recurrence of lung cancer. Of the 99 patients with low NLRs, 10 (10%) died from lung cancer, 19 (19%) from other diseases, and 70 (71%) were still alive. Of the 245 patients with intermediate NLRs, 47 (19%) died from cancer, 43 (18%) from other diseases, and 155 (63%) were still alive. Of the 38 patients

Table 1 Clinicopathological characteristics according to preoperative NLRs

Group		Patients	low NLRs (< 1.5: $n = 99$)	intermediate NLRs (1.5–3.5: $n = 245$)	High NLRs (≥ 3.5: $n = 38$)	P-value
Age (years)	< 75	289	78	182	29	0.675
	≥ 75	93	21	63	9	
Sex	Male	232	57	154	21	0.509
	Female	150	42	91	17	
BMI (Kg/m^2)			22.3 ± 3.0	22.3 ± 3.2	21.0 ± 3.0	0.049
Smoking History	Yes	240	61	156	23	0.895
	No	142	38	89	15	
PS	0–1	355	94	224	37	0.273
	2	27	5	21	1	
Predicted post PFTs[a]	≥ 40	355	95	227	33	0.184
	< 40	27	4	18	5	
Histology	Ad	264	79	166	19	0.003
	Others	118	20	79	19	
Differentiation	Well	125	37	78	10	0.412
	Mod/poor	257	62	167	28	
p-stage	IA	212	62	131	19	0.233
	IB	170	37	114	19	
Child-Pugh Score	5	342	90	220	32	0.539
	≥ 6	40	9	25	6	
eGFR (ml/min/1.73m^2)	≥ 60	301	85	189	27	0.094
	< 60	81	14	56	11	
Albumin (g/dl)			4.1 ± 0.29	4.1 ± 0.35	4.1 ± 0.38	0.798
CRP (mg/dl)			0.14 ± 0.39	0.22 ± 0.43	0.87 ± 2.18	< 0.001

[a]Predicted postoperative values of $FEV_{1.0}$ or DL_{CO} less than 40% are defined as high-risk results of pulmonary function tests

Ad adenocarcinoma, *BMI* body mass index, *PFT* pulmonary function test, *PS* performance status, *p-stage* pathological stage

with high NLRs there were six deaths from cancer (16%), 11 from other diseases (29%) and 21 patients were still alive (55%). Patients with intermediate and high NLRs (i.e., ≥1.5) had a significantly greater risk of death not related to lung cancer than those with low NLRs (HR = 2.23, 95% CI; 1.18–4.66; $P = 0.012$).

There was no difference between the three groups in ratio of receiving chemotherapy or radiation therapy excluding palliative irradiation: Postoperative oral fluoropyrimidine was received in 26% (11/42) of low, 29% (26/89) of intermediate and 44% (4/9) of high NLRs ($P = 0.570$). After detection of lung cancer recurrence, systemic chemotherapy or radiation therapy were performed in 92% (11/12) of low, 77% (44/57) of intermediate and 56% (5/9) of high NLRs ($P = 0.151$).

As shown in Fig. 2a, the 3-, 5- and 10-year survival rates in patients with low, intermediate, and high NLRs were 92, 77, and 59%; 82, 70, and 50%; and 76, 58, and 32%, respectively ($P = 0.034$). The survival rate of patients with low NLRs was significantly higher than that of those with

intermediate (HR =1.507, 95% CI: 1.004–2.331; $P = 0.047$) and high (HR = 2.133, 95% CI: 1.144–3.855, $P = 0.018$) NLRs. Regarding progression, recurrence-free survival is shown in Fig. 2b. The 1-, 3- and 5-year recurrence-free rates were 98, 90 and 86% in patients with low NLRs; 91, 77 and 74% in those with intermediate NLRs; and 92, 77, and 68% in those with high NLRs ($P = 0.033$).

Multivariate analysis of NLR and clinicopathological variables

Univariate analysis and the log-rank test found that sex, age, PS, smoking history, NLR (> 1.5; intermediate, and high), postoperative PFTs, histology, degree of tumor differentiation, lymph-vascular invasion, pathological stage, postoperative complications, and some preoperative comorbidities (i.e., cardiac, cerebral, kidney and liver disease; and a prior history of tumors) were significantly associated with survival (Table 2). Multivariate analysis including the significant variables confirmed sex, age, PS, histology (non-adenocarcinoma), differentiation, lymph-vascular invasion, pathological stage, and a history of prior tumors as independent predictors of overall survival. NLR was not predictive of overall survival.

The analysis of factors that increased risk of recurrence is shown in Table. 3. Univariate analysis and the log-rank test found that sex, age, smoking history, NLR > 1.5, tumor differentiation, lymph-vascular invasion, pathological stage, and preoperative cerebral comorbidity were significantly associated with recurrence. According to multivariate analysis, age, differentiation, lymph-vascular invasion, and pathological stage were independent predictors of overall survival. NLR (HR = 2.03, 95% CI: 1.17–3.79; $P = 0.011$) was a significant risk factor of recurrence as were age, pathological stage, differentiation of resected tumor, and lymph-vascular invasion.

Discussion

We found that an increase in the NLR was associated with systemic inflammation and predicted recurrence in patients with completely resected stage 1 NSCLC. We also found a positive relationship between serum ROS concentration and the NLR in those patients. Numerous physiological variables have been reported as markers of long-term survival following pulmonary resection for lung cancer. These include age, sex, PS, weight loss, sarcopenia, depressed mood, quality of life, smoking, arterial blood gases, Charlson Comorbidity Index score, forced expiratory volume in 1 s ($FEV_{1.0}$), and diffusing capacity of the lungs for carbon monoxide (DLCO) [21–24]. The NLR is often used as an inflammation marker, and its prognostic value in lung cancer has been recently reported [7, 25–27]. The patients in this series with intermediate and high NLRs (i.e., ≥1.5) had a significantly greater risk of death not related to lung cancer than those with low NLRs.

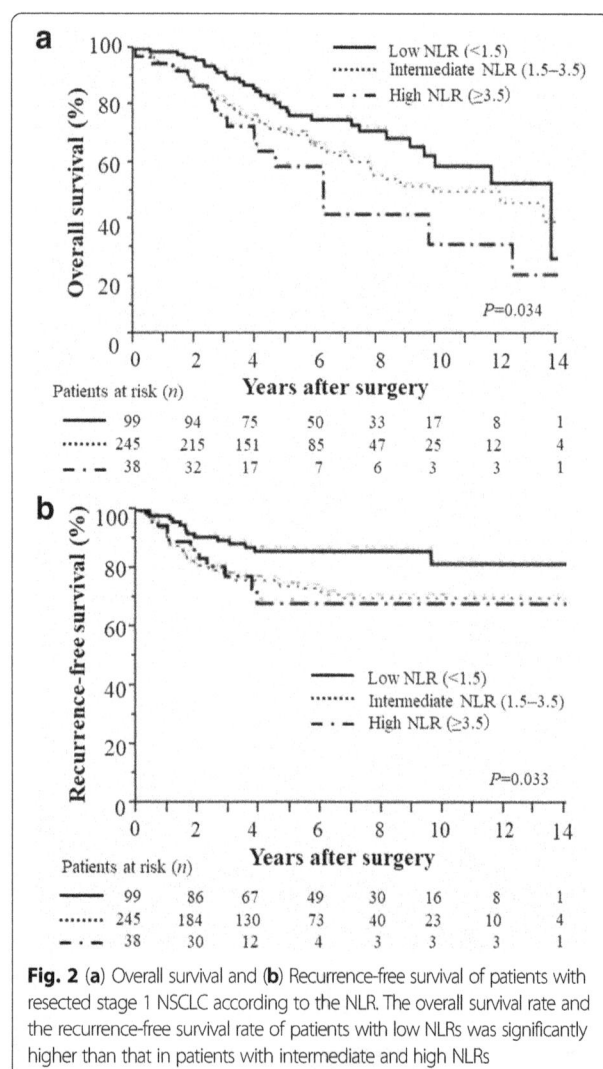

Fig. 2 (**a**) Overall survival and (**b**) Recurrence-free survival of patients with resected stage 1 NSCLC according to the NLR. The overall survival rate and the recurrence-free survival rate of patients with low NLRs was significantly higher than that in patients with intermediate and high NLRs

Table 2 Multivariate analysis of factors predicting overall survival

Factors	Univariate (P-value)	Multivariate (P-value)	Risk ratio	95% CI
Sex (male vs. female)	< 0.001	< 0.001	2.26	1.43–3.65
Age (≥70 years)	< 0.001	< 0.001	2.64	1.81–3.90
PS (2 vs 0–1)	< 0.001	0.026	2.04	1.10–3.56
Smoking	0.002	0.257	–	–
NLR (> 1.5)	0.028	0.316	–	–
Predicted post PFT[a]	0.025	0.058	–	–
Histology (other vs. adenocarcinoma)	0.034	0.021	1.60	1.07–2.41
Differentiation (m/p vs. well)	< 0.001	0.035	1.64	1.03–2.66
Lymph-vascular invasion	0.002	0.029	1.50	1.04–2.16
Pathological stage (IB vs. IA)	< 0.001	0.006	1.68	1.16–2.45
Postoperative complications	0.024	0.449	–	–
Preoperative comorbidities				
Hypertension	0.829	–	–	–
Diabetes mellitus	0.496	–	–	–
eGFR (< 70 mL/min/1.73 m^2)	0.022	0.890	–	–
Child–Pugh classification (B or C)	0.028	0.880	–	–
Cardiac disease	0.011	0.301	–	–
Cerebral disease	0.014	0.876	–	–
Any prior tumors	< 0.001	< 0.001	3.37	2.27–4.96

[a]Predicted postoperative values of $FEV_{1.0}$ or DLCO < 40% are defined as high-risk for PFTs

PS performance status, NLR neutrophil-lymphocyte ratio, PFT pulmonary function test, eGFR estimated glomerular filtration rate, m/p moderate or poor

Previous reports and meta-analyses [7, 25, 26] found that an elevated NLR was a marker of poor prognosis, and was associated with recurrence of lung cancer. In cancer patients, oxidative stress can be caused by various tumor progression mechanisms, such as malignant conversion; tumor cell survival, proliferation, chemo- and radio-resistance, invasion, angiogenesis, metastasis, and stem cell survival [4, 5] However, it is not possible to evaluate oxidative stress within the tumor microenvironment of living organs. Unlike previous studies that enrolled heterogeneous groups including patients with different NSCLC stages, we focused on patients with stage 1 disease. Tumor progression and/or tumor burden were thus limited, and patients with symptoms, treatments, or histories that could influence their inflammatory or nutrition status were excluded. The serum d-ROM results obtained in this study mainly reflected systemic inflammation, with a relatively small contribution by carcinoma-induced inflammation. In patients in good general condition, the level of systemic oxidative stress may correlate with oxidative stress associated with the tumor micro-environment, and vice versa. This oxidative stress-inflammation interaction may induce factors that promote recurrence and tumor progression.

Based on that hypothesis, we measured serum ROMs, an indicator of systemic inflammation, to reveal the relationship with NLRs. We have reported that preoperative serum ROM level was an independent predictive factor for nodal involvement in patients with clinical stage I lung adenocarcinoma [19]. The AUC was 0.763 (95% CI 0.625–0.902), and the ROC curve provided a prognostic cutoff value of approximately 300 U.CARR [19]. In this study, the mean NLR in patients with low ROMs (< 300 U.CARR) was 1.4, a significantly lower value than that in patients with high ROMs. In patients with NLRs less than 1.5, a relatively small proportion of lymphocytes would result in decreased inflammatory stress and less promotion of cancer progression. Important to note, most of patients of Low (< 1.5) NLR (92%) were received systemic chemotherapy after recurrence of cancer in this study, suggesting their good general condition. Overall, NLRs might have both physiological and oncological prognostic value.

An optimal NLR cutoff value of 5 has been used to define high preoperative inflammatory status [12, 26, 27]. However, only four patients in this study had an NLR greater than 5. Therefore we stratified the patients into three groups by the NLRs determined by ROC analysis and then assessed survival in each group. In particular, we focused on low NLRs in patients with completely resected stage 1 NSCLC. The significance of the NLR in early stage NSCLC has recently been reported in stage 1 patients with complete tumor resection [14] or treated with stereotactic radiation therapy [28]. As in our patient population, their

Table 3 Multivariate analysis of factors predicting recurrence-free survival

Factors	Univariate (P-value)	Multivariate (P-value)	Risk ratio	95% CI
Sex (male vs. female)	0.001	0.118	–	–
Age (≥70 years)	< 0.001	< 0.001	2.20	1.38–3.53
PS (2 vs. 0–1)	0.254	–	–	–
Smoking	0.005	0.183	–	–
NLR(> 1.5)	0.009	0.011	2.03	1.17–3.79
Predicted post PFT[a]	0.211	–	–	–
Histology (other vs adenocarcinoma)	0.123	0.090	–	–
Differentiation (m/p vs. well)	0.004	0.038	1.77	1.03–3.18
Lymph-vascular invasion	< 0.001	< 0.001	2.31	1.47–3.66
Pathological stage (IB vs. IA)	< 0.001	0.003	2.09	1.27–3.48
Postoperative complication	0.368	–	–	–
Preoperative comorbidities				
Hypertension	0.846	–	–	–
Diabetes mellitus	0.797	–	–	–
eGFR (< 70 mL/min/1.73 m^2)	0.107	0.647	–	–
Child–Pugh classification (B or C)	0.246	–	–	–
Cardiac disease	0.389	–	–	–
Cerebral disease	0.008	0.367	–	–
Any prior tumors	0.191	0.070	–	–

[a]Predicted postoperative values of $FEV_{1.0}$ or DLCO < 40% is defined as high-risk for PFTs
PS performance status, *NLR* neutrophil-lymphocyte ratio, *PFT* pulmonary function test, *m/p* moderate or poor, *eGFR* estimated glomerular filtration rate

NLR cutoff values (2.5 and 2.98) were lower than those reported in previous studies that enrolled stage I–III patients with surgical resection [25, 26].

The main cause of recurrence after potentially curative surgery might be the growth of micro-metastases which had been established prior to resection. In this study, an NLR > 1.5, reflecting a low peripheral lymphocyte count, predicted recurrence within 3 years. Although there was no significant relation between NLR and initial recurrence site (i.e., local or distant metastasis) in this study (data not shown), Takahashi et al. reported that the proportion of distant metastasis was higher in patients with high NLRs than in those with low NLRs [14]. Peripheral lymphocyte count has also been considered as an important marker of cancer progression and recurrence and as an independent prognostic factor in node-negative NSCLC associated with vascular invasion [15]. Moreover, low lymphocyte counts that accompany chemotherapy in patients with advanced tumors may indicate low treatment effectiveness, and low NLRs may indicate a good response to chemotherapy after detection of recurrence [29]. Furthermore, high NLRs have also been associated with infiltration of tumor by lymphocytes with low CD3+ and high CD5+ expression [30]. The presence and type of lymphocytes in the tumor microenvironment might be useful as a marker of improved therapeutic response to immunotherapy.

Conclusion

In patients with completely resected stage 1 NSCLC, NLR was associated with systemic inflammation and predicted recurrence. Routine monitoring of the NLR may be useful when planning follow-up intervals and considering adjuvant therapy. Further investigation is needed to reveal the significance of relationships between perioperative NLRs in early lung cancer and the tumor microenvironment, inflammation, and host immunity.

Abbreviations
AUC: area under the curve; BMI: body mass index; CRP: C-reactive protein; DLCO: diffusing capacity of the lungs for carbon monoxide; eGFR: estimated glomerular filtration rate; $FEV_{1.0}$: forced expiratory volume in 1 s; NLR: neutrophil-lymphocyte ratio; NSCLC: non-small cell lung cancer; PFTs: pulmonary function tests; PS: performance status; ROMs: reactive oxygen metabolites

Funding
This study was not financially supported.

Authors' contributions
All authors were involved in the preparation of this manuscript. SM performed statistical analysis, and draft the manuscript. NI, TT, and NN conceived of the study, and participated in its design and coordination and helped to draft the manuscript. TT carried out the ROS analysis. SM, NI, TT, HK and NN performed the operation and participated in collecting the data. All authors read and approved the final manuscript.

Competing interests

The authors declare that they have no competing interests.

References

1. Mantovani A, Allavena P, Sica A, Balkwill F. Cancer-related inflammation. Nature. 2008;454(7203):436–44.
2. Christiansen JJ, Rajasekaran AK. Reassessing epithelial to mesenchymal transition as a prerequisite for carcinoma invasion and metastasis. Cancer Res. 2006;66(17):8319–26.
3. Radisky DC, Levy DD, Littlepage LE, Liu H, Nelson CM, Fata JE, et al. Rac1b and reactive oxygen species mediate MMP-3-induced EMT and genomic instability. Nature. 2005;436(7047):123–7.
4. Reuter S, Gupta SC, Chaturvedi MM, Aggarwal BB. Oxidative stress, inflammation, and cancer: how are they linked? Free Radic Biol Med. 2010; 49(11):1603–16.
5. Grivennikov SI, Greten FR, Karin M. Immunity, inflammation, and cancer. Cell. 2010;140(6):883–99.
6. Proctor MJ, McMillan DC, Morrison DS, Fletcher CD, Horgan PG, Clarke SJ. A derived neutrophil to lymphocyte ratio predicts survival in patients with cancer. Br J Cancer. 2012;107(4):695–9.
7. Guthrie GJ, Charles KA, Roxburgh CS, Horgan PG, McMillan DC, Clarke SJ. The systemic inflammation-based neutrophil-lymphocyte ratio: experience in patients with cancer. Crit Rev Oncol Hematol. 2013;88(1):218–30.
8. Paesmans M, Sculier JP, Libert P, Bureau G, Dabouis G, Thiriaux J, et al. Prognostic factors for survival in advanced non-small-cell lung cancer: univariate and multivariate analyses including recursive partitioning and amalgamation algorithms in 1,052 patients. The European lung Cancer working party. J Clin Oncol. 1995;13(5):1221–30.
9. Teramukai S, Kitano T, Kishida Y, Kawahara M, Kubota K, Komuta K, et al. Pretreatment neutrophil count as an independent prognostic factor in advanced non-small-cell lung cancer: an analysis of Japan multinational trial organisation LC00-03. Eur J Cancer. 2009;45(11):1950–8.
10. Sarraf KM, Belcher E, Raevsky E, Nicholson AG, Goldstraw P, Lim E. Neutrophil/lymphocyte ratio and its association with survival after complete resection in non-small cell lung cancer. J Thorac Cardiovasc Surg. 2009; 137(2):425–8.
11. Tomita M, Shimizu T, Ayabe T, Yonei A, Onitsuka T. Preoperative neutrophil to lymphocyte ratio as a prognostic predictor after curative resection for non-small cell lung cancer. Anticancer Res. 2011;31(9):2995–8.
12. Pinato DJ, Shiner RJ, Seckl MJ, Stebbing J, Sharma R, Mauri FA. Prognostic performance of inflammation-based prognostic indices in primary operable non-small cell lung cancer. Br J Cancer. 2014;110(8):1930–5.
13. Zhang H. Clinical significance of preoperative neutrophil-lymphocyte versus platelet-lymphocyte ratio in primary operable patients with non-small cell lung cancer. 2015.
14. Takahashi Y, Horio H, Hato T, Harada M, Matsutani N, Morita S, et al. Prognostic significance of preoperative neutrophil-lymphocyte ratios in patients with stage I non-small cell lung Cancer after complete resection. Ann Surg Oncol. 2015;22(Suppl 3):1324–31.
15. Kobayashi N, Usui S, Kikuchi S, Goto Y, Sakai M, Onizuka M, et al. Preoperative lymphocyte count is an independent prognostic factor in node-negative non-small cell lung cancer. Lung Cancer. 2012;75(2):223–7.
16. Shimizu K, Okita R, Saisho S, Maeda A, Nojima Y, Nakata M. Preoperative neutrophil/lymphocyte ratio and prognostic nutritional index predict survival in patients with non-small cell lung cancer. World J Surg Oncol. 2015;13:291.

17. Zhang H, Xia H, Zhang L, Zhang B, Yue D, Wang C. Clinical significance of preoperative neutrophil-lymphocyte vs platelet-lymphocyte ratio in primary operable patients with non-small cell lung cancer. Am J Surg. 2015;210(3): 526–35.
18. Travis WD, Giroux DJ, Chansky K, Crowley J, Asamura H, Brambilla E, et al. The IASLC lung Cancer staging project: proposals for the inclusion of broncho-pulmonary carcinoid tumors in the forthcoming (seventh) edition of the TNM classification for lung Cancer. J Thorac Oncol. 2008;3(11):1213–23.
19. Tsukioka T, Nishiyama N, Iwata T, Nagano K, Tei K, Suehiro S. Preoperative serum oxidative stress marker as a strong indicator of nodal involvement in clinical stage I lung adenocarcinoma. Int J Clin Oncol. 2012;17(3):250–5.
20. Trotti R, Carratelli M, Barbieri M. Performance and clinical application of a new, fast method for the detection of hydroperoxides in serum. Panminerva Med. 2002;44(1):37–40.
21. Brunelli A, Kim AW, Berger KI, Addrizzo-Harris DJ. Physiologic evaluation of the patient with lung cancer being considered for resectional surgery: diagnosis and management of lung cancer, 3rd ed: American College of Chest Physicians evidence-based clinical practice guidelines. Chest. 2013; 143(5 Suppl):e166S–90S.
22. Moro-Sibilot D, Aubert A, Diab S, Lantuejoul S, Fourneret P, Brambilla E, et al. Comorbidities and Charlson score in resected stage I nonsmall cell lung cancer. Eur Respir J. 2005;26(3):480–6.
23. Mizuguchi S, Iwata T, Izumi N, Tsukioka T, Hanada S, Komatsu H, et al. Arterial blood gases predict long-term prognosis in stage I non-small cell lung cancer patients. BMC Surg. 2016;16(1):3.
24. Tsukioka T, Nishiyama N, Izumi N, Mizuguchi S, Komatsu H, Okada S, et al. Sarcopenia is a novel poor prognostic factor in male patients with pathological stage I non-small cell lung cancer. Jpn J Clin Oncol. 2017;47(4):363–8.
25. Zhao QT, Yang Y, Xu S, Zhang XP, Wang HE, Zhang H, et al. Prognostic role of neutrophil to lymphocyte ratio in lung cancers: a meta-analysis including 7,054 patients. Onco Targets Ther. 2015;8:2731–8.
26. Gu XB, Tian T, Tian XJ, Zhang XJ. Prognostic significance of neutrophil-to-lymphocyte ratio in non-small cell lung cancer: a meta-analysis. Sci Rep. 2015;5:12493.
27. Choi JE, Villarreal J, Lasala J, Gottumukkala V, Mehran RJ, Rice D, et al. Perioperative neutrophil:lymphocyte ratio and postoperative NSAID use as predictors of survival after lung cancer surgery: a retrospective study. Cancer Med. 2015;4(6):825–33.
28. Cannon NA, Meyer J, Iyengar P, Ahn C, Westover KD, Choy H, et al. Neutrophil-lymphocyte and platelet-lymphocyte ratios as prognostic factors after stereotactic radiation therapy for early-stage non-small-cell lung cancer. J Thorac Oncol. 2015;10(2):280–5.
29. Lissoni P, Brivio F, Fumagalli L, Messina G, Ghezzi V, Frontini L, et al. Efficacy of cancer chemotherapy in relation to the pretreatment number of lymphocytes in patients with metastatic solid tumors. Int J Biol Markers. 2004;19(2):135–40.
30. Dirican N, Karakaya YA, Gunes S, Daloglu FT, Dirican A. Association of Intratumoral Tumor Infiltrating Lymphocytes and Neutrophil-to-Lymphocyte Ratio are an independent prognostic factor in non-small cell lung Cancer. Clin Respir J. 2017;11(6):789–96.

31

Percutaneous versus thoracoscopic ablation of symptomatic paroxysmal atrial fibrillation: a randomised controlled trial-the FAST II study

Jesper Eske Sindby[1]*(iD), Henrik Vadmann[2], Søren Lundbye-Christensen[3], Sam Riahi[2], Søren Hjortshøj[2,4], Lucas V A Boersma[5,6] and Jan Jesper Andreasen[1,4]

Abstract

Background: The most efficient first-time invasive treatment, for achieving sinus rhythm, in symptomatic paroxysmal atrial fibrillation has not been established. We aimed to compare percutaneous catheter and video-assisted thoracoscopic pulmonary vein radiofrequency ablation in patients referred for first-time invasive treatment due to symptomatic paroxysmal atrial fibrillation. The primary outcome of interest was the prevalence of atrial fibrillation with and without anti-arrhythmic drugs at 12 months.

Methods: Ninety patients were planned to be randomised to either video-assisted thoracoscopic radiofrequency pulmonary vein ablation with concomitant left atrial appendage excision or percutaneous catheter pulmonary vein ablation. Episodes of atrial fibrillation were defined as more than 30 s of atrial fibrillation observed on Holter monitoring/telemetry or clinical episodes documented by ECG.

Results: The study was terminated prematurely due to a lack of eligible patients. Only 21 patients were randomised and treated according to the study protocol. Thoracoscopic pulmonary vein ablation was performed in 10 patients, and 11 patients were treated with catheter ablation. The absence of atrial fibrillation without the use of anti-arrhythmic drugs throughout the follow-up was observed in 70% of patients following thoracoscopic pulmonary vein ablation and 18% after catheter ablation ($p < 0.03$).

Conclusion: Thoracoscopic pulmonary vein ablation may be superior to catheter ablation for first-time invasive treatment of symptomatic paroxysmal atrial fibrillation with regard to obtaining sinus rhythm off anti-arrhythmic drugs 12 months postoperative.

Keywords: Paroxysmal atrial fibrillation, Catheter ablation, Thoracoscopic, Randomised study

Background

Atrial fibrillation (AF) is characterized by disorganized, rapid, and irregular contraction of the atria. Its effects on hemodynamic and thromboembolic events result in significant morbidity, mortality, impaired quality of life (QOL), hospitalizations, and health-cost. It is the most common sustained cardiac arrhythmia. By 2030, it is estimated that 14–17 millions Europeans will suffer from this arrhythmia, with 120,000 to 215,000 newly diagnosed patients per year [1].

Many patients are first diagnosed with AF when they are admitted to the hospital for AF related event (transient ischaemic attacks (TIA), stroke etc.). Other patients are increasingly affected by their symptoms (dyspnoea, palpitations etc.) with episodes increasing in severity and duration. AF is a progressive disease, where paroxysmal AF (PAF) can transform into persistent AF, long-standing persistent and permanent AF.

* Correspondence: eskesindby@gmail.com
[1]Department of Cardiothoracic Surgery, Aalborg University Hospital, Hobrovej 18-22, 9000 Aalborg, Denmark
Full list of author information is available at the end of the article

The current understanding of the pathophysiology of AF implies that 'triggers' or foci may be located in the pulmonary veins. Furthermore, electrical and structural changes of the atrium itself may serve as a 'substrate' that can perpetuate AF [1].

AF is treated medically with varying results and there is no definitive long-term curative treatment. The main goal aims at reducing symptoms and preventing disabling complications. Treatment normally includes antithrombotic, rhythm, and/or rate management. The decision regarding acute or long-term management depends on severity of the symptoms.

Non-pharmacological interventions have evolved over the last few decades to prevent and treat atrial fibrillation and/or to reduce symptoms. These interventions include catheter ablation (CA), video-assisted thoracoscopic (VATS) ablation and surgical Maze procedures. Surgical incisions or lines made by different energy sources, e.g., radio frequency or cryo-ablation, inhibit the progression of electrical impulses from spreading within the atrium [2].

The rationale for eliminating AF with ablation includes a potential improvement in quality of life [3], a decreased stroke risk [4] and a decreased heart failure risk and improved survival.

The long-term results of different treatments modalities are emerging. However, few randomised trials have been conducted to compare the surgical and CA modalities. The Atrial Fibrillation Catheter Ablation Versus Surgical Ablation Treatment (FAST) study randomized patients with previously failed CA to thoracoscopic pulmonary vein ablation (PVI) or repeat CA, which showed significantly greater efficacy of VATS PVI, but at the price of a significantly higher adverse event rate [5]. Other studies on surgical treatment have shown difference in efficacy depending on whether patients had paroxysmal, persistent, long-standing persistent or permanent AF and which lesion-set was made [6].

The most efficient first-time invasive treatment, for achieving sinus rhythm, in symptomatic paroxysmal atrial fibrillation has not been established. We aimed to compare the results of CA versus VATS pulmonary vein isolation (PVI) as a first invasive treatment in symptomatic paroxysmal AF patients. The primary outcome of interest was the prevalence of AF with and without anti-arrhythmic drugs (AAD) after 12 months.

Methods

The study was designed as a dual-centre, prospective randomised study. Two centres were planned to include and allocate patients 1:1, i.e. the Departments of Cardiology and Cardiothoracic Surgery, Aalborg University Hospital, Denmark; and the Departments of Cardiology and Cardiothoracic surgery, St. Antonius Hospital, Nieuwegein, The Netherlands.

Enrolment began in April 2011 and was planned to end during the spring of 2013, or when the planned number of patients was enrolled. Due to administrative reasons and the relocation of surgical staff, no patients were included at St. Antonius Hospital.

Eligible patients referred to the Department of Cardiology, Aalborg University Hospital, Denmark, were screened, enrolled and randomised through an automatic digital call centre by cardiologists after oral and written informed consent from the patient was obtained.

The Danish Ethics Committee approved the study (VEK project ID: N20110009), and the trial was registered at ClinicalTrials.gov - Identifier: NCT01336075.

Inclusion criteria

Eligible patients were patients with recurrent symptomatic paroxysmal AF. Inclusion criteria were previous failure with one or more AAD (treatment > 30 days) and/or cardioversion or any contraindications against treatment with AADs. ADDs were amiodarone, flecainid, propafenone, sotalol, beta-blockers and dronedarone.

Further inclusion criteria were willingness and ability to attend the scheduled follow-up visits, age between 18 and 75 years, and the provision of signed informed consent.

Exclusion criteria

Exclusion criteria were persistent, long-standing persistent or permanent AF, a previous AF ablation procedure, AF secondary to electrolyte imbalance, thyroid disease, a reversible or non-cardiac cause, severe underlying heart disease (congenital heart disease, significant valvular disease, cardiomyopathy with a left ventricular ejection fraction (LVEF) < 35%, or angina pectoris/ischaemic heart disease), severe enlargement of the left atrium (> 45 mm), the presence of a pacemaker, failure to obtain informed consent, pregnancy or breastfeeding, an inability to undergo transesophegeal echocardiography (TEE), a documented left atrial thrombus, the presence of co-morbid conditions that, in the opinion of the investigator, constitute an increased risk for general anaesthesia or port access, e.g., pleural fibrosis, chronic obstructive pulmonary disease (Forced Expiratory Volume during 1 s. < 1.5 L/s), known internal carotid artery stenosis (> 80%), current enrolment in another clinical trial, life expectancy < 1 year, or previous transient ischaemic attacks (TIA)/stroke.

Procedure

Both CA and VATS PVI are standard treatment options at Aalborg University Hospital. Approximately 200 CA procedures are performed annually by three cardiologists. One surgeon performed all VATS PVI procedures.

VATS PVI

The procedure was performed under general anaesthesia with intravenous medication and the placement of a double-lumen endotracheal tube. TEE was performed in the operating room (OR) to verify the absence of a left atrial thrombus before the start of the operation. The procedure has been described in details by Wolf et al. [7] and Edgerton et al. [8].

Briefly, three ports were introduced on each side. The pericardium was incised from the superior vena cava to the inferior vena cava 2–3 cm anterior and parallel to the phrenic nerve. Blunt dissection around the pulmonary veins (PV) was facilitated by an articulated lighted dissector (Lumitip™ Dissector probe, AtriCure, Inc., Cincinnati, Ohio). Correct positioning of the ablation clamp (Isolator Synergy™ Clamp, AtriCure, Inc., Cincinnati, Ohio) on the atrium and not on the PVs was verified via direct inspection of the device after closing the jaws of the clamp. Bipolar RF energy was applied to electrically isolate the PVs; two to five overlapping lesions were created to ensure isolation. When the conductance of the tissue decreased to less than 0.0025 Siemens, an audible signal was automatically generated to indicate that the lesion was transmural. Stimulation with the Coolrail™ linear pen (AtriCure, Inc., Cincinnati, Ohio) on the PVs and atria confirmed conductance blockade of the area.

A chest tube was placed, the right lung was re-inflated, and the port sites were closed. The technique was repeated on the left side with the addition of division of the ligament of Marshall. The left atrial appendage (LAA) was then excised using a stapling device (EZ 45–60 stapler, Ethicon Endosurgery). LAA exclusion was verified on TEE. Pacing of the PVs during sinus rhythm was performed to ensure conductance blockade of the ablation-lines. No heparin was used during the procedure. If the patient was not in sinus rhythm by the end of the procedure, a synchronized direct-current shock was performed to establish sinus rhythm (SR). Extubation was performed in the OR.

Percutaneous radiofrequency catheter ablation

Combined with computer tomography scan, a complete anatomical image of the left atrium was generated with the CARTO® mapping system (Biosense Webster Inc., Diamond Bar, CA, USA), allowing 3-D non-fluoroscopic navigation in the left atrium. The ablation procedure was performed as described extensively in the literature by Oral et al. [9] and Pappone et al. [10]. Briefly, access to the left atrium was achieved through a standard transseptal puncture using the Brockenbrough technique. Two 8F sheaths were advanced to the left atrium through two separate transseptal punctures. During the procedure, unfractionated heparin was administered to maintain an activated clotting time value > 300 s., measured every 30 min.

Ablation was performed with a 4-mm irrigated tip catheter. Circumferential ablation lines were performed, encircling the left and right PVs in the left atrium, with a demonstration of electrical discontinuity between the PV and the atrium as an endpoint. Electrical discontinuity was demonstrated by means of a Lasso catheter placed in the PVs and/or by the mapping/ablation catheter.

End points

The primary endpoint was freedom from AF/left atrial tachycardia without antiarrhythmic therapy at 6- and 12-month follow-ups as determined by 7 days of Holter monitoring, ECG, and patient interviews. AF recurrence documented by ECG, admission to the hospital due to AF beyond a blanking period from 3 to 12 months were also considered treatment failures in addition to re-intervention.

An episode of AF was defined as more than 30 s of AF observed on Holter monitoring/telemetry or clinical symptoms with ECG documentation of AF.

Secondary endpoints were symptom improvement by the European Heart Rate Association score (EHRA), the absence of AF/left atrial tachycardia with AADs, procedural complications (local haematomas/ecchymosis, thromboembolism, vasovagal reaction, haemothorax, pneumothorax, infection at the entry sites, endocarditis, pulmonary vein stenosis, cardiac perforation or tamponade, complete heart block, air embolism, arrhythmias, vascular damage or insufficiency, pericardial effusion, TIA, pericarditis, phrenic nerve damage, death, sternotomy, pain, pneumonia, or chest pain/discomfort), and reduction of the AF-burden.

Data were collected at follow-up visits at one, three, six and 12 months and from unplanned admissions to the hospital and outpatient clinic. Holter monitoring was performed for 7 days shortly before the follow-up visits at six and 12 months. Information on EHRA-score, medication, AF recurrence and complications were recorded.

Statistical analysis

A power calculation was performed with a significance level of 5% and a power of 90% assuming success rates of 70% and 90% for percutaneous CA and VATS PVI, respectively. Therefore, the study required 79 patients in each arm. Assuming a dropout rate of 10%, the inclusion of 90 patients in each arm was planned.

All continuous variables were reported as means and standard deviations. Comparisons between groups were conducted using an unpaired t-test with a bootstrap calculation of standard error to address potential non-normality and variance inhomogeneity. Categorical variables were reported as numbers and percentages. Comparisons were conducted using Fisher's exact test. EHRA scores over time were analysed using Wald test based on repeated measures

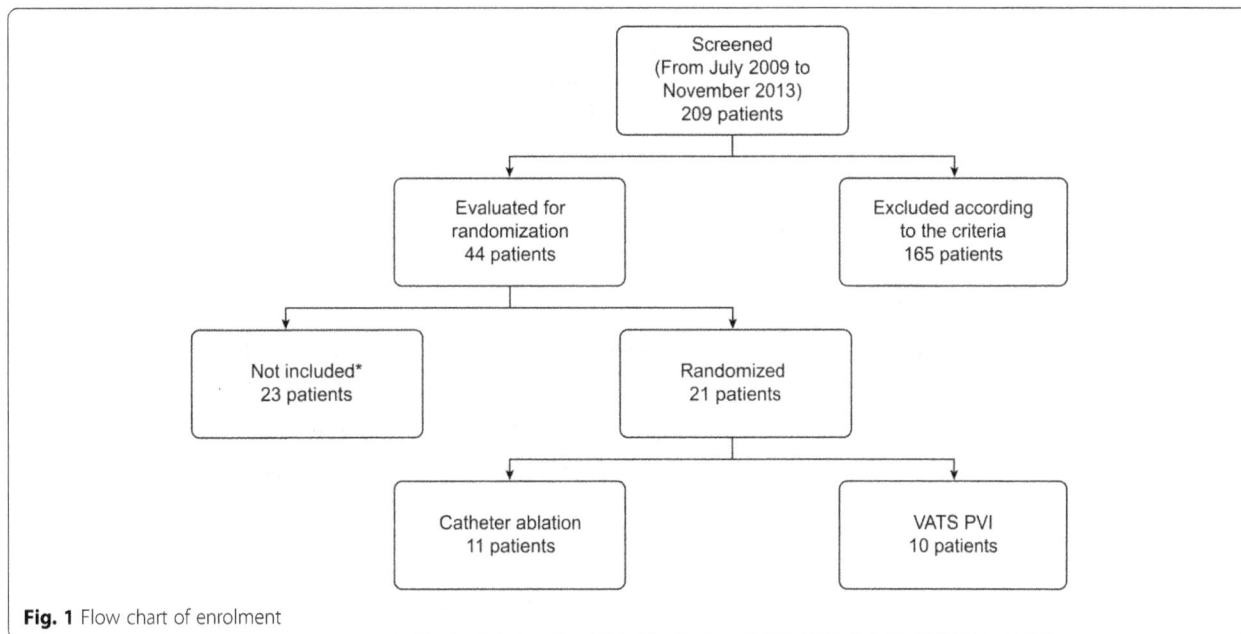

Fig. 1 Flow chart of enrolment

model. Measures of associations with *p*-values (two-tailed) < 0.05 were considered statistically significant. STATA, version 13.1 (StataCorp, College Station, TX, US) was the statistical software used.

Results

The study was terminated in January 2014 as only 21 patients had been enrolled at Aalborg University Hospital. No patients were included in the Dutch centre due to administrative reasons and due to relocation of the surgical staff. Termination of the study was due to a lack of progress in enrolment caused by a lack of patients who fulfilled the inclusion criteria, as well as administrative challenges. The first patient was screened in July 2011, and by November 2013, 209 patients had been screened for possible enrolment in the study.

Figure 1 shows the patient flow diagram.

Of the screened patients, 165 were excluded according to the criteria. Of the remaining 44 patients eligible for randomization, 22 patients declined participation after written and oral study information was provided. A total of 22 patients were randomized. One patient in the PVI group had a malignant looking nodulus on chest x-ray and crossed over to CA group after removal of a pT1aN0M0 adenocarcinoma from the lower right pulmonary lobe. One patient in CA group was excluded after the procedure as it turned out the patient had an underlying atrioventricular nodal re-entrant-tachycardia.

After 6 months of follow-up, one patient in the VATS PVI group declined further participation in the study.

Baseline patient characteristics are shown in Table 1.

Efficacy of CA and VATS PVI

Figure 2a and b shows the success-rates with regard to being in SR at 3-to-6 month, 6-to-12 month and for the entire 3-to-12 month period after the procedure. Figure 2a shows patients off AAD. Figure 2b shows the combination of on and off AAD.

Table 1 Patient characteristics

	CA	VATS PVI
Age at procedure – Years (Mean ± SD)	55.5 (8.1)	53.5 (6.7)
BMI (Mean ± SD)	27.8 (4.4)	28.1 (3.8)
LVEF % (Mean ± SD)	64.5 (4.7)	63.5 (7.1)
LA Diameter – mm (Mean ± SD)	42.2 (3.2)	42.3 (5.1)
DC-conversion pre proc. (Mean ± SD)	2.3 (3.0)	1.5 (3.2)
Sex (Male/Female)	8/3	9/1
Hypertension, n (%)	4 (36.4)	3 (30)
Symptoms - EHRA 2, n (%)	5 (45.5)	5 (50)
Symptoms - EHRA 3, n (%)	6 (54.5)	5 (50)
CHADS2 – score 0, n (%)	4 (36.4)	5 (50)
CHADS2 – score 1, n (%)	4 (36.4)	4 (40)
CHADS2 – score 2, n (%)	3 (27.2)	1 (10)
COPD, n (%)	0	0
Diabetes, n (%)	2 (18.2)	0 (0)
AAD - 0	0	1 (10)
AAD - 1	2 (18.2)	1 (10)
AAD - 2	6 (54.5)	3 (30)
AAD – 3	3 (27.3)	3 (30)
AAD - 4	0	0
AAD - 5	0	2 (20)

A Sinus Rhythm off AAD

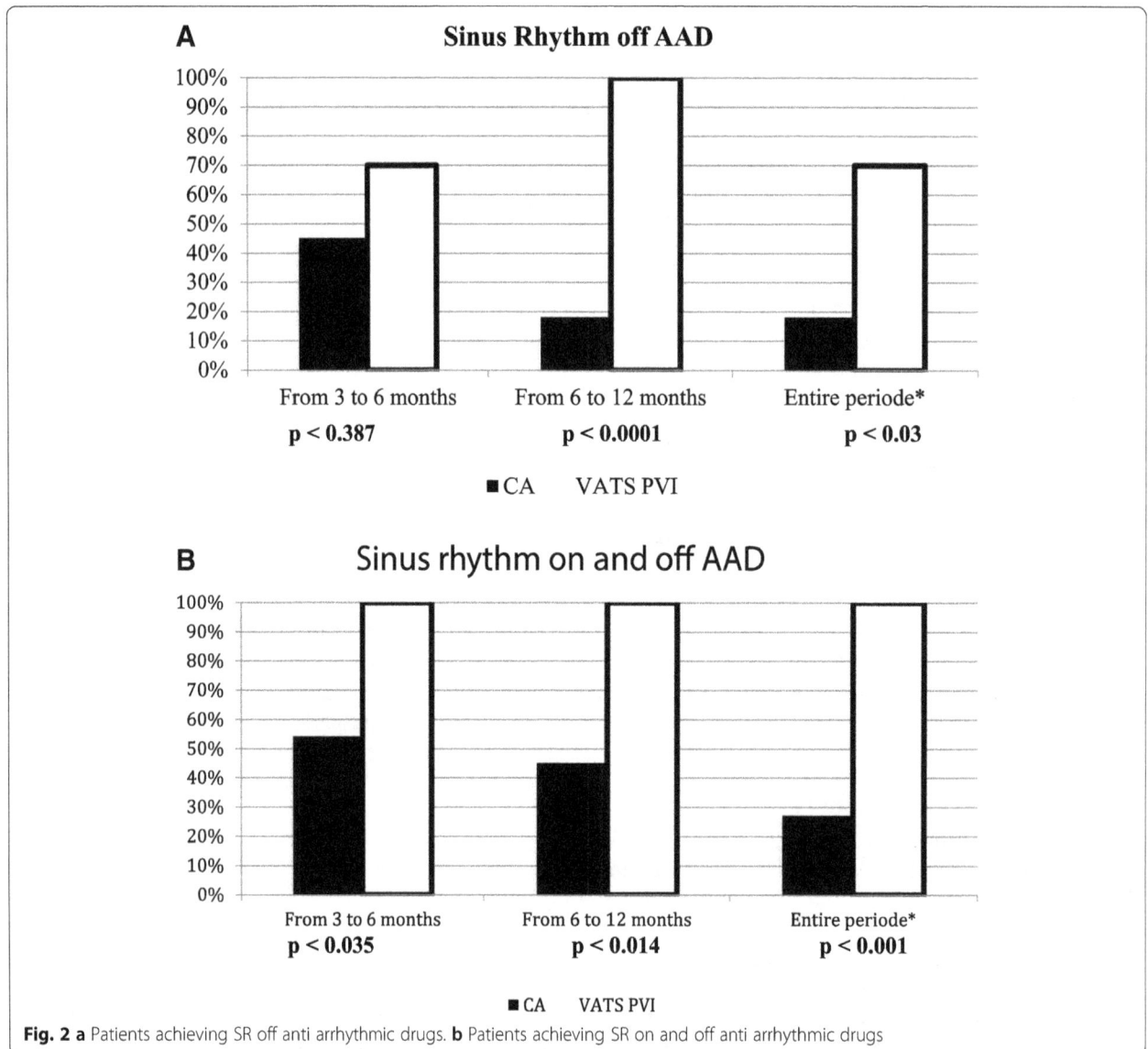

From 3 to 6 months
p < 0.387

From 6 to 12 months
p < 0.0001

Entire periode*
p < 0.03

■ CA   VATS PVI

B Sinus rhythm on and off AAD

From 3 to 6 months
p < 0.035

From 6 to 12 months
p < 0.014

Entire periode*
p < 0.001

■ CA   VATS PVI

Fig. 2 a Patients achieving SR off anti arrhythmic drugs. **b** Patients achieving SR on and off anti arrhythmic drugs

A total of 18% of the patients in the CA group and 70% in VATS PVI group ($p < 0.03$) achieved SR off AAD for the entire postoperative blanking period. For patients both on and off AAD the results were 27% versus 100%, respectively ($p < 0.001$).

The results from Holter monitoring after CA at six and 12 months showed 80% and 70% in SR +/– AADs, respectively. For VATS PVI, the results showed 100% in SR +/– AADs at 6 and 12 months.

At the 6-month follow-up, two patients lacked 7-day Holter monitoring data and two patients lacked Holter monitoring data at the 12-month follow-up. The Holter monitoring data at six and 12 months showed that two and three different patients respectively, all in the CA group, had documented AF.

No patients suffered a stroke, TIA or bleeding complications during the follow-up.

Figure 3 depicts development of symptoms, classified in EHRA-score, from before the procedure to 12 month after.

Safety of CA and VATS PVI (Tables 2 and 3)

Discussion

In this randomised clinical trial, VATS PVI was compared with CA as a first-time invasive treatment for patients with paroxysmal AF. The results from this limited number of patients indicated that VATS PVI might be superior to CA for the first-time invasive treatment of paroxysmal AF relative to the primary endpoint of freedom from AF without AADs at 12 months. However, the VATS PVI procedure resulted in a higher rate of complications and an increased length of hospital stay. Due to the premature termination of the study, no solid conclusions can be drawn.

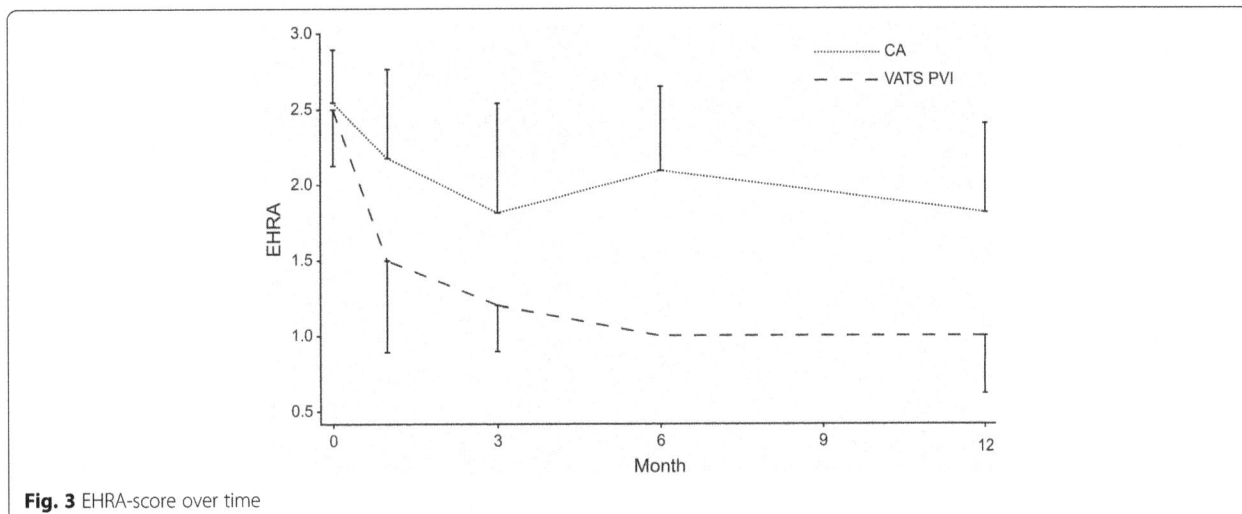

Fig. 3 EHRA-score over time

For the entire follow-up period, VATS PVI was significantly better at achieving SR without AADs.

The optimal follow-up would have been continuous monitoring of the heart rhythm for the entire period as suggested by The Society of Thoracic Surgeons [11]. We present the results from the different time periods along with the scheduled Holter monitoring at 6 and 12 month including the success-rate for the entire follow-up (3 to 12 month) as it somewhat resembles a continuous monitoring.

Our dataset is too small to assess reliable differences in success rates between the different time periods within the CA and VATS PVI groups. Most AF relapses occurred outside the scheduled Holter monitoring period. A 7-day Holter monitoring covers only a small portion of the follow-up period. Similar monitoring issues could be suspected when comparing results from the present study with other studies.

No pre-operative Holter monitoring was performed, so a comparison with 7-day Holter monitoring at six and 12 months could not be done. According to the Holter monitoring data, five patients showed various degrees of AF-burden (from 0.1 to 99.9%) in the CA group.

The Atrial Fibrillation Catheter Ablation Versus Surgical Ablation Treatment (FAST) study [5] randomized patients

with previously failed CA to VATS pulmonary vein isolation (PVI) or repeat CA and showed significantly greater efficacy with VATS PVI, but at the cost of a higher adverse event rate. Their results showed absence of AF without AADs at 12 months at 36,5% for CA and 65,6% for VATS PVI. However, the patients in the FAST-study differed from the patients in the present study in that some had paroxysmal AF, persistent AF and/or an enlarged left atrium and previously failed CA. Patients with an enlarged atria and persistent AF especially, have lower success rates with PVI as the only treatment and could account for the failures in the FAST-study.

A recent review article on VATS PVI by Laar et al. [12] showed an efficacy rate of VATS PVI of 81% at 1 year (SR off AAD), which is similar to our results.

Different strategies for post-procedure monitoring have been applied in many studies and all have their strengths and weaknesses. Mostly, 1- to 7-day Holter monitoring has been used because it is relatively easy to apply and is patient-friendly. Unfortunately, it only covers a small

Table 2 Procedure characteristics

	CA	VATS PVI
Procedure time	174 min	168.5 min
Grey/Radiation	28 Gy (Range 12–61)	0
Admitted – Days	1 (SD 0)	7.6 (Range 3–21)
Removal of LAA	0%	100%
Procedural endpoint achieved	100%	100%

CA Catheter Ablation, *VATS PVI* Video Assisted Thoracoscopic Pulmonary Vein Isolation, *Gy* Grey, *SD* Standard Deviation, *LAA* Left Atrial Appendage

Table 3 Complications

	CA	VATS PVI
Procedure complications	0	1[a]
Complications during hospitalization	0	2[b]
Complications 1 month	1[c]	0
Complications 3 month	0	0
Complications 6 month	1[d]	0
Complications 12 month	0	0

CA Catheter Ablation, *VATS PVI* Video Assisted Thoracoscopic Pulmonary Vein Isolation
[a] The patient was converted to sternotomy due to bleeding. A full Maze IV was performed and the patient was discharged on post-operative day five without any further events; [b] One patient with heart block which resolved spontaneously and one patient with tamponade (relived with percutaneous drainage) and pneumonia; [c] Patient had discomfort in the chest and resolved within a few days without treatment; [d] Re-ablated and pacemaker insertion

fraction of the entire follow-up period. Pappone et al. [10] reported an average of 6 ± 4 AF episodes per month prior to treatment. A 24-h Holter monitoring would have an approximate 20% chance of detecting AF based on those numbers. Jaïs et al. [13] showed 4–30 episodes per month in which the average episode lasted 5.5 h (range 1–12 h). Therefore, Holter monitoring may have a very good positive predictive value but a low negative predictive value in this setting.

In a review article by Kis et al. on CA PVI treatment [14] showed a success rate of 78% (freedom from AF both on and off AADs) based on the majority of the included studies having 24-h Holter monitoring at different time intervals as a reflection of success. In our opinion, this would generally be insufficient to detect asymptomatic episodes of AF.

Because of different follow-up strategies, it is difficult to compare our CA results with others.

We suggest reporting data for the entire follow-up period and following patients for at least 1 year, preferably longer. Insertable Cardiac Monitor devices may be preferred in the future as they are becoming smaller and less expensive, and these devices can detect AF/Arrhythmia on a continuous basis for a longer period depending on the battery capacity [15]. However, there is risk of 'noise' and hence over-estimation of AF/arrhythmia.

Three out of five patients were reluctant to participate in the study, although the reason remained unspecified for the majority. Patients have different preferences and intentions when they come to the specialists; some choose for 100% efficacy, others choose for minimal impact and therefore they do not want to be randomized in a scientific study.

EHRA scores decreased over time in both groups, but improved more in the VATS PVI group than in the CA group, possibly due to the higher success rate of VATS PVI, even though CA has been shown to decrease the frequency and severity of symptoms [13].

The LARIAT-study showed a decrease in AF-burden after ligation of the LAA without any ablation [16]. This finding is of interest in relation to the present study as a major procedural difference between VATS PVI and CA was exclusion of the LAA. In a study by Di Biase et al. [17], it was shown that 27% of failed CA procedures occurred in patients with initiation/trigger points for AF in or around the LAA, which could partly explain the higher success rate with VATS PVI as the LAA is excluded. Romanov et al. [18] have found no difference in success rates when removing the LAA in patients with non-paroxysmal AF.

Ligation of the LAA as the only treatment [19] has shown a persistent decrease in blood pressure (BP) and a short-term reduction in sodium levels. Neuro-hormonal changes are still unclear, but indicate that AF could be much more than just a 'mechanical' problem of irregular heartbeats.

Concerning matters of LAA, one should notice that this study was not designed nor powered for a comparison of ablation lines but in order to compare two invasive treatment procedures.

Complications occurred more often in the surgical group as also shown by others authors [1, 5, 12]. The main reasons for prolonged hospital stays in the present study were pneumonia, temporary heart block and pain management. Complications in the VATS PVI group were dealt with during the hospital stay and none of the patients had problems after discharge. Laar et al. [12] showed a complication rate similar to CA after minor complications e.g. pneumothorax and pleural effusions were excluded from analysis.

Even though the objectives of the procedures are similar, the risk-profiles of CA and VATS PVI are different [1]. To optimize communication with patients, complications may be classified as life-threatening, severe, moderate, minor and unknown as outlined in published guidelines [1]. The risk-profile and long-term benefits of a procedure should be taken into consideration and conveyed to the patient when choosing a treatment strategy.

A major limitation of this study is the low number of patients included, and therefore the study was not powered for firm conclusions.

Conclusion

VATS PVI may be superior to CA for the first-time invasive treatment of symptomatic paroxysmal AF in obtaining freedom from AF without AADs 12 months postoperative. However, a higher rate of complications and longer hospitalization is associated with VATS PVI. Although this was a randomised study, no solid conclusions can be drawn based on the results from this study due to the low number of patients included. A similar study should be carried out in centres with more patients.

Abbreviations

AAD: Anti-arrhythmic drugs; AF: Atrial fibrillation; CA: Catheter ablation; EHRA: European Heart Rate Association score; LAA: Left Atrial Appendage; LVEF: Left ventricular ejection fraction; OR: Operating room; PV: Pulmonary veins; PVI: Pulmonary vein isolation; SR: Sinus rhythm; TEE: Transesophageal echocardiography; TIA: Transient ischaemic attacks; VATS: Video-assisted thoracoscopic

Funding

This study was supported by the Strategic Research Council, Denmark, and the Atrial Fibrillation Study Group, Aalborg University Hospital, Denmark. The funders had no role in study design, data collection and analysis, decision to publish or preparation of the manuscript.

Authors' contributions

JES is the corresponding author and has been responsible for analysis and interpretation of date and drafting and writing of the manuscript. HV made the protocol, conception and design of the study as well as enrolment and acquisition of data. SL-C has made statistical analysis of data. SR has performed a large part of CA procedures and participated in revision of the manuscript. SH, LVAB, JJA has all been involved in drafting and revising the manuscript. All authors read and approved the final manuscript.

Competing interests

L.Boersma have received grants from Medtronic, Boston Scientific and Abbott as a consultant.

Author details

[1]Department of Cardiothoracic Surgery, Aalborg University Hospital, Hobrovej 18-22, 9000 Aalborg, Denmark. [2]Department of Cardiology, Aalborg University Hospital, Aalborg, Denmark. [3]Unit of Clinical Biostatistics, Aalborg University Hospital, Aalborg, Denmark. [4]Atrial Fibrillation Study Group, Aalborg University Hospital, Aalborg, Denmark. [5]Department of Cardiology, St. Antonius Hospital, Nieuwegein, The Netherlands. [6]AMC Amsterdam, University of Amsterdam, Amsterdam, The Netherlands.

References

1. Kirchhof P, Benussi S, Kotecha D, Ahlsson A, Atar D, Casadei B, et al. 2016 ESC guidelines for the management of atrial fibrillation developed in collaboration with EACTS. Eur Heart J. 2016. https://doi.org/10.1093/eurheartj/ehw210.
2. Cox JL, Schuessler RB, Boineau JP. The development of the maze procedure for the treatment of atrial fibrillation. Semin Thorac Cardiovasc Surg. 2000; 12:2–14.
3. Biviano AB, Hunter TD, Dandamudi G, Fishel RS, Gidney B, Herweg B, et al. Healthcare utilization and quality of life improvement after ablation for paroxysmal AF in younger and older patients. Pacing Clin Electrophysiol PACE. 2017;40:391–400.
4. Oral H, Chugh A, Özaydın M, Good E, Fortino J, Sankaran S, et al. Risk of thromboembolic events after percutaneous left atrial radiofrequency ablation of atrial fibrillation. Circulation. 2006;114:759–65.
5. Boersma LVA, Castella M, van BW, Berruezo A, Yilmaz A, Nadal M, et al. Atrial fibrillation catheter ablation versus surgical ablation treatment (FAST) a 2-center randomized clinical trial. Circulation. 2012;125:23–30.
6. Je HG, Shuman DJ, Ad N. A systematic review of minimally invasive surgical treatment for atrial fibrillation. Eur J Cardiothorac Surg. 2015;48:531–41.
7. Wolf RK, Schneeberger EW, Osterday R, Miller D, Merrill W, Flege JB, et al. Video-assisted bilateral pulmonary vein isolation and left atrial appendage exclusion for atrial fibrillation. J Thorac Cardiovasc Surg. 2005;130:797–802.
8. Edgerton JR, Jackman WM, Mack MJ. A new epicardial lesion set for minimal access left atrial maze: the Dallas lesion set. Ann Thorac Surg. 2009; 88:1655–7.
9. Oral H, Pappone C, Chugh A, Good E, Bogun F, Pelosi FJ, et al. Circumferential pulmonary-vein ablation for chronic atrial fibrillation. N Engl J Med. 2006;354: 934–41.
10. Pappone C, Augello G, Sala S, Gugliotta F, Vicedomini G, Gulletta S, et al. A randomized trial of circumferential pulmonary vein ablation versus antiarrhythmic drug therapy in paroxysmal atrial fibrillation: the APAF Study. J Am Coll Cardiol. 2006;48:2340–7.
11. Shemin RJ, Cox JL, Gillinov AM, Blackstone EH, Bridges CR, Workforce on evidence-based surgery of the Society of Thoracic Surgeons. Guidelines for reporting data and outcomes for the surgical treatment of atrial fibrillation. Ann Thorac Surg. 2007;83:1225–30.
12. Laar C, Kelder J, van Putte BP. The totally thoracoscopic maze procedure for the treatment of atrial fibrillation. Interact CardioVasc Thorac Surg. 2017; 24(1):102–11 https://doi.org/10.1093/icvts/ivw311.
13. Jaïs P, Cauchemez B, Macle L, Daoud E, Khairy P, Subbiah R, et al. Catheter ablation versus antiarrhythmic drugs for atrial fibrillation CLINICAL PERSPECTIVE. Circulation. 2008;118:2498–505.
14. Kis Z, Muka T, Franco OH, Bramer WM, De Vries LJ, Kardos A, et al. The short and long-term efficacy of pulmonary vein isolation as a sole treatment strategy for paroxysmal atrial fibrillation: a systematic review and meta-analysis. Curr Cardiol Rev. 2017;13:199–208. https://doi.org/10.2174/1573403X13666170117125124.
15. Diederichsen SZ, Haugan KJ, Køber L, Højberg S, Brandes A, Kronborg C, et al. Atrial fibrillation detected by continuous electrocardiographic monitoring using implantable loop recorder to prevent stroke in individuals at risk (the LOOP study): rationale and design of a large randomized controlled trial. Am Heart J. 2017;187:122–32.
16. Lakkireddy DR, Earnest M, Janga P, Reddy M, Vallakati A, Nath J, et al. Effect of endoepicardial percutaneous left atrial appendage ligation (lariat) on arrhythmia burden in patients with atrial fibrillation. J Am Coll Cardiol. 2013; Available from: https://doi.org/10.1016/S0735-1097(13)60385-X. [cited 31 Oct 2017].
17. Biase LD, Burkhardt JD, Mohanty P, Sanchez J, Mohanty S, Horton R, et al. Left Atrial Appendage. Circulation. 2010;122:109–18.
18. Romanov A, Pokushalov E, Elesin D, Bogachev-Prokophiev A, Ponomarev D, Losik D, et al. Effect of left atrial appendage excision on procedure outcome in patients with persistent atrial fibrillation undergoing surgical ablation. Heart Rhythm. 2016;13:1803–9.
19. Maybrook R, Pillarisetti J, Yarlagadda V, Gunda S, Sridhar ARM, Deibert B, et al. Electrolyte and hemodynamic changes following percutaneous left atrial appendage ligation with the LARIAT device. J Interv Card Electrophysiol Int J Arrhythm Pacing. 2015;43:245–51.

Permissions

The contributors of this book come from diverse backgrounds, making this book a truly international effort. This book will bring forth new frontiers with its revolutionizing research information and detailed analysis of the nascent developments around the world.

We would like to thank all the contributing authors for lending their expertise to make the book truly unique. They have played a crucial role in the development of this book. Without their invaluable contributions this book wouldn't have been possible. They have made vital efforts to compile up to date information on the varied aspects of this subject to make this book a valuable addition to the collection of many professionals and students.

This book was conceptualized with the vision of imparting up-to-date information and advanced data in this field. To ensure the same, a matchless editorial board was set up. Every individual on the board went through rigorous rounds of assessment to prove their worth. After which they invested a large part of their time researching and compiling the most relevant data for our readers.

The editorial board has been involved in producing this book since its inception. They have spent rigorous hours researching and exploring the diverse topics which have resulted in the successful publishing of this book. They have passed on their knowledge of decades through this book. To expedite this challenging task, the publisher supported the team at every step. A small team of assistant editors was also appointed to further simplify the editing procedure and attain best results for the readers.

Apart from the editorial board, the designing team has also invested a significant amount of their time in understanding the subject and creating the most relevant covers. They scrutinized every image to scout for the most suitable representation of the subject and create an appropriate cover for the book.

The publishing team has been an ardent support to the editorial, designing and production team. Their endless efforts to recruit the best for this project, has resulted in the accomplishment of this book. They are a veteran in the field of academics and their pool of knowledge is as vast as their experience in printing. Their expertise and guidance has proved useful at every step. Their uncompromising quality standards have made this book an exceptional effort. Their encouragement from time to time has been an inspiration for everyone.

The publisher and the editorial board hope that this book will prove to be a valuable piece of knowledge for researchers, students, practitioners and scholars across the globe.

List of Contributors

Jae Hang Lee, Jin-Ho Choi and Eung-Joong Kim
Department of thoracic and cardiovascular surgery, Dongguk University Ilsan Hospital, Goyang, Gyeonggi, South Korea

Nizar Abbas
Department of thoracic surgery, Al-Assad University Hospital, Damascus, Syrian Arab Republic

Sarah Zaher Addeen, Fatima Abbas, Tareq Al Saadi, Ibrahem Hanafi, Mahmoud Alkhatib and Tarek Turk
Faculty of Medicine, University of Damascus, Damascus, Syrian Arab Republic

Ahmad Al Khaddour
Cardiothoracic surgeon, Damascus University Hospital, Damascus, Syria

Pey-Jen Yu, Allan Mattia, Hugh A. Cassiere, Rick Esposito, Frank Manetta and Alan R. Hartman
Department of Cardiovascular and Thoracic Surgery, Hofstra Northwell School of Medicine, 300 Community Drive, 1DSU, Manhasset, NY 11030, USA

Nina Kohn
The Feinstein Institute for Medical Research, Manhasset, NY, USA

Meishuang Li, Yanan Wang, Yulong Chen and Zhenfa Zhang
Department of Lung Cancer, Tianjin Medical University Cancer Institute and Hospital, Huanhu West Road, Tianjin 300060, China
National Clinical Research Center for Cancer, Key Laboratory of Cancer Prevention and Therapy, Tianjin 300060, China
Tianjin's Clinical Research Center for Cancer, Tianjin 300060, China.
Tianjin Lung Cancer Center, Tianjin 300060, China

Sanaz Amin, George Krasopoulos and David P. Taggart
University of Oxford, Oxford, UK
Department of Cardiovascular Surgery, Oxford University Hospitals Trust, Oxford, UK

Raphael S. Werner
Department of thoracic surgery, Faculty of Medicine, University of Zurich, Zurich, Switzerland

Per Lav Madsen
Department of Cardiology, Copenhagen University Hospital, Herlev, Denmark

Natsumi Nomoto and Toshiko Konda
Department of Clinical Technology, Kobe City Medical Center General Hospital, 2-1-1 Minatojima-Minamimachi, Chuo-ku, Kobe 650-0047, Japan

Tomoko Tani
Basic Medical Science, Kobe City College of Nursing, 3-4 Gakuennishi-machi, Nishi-ku, Kobe 651-2103, Japan

Kitae Kim, Takeshi Kitai, Mitsuhiko Ota, Shuichiro Kaji and Yutaka Furukawa
Department of Cardiovascular Medicine, Kobe City Medical Center General Hospital, 2-1-1 Minatojima-Minamimachi, Chuo-ku, Kobe 650-0047, Japan

Yukihiro Imai
Department of Pathology, Kobe City Medical Center General Hospital, 2-1-1 Minatojima-Minamimachi, Chuo-ku, Kobe 650-0047, Japan

Yukikatsu Okada
Department of Cardiovascular Surgery, Kobe City Medical Center General Hospital, 2-1-1 Minatojima-Minamimachi, Chuo-ku, Kobe 650-0047, Japan

Haiqi He, Qifei Wu, Zhe Wang, Yong Zhang, Nanzheng Chen, Junke Fu and Guangjian Zhang
Department of thoracic surgery, The First Affiliated Hospital of Xi'an Jiaotong University, 277 West Yanta Road, Xi'an, Shaanxi 710061, China

Takashi Anayama, Kentaro Hirohashi, Ryohei Miyazaki, Hironobu Okada, Nobutaka Kawamoto, Marino Yamamoto and Kazumasa Orihashi
Division of Thoracic Surgery, Department of Surgery II, Kochi Medical School, Kochi University, Kohasu Oko Nankoku Kochi 783-8505, Japan

Takayuki Sato
Department of Circulation Control, Kochi Medical School, Kochi University, Kohasu Oko Nankoku Kochi 783-8505, Japan

Huai-Yu Wang, Yan-Jun Zhu, Jie Liu and Ying-Hui Liu
Thoracic Surgery Department of General Hospital of Air-Force PLA, No.30 Fucheng Road, Haidian District, Beijing PC: 100142, China

Li-Wei Li
Nuclear Medicine Department of General Hospital of Air-Force PLA, No.30 Fucheng Road, Haidian District, Beijing 100142, China

Philippe Grieshaber, Tobias Schneider, Coskun Orhan, Peter Roth, Bernd Niemann and Andreas Böning
Department of Adult and Pediatric Cardiovascular Surgery, University Hospital Giessen, Rudolf-Buchheim-Str. 7, DE-35392 Giessen, Germany

Lukas Oster
Department of Anaesthesiology, Sana Hospital Berlin-Lichtenberg, Berlin, Germany

Victoria Johnson
Department of Cardiology and Angiology, University Hospital Giessen, Giessen, Germany

Kai Qian, Yong-Geng Feng, Jing-Hai Zhou, Ru-Wen Wang, Qun-You Tan and Bo Deng
Department of Thoracic Surgery, Institute of Surgery Research, Daping Hospital, Army Medical University, Chongqing 400042, People's Republic of China

Enzhi Yin, Masateru Uchiyama and Masanori Niimi
Department of Surgery, Teikyo University, 2-11-1 Kaga, Itabashi-ku, Tokyo 173-8605, Japan

Enzhi Yin
Department of Cardiovascular Surgery, The 2nd Affiliated Hospital of Harbin Medical University, Harbin, China

Shigefumi Matsuyama
Department of Cardiovascular Surgery, New Tokyo Hospital, Chiba, Japan
Department of Cardiovascular Surgery, Teikyo University, Tokyo, Japan

Masateru Uchiyama and Kento Kawai
Transplantation Research Immunology Group, Nuffield Department of Surgical Sciences, University of Oxford, John Radcliffe Hospital, Oxford, UK

Xuhua Shi, Yongfeng Zhang and Yuewu Lu
Department of Rheumatology and Immunology, Beijing Chao-Yang Hospital, Capital Medical University, 8 Gongren Tiyuchang Nanlu, Chaoyang District, Beijing 100020, China

Chong Zhang, Yuequn Niu, Li Yu, Wang Lv, Haichao Xu, Abudumailamu Abuduwufuer, Jinlin Cao and Jian Hu
Department of Thoracic Surgery, First Affiliated Hospital of Zhejiang University, No. 79 Qingchun Road, Zhejiang, Hangzhou 310003, China

Tae Hwan Park, Jang Won Lee and Chan Woo Kim
Department of Plastic and Reconstructive Surgery, CHA Bundang Medical Center, CHA University, 59 Yatap-ro, Bundang-gu, Seongnam, Gyeonggi 13496, Republic of Korea

Kaoru Kaseda and Keisuke Asakura
Department of Thoracic Surgery, Sagamihara Kyodo Hospital, 2-8-18 Hashimoto, Midori-ku, Sagamihara, Kanagawa 252-5188, Japan

Akio Kazama
Department of Pathology, Sagamihara Kyodo Hospital, 2-8-18 Hashimoto, Midori-ku, Sagamihara, Kanagawa 252-5188, Japan

Yukihiko Ozawa
Yuai Clinic, 1-6-2 Kitashinyokohama, Kohoku-Ku, Yokohama, Kanagawa 223-0059, Japan

Zhi-Nuan Hong, Qiang Chen, Ze-Wei Lin, Gui-Can Zhang, Liang-Wan Chen, Qi-Liang Zhang and Hua Cao
Department of Cardiovascular Surgery, Union Hospital, Fujian Medical University, Fuzhou 350001, People's Republic of China

Younes Moutakiallah, Mahdi Aithoussa, Noureddine Atmani, Aniss Seghrouchni and Abdelatif Boulahya
Cardiac surgery department, Mohammed V teaching military hospital, Hay Riyad, PB 10100, Rabat, Morocco

Azeddine Moujahid and Abdedaïm Hatim
Intensive care of cardiac surgery, Mohammed V teaching military hospital, Rabat, Morocco

Iliyasse Asfalou and Zouhair Lakhal
Cardiology department, Mohammed V teaching military hospital, Rabat, Morocco

Younes Moutakiallah, Mahdi Aithoussa, Noureddine Atmani, Aniss Seghrouchni, Azeddine Moujahid, Abdedaïm Hatim, Iliyasse Asfalou, Zouhair Lakhal and Abdelatif Boulahya
Faculty of medicine and pharmacy, Mohammed V university, Rabat, Morocco

Naoki Hashiyama and Makoto Mo
Department of Cardiovascular Surgery, Yokohama Minami-kyosai Hospital, Mutsuurahigashi 1-21-1, Kanazawa-ku, Yokohama 236-0037, Japan

Motohiko Goda, Yukihisa Isomatsu, Shinichi Suzuki and Munetaka Masuda
Department of Cardiovascular Surgery, Yokohama City University Hospital, Fukuura 3-9, Kanazawaku, Yokohama 236-0004, Japan

Munetaka Masuda
Cardiovascular Center, Yokohama City University Medical Center, Yokohama, Japan

Takahiro Nishida
Department of Cardiovascular Surgery, Yokohama Citizen's Municipal Hospital, Yokohama, Japan

Uzma Shahid, Joveria Farooqi and Erum Khan
Section of Microbiology, Department of Pathology and Laboratory Medicine, Aga Khan University, Karachi, Pakistan

Hasanat Sharif
Section of Cardiothoracic Surgery, Department of Surgery, Aga Khan University, Karachi, Pakistan

Bushra Jamil
Section of Infectious Diseases, Department of Medicine, Aga Khan University, Karachi, Pakistan

Manuel Giraldo-Grueso
Vascular Function Research Laboratory, Fundación Cardioinfantil- Instituto de Cardiologia, Bogotá, Colombia

Néstor Sandoval-Reyes and Jaime Camacho
Cardiac Surgery, Fundación Cardioinfantil-Instituto de Cardiologia, Bogotá, Colombia

Ivonne Pineda
Cardiac Surgery Department, Fundación Cardioinfantil-Instituto de Cardiologia, Bogotá, Colombia

Juan P. Umaña
Director Cardiovascular Medicine, Cardiac Surgery Department, Fundación Cardioinfantil- Instituto de Cardiologia, Bogotá, Colombia

Mohamed Fouad Ismail, Tamer E. Hamouda, Azzahra Edrees, Abdulbadee Bogis, Nashwa Badawy, Alaa B. Mahmoud, Ahmed Farid Elmahrouk and Ahmed A. Jamjoom
Cardiothoracic Surgery Department, King Faisal Specialist Hospital and Research Center, MBC J-16, Jeddah 21499, Saudi Arabia

Mohamed Fouad Ismail
Cardio-thoracic Surgery Department, Mansoura University, Mansoura, Egypt

Amr A. Arafat, Alaa B. Mahmoud and Ahmed Farid Elmahrouk
Cardiothoracic Surgery Department, Tanta University, Tanta, Egypt

Tamer E. Hamouda
Cardio-thoracic Surgery Department, Benha University, Benha, Egypt

Amira Esmat El Tantawy and Nashwa Badawy
The Department of Pediatrics, Faculty of Medicine Cairo University, Cairo, Egypt

Huan Wang, Weijian Zheng, Weiping Fang, Gaige Meng, Lei Zhang, Yannan Zhou, Erwei Gu and Xuesheng Liu
Department of Anesthesiology, the First Affiliated Hospital of Anhui Medical University, No. 218 Jixi Road, Hefei, Anhui 230022, People's Republic of China

Motohiko Goda and Bart Meuris
Department of Cardiac Surgery, University Hospitals Leuven, Leuven, Belgium

Tomoyuki Minami, Kiyotaka Imoto and Keiji Uchida
Cardiovascular Center, Yokohama City University Medical Center, Yokohama, Japan

Motohiko Goda and Munetaka Masuda
Department of Cardiovascular Surgery, Yokohama City University Hospital, Yokohama, Japan

Andreas Keyser, Simon Schopka, Maik Foltan and Christof Schmid
Department of Cardiothoracic Surgery, University Medical Center Regensburg, Franz-Josef-Strauss-Allee 11, 93053 Regensburg, Germany

Carsten Jungbauer
Department of Internal Medicine II/Cardiology, University Medical Center, Regensburg, Germany

Peng Zhu, Songlin Du, Yu Hu, Li Liu and Shaoyi Zheng
Department of Cardiovascular Surgery, NanFang hospital, Southern Medical University, 1838 North Guangzhou Avenue, Guangzhou 510515, People's Republic of China

Shijun Chen and Shaobin Zheng
Department of Urinary Surgery, NanFang hospital, Southern Medical University, GuangZhou, People's Republic of China

Suresh Giritharan, Kareem Salhiyyah, Geoffrey M. Tsang and Sunil K. Ohri
Wessex Cardiac Centre, University Hospitals Southampton, Tremona Road, Southampton SO16 6YD, UK

Suresh Giritharan
Southampton, UK

Hiroshi Sato
Department of Cardiovascular Surgery, Sapporo Medical University School of Medicine, S1W16, Chuo-ku, Sapporo 060-8543, Japan

Masanori Nakamura, Takeshi Uzuka and Mayo Kondo
Department of Cardiovascular Surgery, Sapporo
City General Hospital, N11W13, Chuo-ku, Sapporo
060-8604, Japan

J. Palussière
Department of Interventional Radiology, Institut
Bergonié, 229 Cours de l'Argonne, 33000 Bordeaux,
France

F. Chomy
Department of Medical Oncology, Institut Bergonié,
229 Cours de l'Argonne, 33000 Bordeaux, France

M. Savina, C. Bellera and S. Mathoulin-Pelissier
Department of Clinical and Epidemiological Research,
Institut Bergonié, 229 Cours de l'Argonne, 33000
Bordeaux, France

T. de Baere
Department of Interventional Imaging, Institut Gustave
Roussy, 114 Rue Edouard Vaillant, 94800 Villejuif,
Paris, France

J. Y. Gaubert
Department of Imaging, CHU Timone, 264 Rue Saint-
Pierre, 13385 Marseille, France

A. Renault and O. Bonnefoy
Department of Imaging, CHU Pau, 4 Boulevard
Hauterive, 64000 Pau, France

F. Laurent
Department of Imaging, CHU Haut Lévêque, Avenue
Magellan, 33600 Pessac, France

C. Meunier
Department of Imaging, CHU Rennes, 2 rue Henri Le
Guilloux, 35033 Rennes, France

**Shinjiro Mizuguchi, Nobuhiro Izumi, Takuma
Tsukioka, Hiroaki Komatsu and Noritoshi Nishiyama**
Department of Thoracic Surgery, Osaka City University
Hospital, 1-4-3 Asahimachi, Abeno-ku, Osaka 545-
8585, Japan

Jesper Eske Sindby and Jan Jesper Andreasen
Department of Cardiothoracic Surgery, Aalborg
University Hospital, Hobrovej 18-22, 9000 Aalborg,
Denmark

Henrik Vadmann, Sam Riahi and Søren Hjortshøj
Department of Cardiology, Aalborg University
Hospital, Aalborg, Denmark

Søren Lundbye-Christensen
Unit of Clinical Biostatistics, Aalborg University
Hospital, Aalborg, Denmark

Søren Hjortshøj and Jan Jesper Andreasen
Atrial Fibrillation Study Group, Aalborg University
Hospital, Aalborg, Denmark

Lucas V A Boersma
Department of Cardiology, St. Antonius Hospital,
Nieuwegein, The Netherlands
AMC Amsterdam, University of Amsterdam,
Amsterdam, The Netherlands

Index